FOUNDATIONS OF ĀYURVEDA, VOLUME I

Essentials of Professional Āyurveda

Vaidya (Dr.) Jessica Vellela, BAMS
Vaidya (Dr.) Prasanth Dharmarajan, PhD (Ayu)

ĀYU ACADEMY LLC

1001 S. Main St. STE 500
Kalispell, MT 59901

https://www.ayu.academy

FOUNDATIONS OF ĀYURVEDA, VOLUME I
Essentials of Professional Āyurveda

Author
Vaidya (Dr.) Jessica Vellela, BAMS

Contributor
Vaidya (Dr.) Prasanth Dharmarajan, PhD (Ayu)

Third Edition

Notice - Disclaimer

Knowledge and best practices in the field of Āyurveda regularly change as new research and experience broaden the understanding of the subject. Adaptable changes with research methods, professional practice and/or management protocols may become necessary. Every effort has been made to ensure that the content provided in this publication is accurate and complete at the time of publishing. However, this is not an exhaustive treatment of the subject. No liability is assumed for losses or damages due to the information provided. Interpretation and application of information from this publication is solely the responsibility of the reader. Always consult an appropriate professional with any questions related to legal, medical or healthcare issues.

Previous editions copyrighted 2018, 2019, 2020

ISBN: 978-1-950876-10-5

To all of our teachers,

and their teachers,

and the teachers before them

Special thanks to the

SVASTHA ĀCHĀRYA STUDENTS

who helped make this book and

higher standards of Āyurveda a reality.

यथा खरश्चन्दनभारवाही भारस्य वेत्ता न तु चन्दनस्य |
एवं हि शास्त्राणि बहून्यधीत्य चार्थेषु मूढाः खरवद्वहन्ति || ४ ||

सु. सू. ४|४

Yathā kharaśhchandanabhāravāhī bhārasya vettā na tu chandanasya |
Evaṁ hi śhāstrāṇi bahūnyadhītya chārtheṣhu mūḍhāḥ kharavadvahanti ||4||

Su. Sū. 4/4

"A donkey suffers under the weight of sandalwood without enjoying its fragrance just as those who study too many streams of knowledge suffer from missing their practical effect."

Table of Contents

UNIT I

Introduction to
Traditional Āyurvedic Medicine (TAM)

Chapter 1 : Introduction

KEY TERMS

anādi Āyurveda Charaka Saṁhitā Hinduism

Āyurveda is a advanced and well-developed holistic health care system. It has been practiced for thousands of years in the Indian subcontinent and Southeast Asia.

Over this time, it has influenced the development and practice of neighboring traditional medical systems in China, Tibet, the Middle East and other regions of the world. It is considered to be the longest, continuously practiced health care system known today.

Āyurveda is capable of operating as a primary health care system as is seen in India, Sri Lanka, Nepal and several other countries today. Historical records bear out that its practices spanned a gamut of specialities, many of which are currently recognized in Western medical practice.

These include Internal Medicine, Surgery and Emergency Medicine, HEENT (Head, Ear, Eyes, Nose and Throat), Obstetrics and Gynecology, Pediatrics, Toxicology and Reproductive Medicine. Classical Āyurvedic specialities such as Rasāyana (Regenerative Medicine) are considered emerging fields in medicine.

Āyurveda is also capable of being practiced in conjunction with other health care systems, modalities and approaches. From this perspective, it is often recognized or classified as Integrative Medicine, Traditional Medicine, Complementary or Alternative Medicine. Similarities in practice exist between Āyurveda and several fields of medicine.

According to the American Board of Integrative Medicine® (ABOIM) and the Consortium of Academic Health Centers for Integrative Medicine, "Integrative medicine ... is the practice of medicine that reaffirms the importance of the relationship between practitioner and patient, focuses on the whole person, is informed by evidence, and makes use of all appropriate therapeutic approaches, health care professionals, and disciplines to achieve optimal health and healing." (American Board of Physician Specialties. n.d.).

The foundation of integrative medicine is strongly in line with core tenets of Āyurveda and echoes Āyurveda's long-standing practice. Commonalities like this exist between Āyurveda and many of today's most popular medical and healing modalities.

ĀYURVEDA: TRADITIONAL MEDICINE

The Sanskrit term "Āyurveda" refers to the traditional, indigenous system of medicine practiced in the Indian subcontinent and recorded over the past two to three thousand years. The phrases "Āyurvedic medicine" and "Traditional Āyurvedic medicine (TAM)" are also used today and may informallly differentiate the medical practice of Āyurveda as compared to self-care practices that are managed by individuals at home.

Traditionally, Āyurveda was referred to as "Āyurveda" in whole and in part. This single name has historically covered its complete, broad range of applications.

The origins of Āyurveda as a distinct health

care system date back at least 3,000 years in written history. Its practice through oral tradition likely spans much further with some claims that it dates back 10,000 years or more.

Logically, it would make sense to consider the possibility of some form of Āyurveda existing from the earliest times of mankind because managing and preventing disease is always a basic survival requirement. The Charaka Saṁhitā supports this view by stating that Āyurveda is "*anādi*," (Cha. Sū. 30/27) meaning that it is timeless, with no beginning or end. Āyurveda describes the inherent laws of nature and the laws of life itself and so it must have existed since the beginning of life.

The source, generation, creation or discovery of Āyurveda is an area ripe with speculation. Historical data provides some extent of plausible explanation, but not enough to confidently determine a single, irrefutable answer.

The long-standing practice of the science is deeply woven into current Hindu traditions with vibrant accounts of mythology, culture and history. Personified deities enliven the science and help reinforce a deeply human understanding of principles and practice.

Over many centuries of refinement, Āyurveda developed and adapted its science to spread into virtually every aspect of Hindu culture and life. Early practitioners of Āyurveda recognized the importance of simple, holistic, sustainable and effective means of disease prevention and management. To promote these methods among the public and gain easy acceptance, Āyurveda was infused into cultural activities as a means of public health protection.

Traditionally, the practice of Āyurveda strives to "maintain the health of the healthy, and cure the diseases of the sick," (Cha. Sū. 30/26).

To accomplish these goals successfully, a wide range of therapeutic interventions are applied from intense, methodical bio-purification protocols to simple, targeted dietary and lifestyle modifications.

Additionally, the vast knowledge of single herbs, purified metals, minerals, animal products and even poisonous substances is utlized and manipulated to produce safe, efficacious medicines in simple and complex, compound formulations.

Myths and misconceptions

Globally, many popular beliefs exist about what Āyurveda is and what it is not. Miscommunication, misunderstanding and misinterpretations due to cultural, religious, environmental and seasonal influences have created major discrepancies in professional and public spheres.

By its own nature, Āyurveda is a science which is adaptable, logical and practical for any people, place or time period on earth. However, all too often, practitioners and the public learn to associate their application of the science as its defined limit. These perspectives have created challenges in spreading the full extent and capacity of the science.

As Āyurveda has gained popularity and recognition outside of the Indian subcontinent, its proponents have spread its name and fame. Many have extolled its healing benefits through popular, "feel-good" methods. However, the depth and strength of Āyurveda's clinical practice has not been well established outside of India.

This has led to many common misconceptions including beliefs that Āyurveda is "mind-body medicine," "plant medicine," "Indian medicine," "Hinduism," "religious medicine," "a diet and lifestyle approach," "medicine without side effects," "a vegetarian diet," "slow to see results," and even "having no side effects."

It is also commonly seen that the minor aspects of spirituality are taken out of context and considered the primary focus of Āyurveda. In this regard, some consider it to be a "spiritual healing system," "self-healing system," or "innate knowledge divined by intuition or higher powers."

Āyurveda is also easily employed to serve the beauty and relaxation industries through spas, massage centers, resorts and similar establishments. While Āyurveda can be very effective in these capacities, they represent a very small portion of its full scope.

Generally, considering Āyurveda from only one or some of these aspects only serves to diminish the advancement of the science and practice. These perspectives often obscure the fact that Āyurveda is a complex science. It evolved through human effort, long-term research and development, discoveries, advancements and refinement over thousands of years.

Limiting the purview of Āyurveda to one or some of the above assumptions only serves to limit its scope of practice. These limitations are often seen more predominantly among non-professional spheres and have been difficult to overcome because of deep cultural ties, an attachment to the science being "ancient," "mystical" or "magical" and lack of perception of forward movement.

TEST YOURSELF

Learn, review and memorize key terms from this section.

anādi

Āyurveda

Charaka Saṁhitā

Hinduism

ĀYURVEDA: AN EMERGING PRIMARY HEALTH CARE SYSTEM

Āyurveda holds tremendous potential to grow and adapt itself to widespread, modern, international practice as a primary health care system.

With the tools and technologies available today, the science can be studied on a global scale and advanced to provide highly customized applications for a wide range of subpopulations, cultures and geographical locations.

For millennia, Āyurveda has provided profound levels of health and happiness for various cultures. It continues to do so today for millions worldwide and has the potential to reach many more.

The demand for effective, affordable and sustainable health care is high today. Āyurveda can provide reliable, preventive care and management for a wide range of acute and chronic disorders. It can integrate with surgery and emergency care to improve outcomes. It should be considered a primary health care solution for local and global communities.

Chapter 1: Review

ADDITIONAL READING

Utilize these references to expand your understanding of the concepts in this chapter.

CLASSICS		1st read	2nd read
Charaka	Cha. Sū. 30/26-27		

REQUIRED READING	Chapters
Modern and Global Ayurveda	1, 3, 4, 5

OPTIONAL READING	Format
Special Issue - Postcolonial Technoscience	Essay

References

American Board of Physician Specialties. (n.d.). Integrative Medicine Defined. Retrieved from http://www.abpsus.org/integrative-medicine-defined.

Śarmā, R. K., & Dāsa, B. Agniveśha's Charaka Saṃhitā. Varanasi: Chowkhamba Sanskrit Series Office; Reprint Edition. 2016. Cha. Sū. 30/.

Murthy, K. R. Srikantha. Vāgbhaṭa's Aṣhṭāṅga Hṛdayam. Chowkhamba Kṛṣhṇadas Academy, Varanasi. Reprint Edition. 2016. AH. Sū. 1/.

Wujastyk, D., Smith, F. (2008). (Eds.). Modern and Global Ayurveda: pluralism and paradigms. Albany, NY: State University of New York Press.

Benchmarks for Training in Ayurveda. (2010). Geneva, Switzerland: World Health Organization.

WHO Traditional Medicine Strategy: 2014-2023. (2013). Geneva, Switzerland: World Health Organization.

QUESTIONS & ANSWERS

Record your questions for this chapter here for further research and discussion.

Question:

Answer:

Question:

Answer:

Question:

Answer:

SELF-ASSESSMENT

1. As an advanced health care system, which of the following recognized medical specialties does Āyurveda include?
   a. Emergency medicine
   b. Obstetrics
   c. Regenerative medicine
   d. Toxicology
   e. All of the above

2. Which is considered the longest, continually practiced health care system known today?
   a. Āyurveda
   b. Traditional Chinese Medicine
   c. Tibetan Medicine
   d. Platonic Medicine
   e. None of the above

3. Āyurveda can collaborate as part of Integrative Medicine because it
   a. can be practiced in tandem with health care modalities.
   b. can operate as a primary health care system.
   c. has spread to almost every aspect of Hindu culture and life.
   d. is the longest continuously practiced health care system.
   e. is woven into various traditions and mythologies.

4. Traditionally, Āyurveda refers to
   a. a system of health care
   b. indigenous medicine of the Indian subcontinent
   c. medical traditions spanning India, Tibet and South-east Asia
   d. Both A and B
   e. All of the above

5. According to Charaka, Āyurveda originated
   a. 5,000 years ago
   b. at the beginning of mankind
   c. in Bhagavad Gītā
   d. in China
   e. in the Charaka Saṁhitā

6. To maintain health and cure disease, Āyurveda employs
   a. bio-purification
   b. complex formulations
   c. dietary modifications
   d. manipulation of animal products
   e. All of the above

7. Āyurveda could best be described as
   a. a spiritual healing system
   b. having no side effects
   c. relaxation therapy
   d. All of the above
   e. None of the above

8. Why is Āyurveda considered a complex system of health care?
   a. It has a long history of research and development.
   b. It has evolved through human efforts, discoveries and advancements.
   c. It has refined itself over thousands of years.
   d. All of the above
   e. None of the above

9. Why has It been challenging for Āyurveda to become a modern, primary health care system?
   a. It cannot be personalized.
   b. It is limited to the Indian subcontinent.
   c. It is only suitable for vegetarians.
   d. Both A and B
   e. None of the above

10. Āyurveda is
   a. affordable
   b. preventative
   c. sustainable
   d. Both A and B
   e. All of the above

Chapter 2 : Defining Āyurveda

KEY TERMS

ahita	duḥkha	paribhāṣhā	Suśhruta
āyuḥ	guṇa	paryāya	sampradāya
Āyurveda	hita	pramāṇa	sūtra
āyuṣhya	iti	śhākhā	sūtrasthāna
cha	jñāna	sampradāya	tantra
Charaka sampradāya	karma	śhāstra	vā
Devanāgarī	lakṣhaṇa	śhloka	veda
dravya	māna	sukha	vidyā

The literal meaning of the word Āyurveda translates to "the science or knowledge of life."

Āyurveda is a Sanskrit term composed of two parts:

āyuḥ	life
veda	science, or knowledge

The phonological rules of Sanskrit, called *sandhi*, render the compound term as:

Āyurveda	आयुर्वेद
not Āyuḥveda	आयुःवेद

DEFINITIONS OF ĀYURVEDA

Āyurveda is a systematic, scientific body of knowledge which encompasses holistic, medicine, disease prevention and complete health care. Āyurveda is capable of using any substance for medicinal purposes.

It includes a large, complex body of knowledge based on constant natural laws. It contains full instructions for holistic, personalized health care, disease management, regenerative treatment principles and health promotion with the ambitious goal to live the healthiest life possible in both quantity and quality.

It includes instructions from pre-pregnancy planning to inevitable death and is considered the longest, continuously practiced health care system known today.

From a very practical perspective, Āyurveda can be considered a life-long owner's manual. Following its instructions, one can promote their capacity to experience a long, happy and meaningful life.

Classically, Āyurveda is defined in several ways. This variety of definitions allows its key purposes and applications to be described effectively to specific audiences.

Current definitions of Āyurveda are still in their nascent stages in English and other non-Indian languages. Expect these definitions to undergo continous refinement as the profession develops.

Review these definitions and consider their significance and application today.

Current definitions

ĀYU Council defines Āyurveda as (Āyurveda, 2019):

> "**Āyurveda**" is a holistic health care system that prioritizes the individual's role and responsibility for personal health through proper living and prevention. It includes scientific practices, protocols and

methods to remove, alleviate and manage acute and chronic health disturbances from their root. It originated in the Indian subcontinent where it continues to be the longest continuously practiced health care system known today.

As the practice of Āyurveda is often more appropriate when localized to the people, place and time, ĀYU Council also defines American Āyurveda (Āyurveda, 2019).

"**American Āyurveda**" is the application and practice of Āyurveda in the United States of America. It is based on the scientific foundations of Āyurveda and analyzes current outcomes to research, advance and improve all aspects of practice appropriately for the current time, place and people.

Additionally, a few significant distinctions within Āyurveda have become better defined as practices grow and expand. Often, these are based on varied traditional practices and geographical locations, particularly within the Indian subcontinent. In the introduction of Modern and Global Ayurveda, Frederick M. Smith and Dagmar Wujastyk define these significant phrases (Wujastyk, Smith, 2008).

"**Modern Ayurveda**" is here understood to be geographically set in the Indian subcontinent and to commence with the processes of professionalization and institutionalization brought about in India by what has been called the nineteenth-century revivalism of Ayurveda (Leslie 1998; Brass 1972; Jeffery 1988). Modern Ayurveda is characterized by a tendency toward the secularization of ayurvedic knowledge and its adaptation to biomedicine, and at the same time by attempts to formulate a unitary theory based on doctrines found in the classical ayurvedic texts.

"**Global Ayurveda**," on the other hand, refers to ayurvedic knowledge that has been transmitted to geographically widespread areas outside of India. Here we may differentiate three broad "lineages" of ayurvedic globalization: the first is characterized by a focus on the ayurvedic pharmacopoeia, beginning with the dissemination of ayurvedic botanical and pharmaceutical lore in the sixteenth century. The study of ayurvedic pharmacopoeia has developed into a full-blown scientific discipline as well as into a hugely profitable pharmaceutical industry in a global market. In line with the ideologies of modern Ayurveda, interest groups concerned with ayurvedic pharmacopoeia stress the "scientific" bases of ayurveda and promote a secularized discipline stripped of its religious and spiritual connotations.

The second lineage of global Ayurveda is identified in the more recent trend of a globally popularized and acculturated Ayurveda, which tends to emphasize and reinterpret, if not reinvent, the philosophical and spiritual aspects of Ayurveda. This type of Ayurveda has been dubbed "New Age Ayurveda" (Zysk 2001; Reddy 2000). ... A third, independent line of global Ayurveda originated in the context of the then-new scholarly discipline of Indic Studies in the early nineteenth century, when Orientalist scholars began to take interest in ayurvedic literature. While the first scholarly documentation on Indian medicine in the form of botanical encyclopedias was not concerned with the conceptual framework of Ayurveda, these scholars were interested in preserving, or even reviving, knowledge of Ayurveda as a historical and philological discipline. … Their work, however, seems never to have been directed at making practical use of the knowledge gained from the texts in regard to the more theoretical aspects underlying ayurvedic medicine. However, scholarly editions and translations of Sanskrit medical works have been important contributions to formalized ayurvedic education and research.

"**New Age Ayurveda**" (Zysk 2001; Reddy 2000). Zysk defines its characteristics as follows:

1. attributing a remote age to Ayurveda and making it the source of other medical systems
2. linking Ayurveda closely to Indian spirituality, especially Yoga
3. making Ayurveda the basis of mind-body medicine
4. claiming the "scientific" basis of Ayurveda and its intrinsic safety as a healing modality

Another important characteristic of New Age Ayurveda (which it shares with some forms of modern Ayurveda in urban settings) is a shift in self-representation from reactive medicine that cures ills to preventive medicine that offers a positive lifestyle index.

New Age Ayurveda is particularly prominent in the United States, and increasingly in Northern Europe. Furthermore, it has been re-imported into India in the shape of "wellness" tourism that caters both to foreign tourists and urban, middle-class Indians. … Thus paradoxically, despite its emphasis on spirituality, New Age Ayurveda has given rise to a new commercialized form of Ayurveda, emphasizing wellness and beauty as fundamental components of good health. Its commercial offerings encompass a range of cosmetic and massage treatments provided in beauty salons and spas, over-the-counter products (mostly cosmetics and nutritional supplements), and do-it-yourself or self-help literature (i.e., guides on beauty treatments, nutrition, and fitness). Selby (2005) describes how Ayurveda, twinned or even merged with yoga into "Ayuryoga," has become a branded commodity in North American spa culture. While the unprotected name "Ayurveda" is used freely in this context, it is not necessarily used to denote a real connection with premodern ayurvedic knowledge but often rather seems to stand for vague notions of "exotic" or "Eastern" self-cultivation. Thus we may find a spa offering a full-day treatment entitled "Ayurvedic Bliss," which in this case mean "Luxury Spa Pedicure, Aromatherapy Salt Glow Body, Exfoliation and Hot Stone Back Massage," treatments that are not found in classical ayurvedic texts. As Sita Reddy (2004) has pointed out, images of the "exotic East" play a crucial role in certain sectors of the marketing of ayurvedic products or treatments.

ĀYU Council defines professional Āyurveda as (Āyurveda, 2019):

"**Professional Āyurveda**" is the practice and application of Āyurveda by a qualified professional using targeted, therapeutic intervention to produce a specific health outcome.

In India, a qualified Āyurvedic Doctor is one who has completed the minimum level of Āyurvedic medical education of at least 5.5 years at a state-recognized institution. Graduation confers the degree of Bachelor of Āyurvedic Medicine & Surgery with the title of Āyurveda Āchārya. Outside of India, the regulations for establishing qualified professionals vary widely by country and generally do not adhere to a standard curriculum.

TEST YOURSELF

Learn, review and memorize key terms from this section.

āyuḥ

____

Āyurveda

____

veda

____

PARIBHĀṢHĀ

Classical definitions of Āyurveda are found throughout the Āyurvedic medical compendia. Key definitions are available from the oldest surviving treatises to the latest classical works.

Classical definitions are recorded in the texts in lines called *śhlokas* in Sanskrit using the *Devanāgarī* script. Here, these definitions are provided in their original script followed by their ĀYUT transliteration which allows for easier reading and pronunciation through the Roman alphabet. Finally, the word-for-word meaning and translation is stated below the *śhloka*.

This format intends to provide the student with the tools necessary for deconstructing each *śhloka* in a meaningful way. Practice and repetition with each statement is an advanced learning tool for understanding, conceptualizing and interpreting the full science of classical Āyurveda.

Each of these definitions provides insight into the purview and scope of Āyurveda in important ways. Although they may be easy to understand from a high-level, superficial perspective, the true depth of meaning often requires years of study and practice to fully reveal itself.

These definitions, just like all classical references, should be reviewed and analyzed regularly throughout the duration of this course and throughout one's career. As the student's knowledge grows with practical application, the classics will present new perspectives and interpretations in various contexts.

Review a few of the significant *śhlokas* from the major classical authors, Charaka and Suśhruta.

Definition #1

<u>Āyurveda as a means for healthy life</u>

This definition from Charaka is likely the best, well-known classical definition of Āyurveda.

हिताहितं सुखं दुःखमायुस्तस्य हिताहितम्
।
मानं च तच्च यत्रोक्तमायुर्वेदः स उच्यते ॥
४१

च. सू. १।४१

Hitāhitaṁ sukhaṁ duḥkhamāyustasya hitāhitam |
Mānam cha tachchha yatroktamāyurvedaḥ sa uchyate || 41

Cha. Sū. 1/41

Hita (That which is good or appropriate for an individual), *ahitaṁ* (that which is inappropriate for an individual), *sukhaṁ* (contentment, or general satisfaction), *duḥkham* (and discontentment, or general dissatisfaction) *āyustasya hitāhitam* (and all which is appropriate or inappropriate for quality and duration of life) *mānam* (can be measured) *cha tachchha yatra-uktam* (and explained [in terms of their characteristics and functions]) *āyurvedaḥ* (by Āyurveda), *sa uchyate* (so it is told).

In a succinct definition, Charaka is able to capture and convey many detailed aspects of Āyurveda. The science has the capacity to clearly identify, describe and measure all factors which contribute to individual and personalized health, happiness and longevity, or otherwise.

Definition #2

Āyurveda and its principles and purpose

This definition from Charaka is more elaborate and rightfully placed in the final chapter of *sūtrasthāna*.

सुखासुखतो हिताहिततः प्रमाणाप्रमाणतश्च;
यतश्चायुष्याण्यनायुष्याणि च
द्रव्यगुणकर्माणि वेदयत्यतोऽप्यायुर्वेदः ।
तत्रायुष्याण्यनायुष्याणि च द्रव्यगुणकर्माणि
केवलेनोपदेक्ष्यन्ते तन्त्रेण || २३

च. सू. ३०|२३

Sukhāsukhato hitāhitataḥ
pramāṇāpramāṇataśhcha;
yataśhchāyuṣhyāṇyanāyuṣhyāṇi cha
dravyaguṇakarmāṇi vedayatyato '
pyāyurvedaḥ |
Tatrāyuṣhyāṇyanāyuṣhyāṇi cha
dravyaguṇakarmāṇi
kevalenopadekṣhyante tantreṇa || 23

Cha. Sū. 30/23

Sukha (That which creates satisfaction) *asukhato* (or dissatisfaction), *hita* (that which is healthy) *ahitataḥ* (or unhealthy), *pramāṇa* (and their proper measurement) *apramāṇata-śhcha* (or improper measurement), *yata-śhcha-āyuṣhyāṇya* (which determine the effects and capacity to produce a full-quality lifespan) *na-āyuṣhyāṇi* (or reduced lifespan) *cha dravya-guṇa-karmāṇi* (according to the scientific principles of *dravya*, *guṇa* and *karma*) *vedayatyato api āyurvedaḥ* (is known through Āyurveda, its science and body of knowledge.)

Tatra-āyuṣhyāṇya (Thus, these factors capable of producing a full-quality) *na-āyuṣhyāṇi* (or reduced lifespan,) *cha dravya-guṇa-karmāṇi* (and their scientific principles of *dravya*, *guṇa* and *karma*) *kevalena-upadekṣhyante* (are discussed individually) *tantreṇa* (throughout this entire treatise.)

Definition #3

Āyurveda as longevity science

आयुरस्मिन् विद्यते, अनेन वाऽऽयुर्विन्दन्ति
इत्यायुर्वेदः । १५

सु. सू. १|१५

Āyurasmin vidyate, anena vā ' '
yurvindanti ityāyurvedaḥ | 15

Su. Sū. 1/15

Āyur-asmin vidyate (As it allows one to become proficient with the knowledge of life) anena vā (and) āyurvindanti (it creates and achieves a full, complete life or lifespan), Iti-āyurvedaḥ (it is called Āyurveda.)

Suśhruta privdes the shortest definition while still capturing the extensive reach of the science and its practices.

TEST YOURSELF

Learn, review and memorize key terms from this section.

ahita

____

āyuṣhya

____

cha

____

Devanāgarī
dravya
duḥkha
guṇa
hita
iti
karma
māna
paribhāṣhā
pramāṇa
śhloka
sukha
sūtrasthāna
vā

PARYĀYA

Classical Āyurvedic literature contains many synonyms in addition to numerous definitions. Synonyms are called *paryāya* in Sanskrit. The extensive number of synonyms confirms the highly developed nature of Sanskrit and its capacity to describe concepts from multiple perspectives.

In classical Āyurveda, synonyms are used to relate specific terminologies to broad and detailed concepts. Many of these concepts do not exist in the realm of Western science and have no direct, comparable translations. This results in multiple Sanskrit synonyms often being translated using the same English term which easily causes confusion.

To better understand these terminologies, consider that synonyms provide pathways to convey context, additional meanings and intentions of the original term. Synonyms are found abundantly throughout the texts to elaborate the scope and provide the reader with a fuller and richer understanding.

Charaka provides a list of synonyms for the term Āyurveda at the close of the first section of *sūtrasthāna* (Cha. Sū. 30/31-32). Review these terms to better understand the classical methodology, application and scope of Āyurveda.

Śhākhā

Śhākhā is defined as:

1. Any branch, specialty, or school of thought within a scientific body of knowledge
2. A limb of the body, or peripheral channel

On a broad level, Āyurveda is a branch of the Vedas. It is similar to a supplementary addendum, or additional, later development. In this context Āyurveda is an *upaveda*.

Additionally, within Āyurveda itself exist many specialities and several schools of thought. In this context, *śhākhā* refers to any of these speciality branches of clinical application such as *Kāya-chikitsā* (Internal Medicine), *Śhalya-tantra* (Surgery), or its major schools of thought, including the:

1. *Charaka sampradāya*

   Charaka's school of thought focusing on Internal Medicine

2. *Suśhruta sampradāya*

Suśhruta's school of thought focusing on Surgery

Vidyā

Vidyā is defined as:

1. Factual knowledge gained through active study, acquisition, learning, discovering or searching which can be developed and expanded over time

This implies that the body of Āyurvedic principles is a researched and developed science which requires extensive study and practice to apply.

Sūtra

Sūtra is defined as:

1. To sew; that which acts as the thread holding material together
2. A short sentence, rule, aphorism or statement; any work containing such statements.

The Āyurvedic treatises are compilations of rules and statements which teach the principles and practice of the science. The term *sūtra* can indicate a single line (usually an encapsulated principle or aphorism) from the text. *Sūtra* may also be short for *Sūtrasthāna*, typically the first section of the older classical *saṁhitās*, or treatises.

Jñāna

Jñāna is defined as:

1. Intellectual knowledge gained through the process of knowing or becoming acquainted with something
2. Knowledge generated through logic and practical application

The process of gaining knowledge through logic and application is a standard method of learning and practicing Āyurveda.

Śhāstra

Śhāstra is defined as:

1. A recorded work that deals with a scientific body of knowledge or subject matter in detail
2. Any tool, book, material, learning resource or instrument capable of teaching a subject matter in detail

The Āyurvedic treatises are detailed works containing instructions and explanations on the scientific body of knowledge of Āyurveda and act as the tools and resources for students to learn the subject properly. These include the Charaka Saṁhitā, Suśhruta Saṁhitā and many other classical texts. In India, these are actively and regularly applied in clinical practice today.

Lakṣhaṇa

Lakṣhaṇa is defined as:

1. Any distinguishing characteristic or attribute of anything
2. A sign or symptom of a disease; when primary or heralding, a *pradhāna lakṣhaṇa*
3. A definition or reference which delineates a specific understanding of a topic, event or instance

Āyurveda as an applied science focuses on the characteristics, attributes and qualities of an individual in order to maintain health and eliminate disease. These characteristics, or *lakṣhaṇas*, manifest in healthy and unhealthy states in various ways.

Tantra

Tantra is defined as:

1. Chapters of any type of scientific work
2. A leading, principle or essential part

3. A means or phrase which leads to two or more results, ambiguity (see also, *tantrayukti*)

The body of knowledge of Āyurveda is stored in authoritative texts which are organized into sections and chapters to form the means of study of the science.

Just as the definitions of Āyurveda may take years to unfold their various levels of meaning and understanding, synonyms can behave in a similar way. Gaining a fuller and deeper understanding of these meanings will come by reading the terms in various contexts throughout the classical texts.

TEST YOURSELF

Learn, review and memorize key terms from this section.

Charaka sampradāya

jñāna

lakṣhaṇa

paryāya

śhākhā

sampradāya

śhāstra

Suśhruta sampradāya

sūtra

tantra

vidyā

Chapter 2: Review

ADDITIONAL READING

Utilize these references to expand your understanding of the concepts in this chapter.

CLASSICS		1st read	2nd read
Charaka	Cha. Sū. 1/41 Cha. Sū. 30/		
Suśhruta	Su. Sū. 1/		

References

"Āyurveda." ĀYU Council, 2019, https://www.ayucouncil.org/ayurveda/.

Wujastyk, D., Smith, F. (2008). (Eds.). *Modern and Global Ayurveda: pluralism and paradigms.* Albany, NY: State University of New York Press.

QUESTIONS & ANSWERS

Record your questions for this chapter here for further research and discussion.

Question:

Answer:

Question:

Answer:

Question:

Answer:

SELF-ASSESSMENT

1. The Sanskrit term Āyurveda is formed by _____ and *veda*.
   a. *āhuṣh*
   b. *āyud*
   c. *āyuḥ*
   d. *ayur*
   e. None of the above

2. What characterizes New Age Āyurveda?
   a. Āyurveda is mind-body medicine.
   b. Āyurveda is the sister science of Yoga.
   c. Āyurveda is the source of other medical systems.
   d. All of the above
   e. None of the above

3. *Paribhāṣhā* means
   a. definition
   b. recorded work
   c. synonym
   d. to discuss
   e. to sew

4. Classical definitions of Āyurveda
   a. are based on Integrative Medicine
   b. are vaguely defined by Charaka
   c. equate health with happiness
   d. highlight the need for Āyurvedic doctors
   e. place priority on self-care

5. A qualified Āyurvedic professional is
   a. a graduate of a state-recognized institution in India
   b. a practitioner of any lineage-based Āyurveda
   c. a holistic healer recognized by AYUSH
   d. All of the above
   e. None of the above

6. Attempting to unify classical Āyurvedic theory and practice is seen primarily in
   a. American Āyurveda
   b. Global Āyurveda
   c. Modern Āyurveda
   d. New Age Āyurveda
   e. Professional Āyurveda

7. Which of the following can be considered *śhāstra*?
   a. Āyurveda
   b. Charaka Saṁhitā
   c. Suśhruta Saṁhitā
   d. All of the above
   e. None of the above

8. Classical Āyurvedic literature contains
   a. *jñāna*
   b. *lakṣhaṇas*
   c. *sūtras*
   d. *vidyā*
   e. All of the above

9. Which synonym of Āyurveda best reflects the descriptive nature of the science?
   a. *jñāna*
   b. *lakṣhaṇa*
   c. *śhākhā*
   d. *sampradāya*
   e. *tantra*

10. The specialty branch of surgery is
    a. the *Charaka sampradāya*
    b. *śhākhā*
    c. the *Suśhruta sampradāya*
    d. Both A and B
    e. Both B and C

Chapter 3 : Purpose and goals

KEY TERMS

ārogya	kāma	puruṣha	svāsthya
artha	mokṣha	puruṣhārtha	uttama
ātura	mūla	roga	vikāra
cha	praśhamana	svastha	vyādhi
dharma	prayojana		

Consensus among classical authors shows that Āyurveda has two specific purposes:

1. To maintain health
2. To eliminate disease

These are most commonly cited as the classical goals of Āyurveda in training and practice. They can be applied in many forms depending on the unique needs of each situation. For example, health maintenance is a daily, individual responsibility, while disease management falls under the purview of professional practice.

The two major schools of thought, the *Charaka sampradāya* and the *Suśhruta sampradāya*, agree on the main purposes and goals of Āyurveda.

Review the major references and compare and contrast them. Consider the purposes and goals from multiple perspectives including therapeutic, professional and personal.

TO PROTECT HEALTH AND ALLEVIATE DISEASE

Charaka's primary purpose of Āyurveda is to protect health and alleviate disease. This reference is provided in the final chapter of *sūtrasthāna* indicating its relevance in professional practice.

प्रयोगनं चास्य स्वस्थस्य
स्वास्थ्यरक्षणमातुरस्य विकारप्रशमनं च ।
२६

च. सू. ३०।२६

Prayojanaṁ chāsya svasthasya
svāsthyarakṣhaṇamāturasya
vikārapraśhamanaṁ cha | 26

Cha. Sū. 30/26

Prayojanaṁ (The purpose of Āyurveda is) *chāsya svasthasya svāsthya-rakṣhaṇam* (to maintain [literally, protect] the health of the healthy), *cha* (and) *āturasya vikāra-praśhamanaṁ* (to alleviate the disorders of the sick [literally, those who are suffering]).

TEST YOURSELF

Learn, review and memorize key terms from this section.

ātura

____

praśhamana

____

prayojana

____

svastha

____

svāsthya

____

vikāra

MANAGEMENT AND OUTCOMES

Suśhruta begins his treatise with a direct statement explaining the methods to attain goals of Āyurveda in clinical practice.

इह खल्वायुर्वेदप्रयोजनं - व्याध्युपसृष्टानां व्याधिपरिमोक्षः, स्वस्थस्य रक्षणं च ॥ १४

सु. सू. १।१४

Iha khalvāyurvedaprayojanaṁ - vyādhyupasṛṣhṭānāṁ vyādhiparimokṣhaḥ, svasthasya rakṣhaṇaṁ cha || 14

Su. Sū. 1/14

Iha khalvāyurveda-prayojanaṁ (And so, the purpose of Āyurveda is) *vyādhy-upasṛṣhṭānāṁ* (to eradicate [literally, throw off] disease) *vyādhi-parimokṣhaḥ*, (to relieve [literally, liberate one from] disease) *ca* (and) *svasthasya rakṣhaṇaṁ* (to protect the healthy).

TEST YOURSELF

Learn, review and memorize key terms from this section.

vyādhi

TO ACHIEVE LIFE GOALS

Charaka begins his treatise slightly differently. Here, he takes a more philosophical and personal perspective on achieving the goals of Āyurveda. These goals highlight the societal ideologies prevalant at his time and amongst his community.

धर्मार्थकाममोक्षाणामारोग्यं मूलमुत्तमम् ॥
रोगास्तस्यापहर्तारः श्रेयसो जीवितस्य च ।
१५

च. सू. १।१५

Dharmārthakāmamokṣhāṇāmārogyaṁ mūlamuttamam ||
Rogāstasyāpahartāraḥ śhreyaso jīvitasya cha | 15

Cha. Sū. 1/15

Ārogyaṁ (Complete absence of disease) *mūlam-uttamam* (is the ultimate root, or best way to achieve one's) *dharma* (duty, obligation or act which is borne as a responsibility by an individual), *artha* (any thing, something produced, material gain as a result of effort, or that which a person works for), *kāma* (enjoyment or pleasure, especially to be able to enjoy the fruits of one's labor) *mokṣhāṇām* (emancipation, liberation, release from worldly existence; setting free; transmigration). *Cha* (And) *rogāstasyāpahartāraḥ* (that which takes away, removes or eradicates disease [ie, Āyurveda]) *śhreyaso jīvitasya* (creates the best life possible).

These four life achievements are classically referred to as the *puruṣhārthas*. This term indicates the *artha* (goals, purposes, results) that each *puruṣha* (individual person) naturally wants to achieve.

Traditionally, the *puruṣhārthas* are considered a fundamental doctrine of Vedic philosophy and are found in prevalent practice in Hinduism today. Further study of Āyurveda reveals that these can be applied for general life guidance. In that capacity, they provide structure for individuals to plan major life stages.

It is important to note that with each of these intended purposes, the Sanskrit terms used are very specific. They convey distinct, precise meanings on how to remove disease. Therapeutic management in Āyurveda includes a wide range of methodologies and protocols that are intended to be performed based on detailed specifications.

The efforts towards gaining and maintaining health are so that the individual may fulfill their duties and obligations, and enjoy the fruits of their labor. Good health is the root of good action and the ability to complete goals. It is intended to be put to good use so individuals can achieve their goals, satisfy their desires and contribute to a healthy community and society.

TEST YOURSELF

Learn, review and memorize key terms from this section.

ārogya

artha

ca

dharma

kāma

mokṣha

mūla

puruṣha

puruṣhārtha

roga

uttama

Chapter 3: Review

ADDITIONAL READING

Utilize these references to expand your understanding of the concepts in this chapter.

CLASSICS		1st read	2nd read
Charaka	Cha. Sū. 1/15 Cha. Sū. 30/		
Suśhruta	Su. Sū. 1/		

References

Śarmā, R. K., & Dāsa, B. Agniveśha's Charaka Saṃhitā. Varanasi: Chowkhamba Sanskrit Series Office; Reprint Edition. 2016. Cha. Sū. 1/, 30/.

Singhal, G.D., et al. Suśhruta Saṁhitā of Suśhruta. Chaukhamba Sanskrit Pratiśhthan, Reprint Edition. 2015. Sū. Sū. 1/.

QUESTIONS & ANSWERS

Record your questions for this chapter here for further research and discussion.

Question:

Answer:

Question:

Answer:

Question:

Answer:

SELF-ASSESSMENT

1. To fulfill the purposes of Āyurveda, "*svasthasya svāsthya-rakṣhaṇam*," which common maxim could be applied?
   a. Early to bed, early to rise
   b. Eat to live, don't live to eat
   c. Health is wealth
   d. All of the above
   e. None of the above

2. *Vyādhi* refers to
   a. a goal of Āyurveda
   b. a personal life goal
   c. an individual
   d. disease
   e. liberation, transmigration

3. Which of the following prevents achievement of the *puruṣhārthas*?
   a. *artha*
   b. *dharma*
   c. *kāma*
   d. *mokṣha*
   e. *roga*

4. Suśhruta explains two methods to achieve the therapeutic goals of Āyurveda. They are
   a. disease prevention
   b. eradication or expulsion of disease
   c. relief or pacification of disease
   d. Both A and B
   e. Both B and C

5. Charaka's professional purpose of Āyurveda first states
   a. disease management
   b. disease prevention
   c. personal commitment
   d. root cause resolution
   e. None of the above

6. The *uttama mūla* for achieving life goals is
   a. *ārogya*
   b. *artha*
   c. *dharma*
   d. *kāma*
   e. *mokṣha*

7. According to Charaka, enjoyment of the fruits of one's labor should happen after
   a. *artha*
   b. *dharma*
   c. *kāma*
   d. *mokṣha*
   e. All of the above

8. Individual responsibility for health is primarily
   a. for disease management
   b. for eradicating disease from the root
   c. for health maintenance
   d. for maximum satisfaction in life
   e. for producing offspring

9. Classically, the goals of Āyurveda meet the needs of
   a. individuals
   b. professional practice
   c. society
   d. All of the above
   e. None of the above

10. The terms *roga* and *ārogya* are
   a. antonyms
   b. homonyms
   c. synonyms
   d. All of the above
   e. None of the above

Chapter 4 : Scope

KEY TERMS

Agada Tantra	karma	sampradāya	Vāstu
Bhūtavidya	Kaumāra-bhṛtya	śharīra	vidhi
Charaka sampradāya	Kāya-chikitsā	śhāstra	Viṣha-gara
hetu	Rasāyana	Suśhruta sampradāya	vyādhi
Jyotiṣha	Śhālākya-tantra	Vājīkaraṇa	Yoga
kāla	Śhalya-tantra		

The science of Āyurveda has several methods for structuring and classifying its knowledge and methodologies. These frameworks establish the scope of practice and delinate its specialities.

GENERAL OVERVIEW

Charaka provides a framework for the general overview of study and practice at the end of *sūtrasthāna.* He states that throughout the complete text, the knowledge of Āyurveda can be grouped in the following categories covering the scope of the science (Cha. Sū. 30/32).

Note that these categories are not exclusive. Knowledge may be appropriately classified into more than one category simultaneously. Compare Charaka's format to those of later authors and note the progression of development of the overall science.

Śharīra	The human body and its study
Vṛtti	Physiology, the study of the functions of the body
Hetu	Etiology, the causative factors for deviation from a healthy state
Vyādhi	Pathology, the study of disease
Karma	Therapeutics, the application of specific management protocols
Kārya	The goal of achievement of good health
Kāla	The influence of time in health, including measurable time (seasons) and stages of disease
Kartṛ	The Vaidya, the one who directs specific actions towards the therapeutic goal
Karaṇa	Wholesome factors and therapies
Vidhi	Rules, laws, methodologies, standard procedures and application

Several terms used in Charaka's framework are commonly found throughout Āyurvedic literature. However, these are all terms with multiple meanings which vary based on context. Here, Charaka has used them to specifically describe their application in fulfilling the purposes and goals of Āyurveda.

TEST YOURSELF

Learn, review and memorize key terms from this section.

hetu

____

kāla

karma

śharīra

vidhi

vyādhi

AṢHṬĀṄGA ĀYURVEDA

The scope of Āyurveda is most popularly known through its eight clinical branches, called the *Aṣhṭāṅga Āyurveda*. This classification has been consistently defined by major authors with minor differences in naming and order of priority. Each author lists the eight branches in an order appropriate to their school of thought.

The branches of the sciences are explained in Charaka Saṁhitā, *sūtrasthāna* 30/28 and Suśhruta Saṁhitā, *sūtrasthāna* 1/7-8.

In addition to thoroughly learning the *Aṣhṭāṅga Āyurveda*, Suśhruta emphasizes the importance of learning related *śhāstras*, or sciences, treatises or texts (Su. Sū. 4/7). Although the knowledge of one *śhāstra* may be sufficient for understanding its scope, it will have limitations.

Related knowledge clarifies and deepen one's understanding for broader application. The explanations and details provided through other specialized treatises help accomplish this goal and inform the student about related professionals who may be able to provide insight and support during practice.

The additional areas of study that Suśhruta refers to primarily include other branches and specializations within Āyurveda, particularly the *Charaka sampradāya* (Su. Sū. 34/14).

Aṅga Branch	Order in *Charaka*	Order in *Suśhruta*	Description of specialty (Su. Sū. 1/8)
Kāya-chikitsā	1	3	Internal Medicine Deals with diseases like fever, hemorrhage, wasting, epilepsy, leprosy, skin, insanity, urinary abnormalities, diabetes, diarrhea, dysentery
Śhālākya-tantra	2	2	Ophthalmology & Otorhinolaryngology Diseases affecting regions above clavicle, ears, eyes, oral and nasal cavities
Śhalya-tantra	3	1	Surgery Removal of foreign bodies, the use of blunt and sharp instruments, alkali treatment, cauterization, management of wounds and surgical conditions
Vājīkaraṇa	8	8	Virility and Fertility Deals with disorders of reproduction and enhancing sexual potency and pleasure
Bhūta-vidya	5	4	Study of the management of mental afflictions (may be similar to Psychiatry) Deals with mental disorders attributable to many causes, including supernatural activity, and diseases of *bhūtas*, or "has been" imprints of life (Cole, 2012)
Kumāra-bhṛtya or *Kaumāra bhṛtya*	6	5	Obstetrics and Pediatrics Pregnancy, delivery, and management of children from conception through puberty, purification of breast milk and care of the wet nurse
Rasāyana	7	7	Regenerative treatment principles Deals with restoring normal form and function, maintaining youth, increasing longevity, intellectual capacity, strength and health
Viṣha-gara	4	n/a	Toxicology Synonymous with *Agada-tantra*
Agada-tantra	n/a	6	Toxicology Deals with the signs, symptoms and management of poisoning from insects, animals or any source

The recommendation to study allied *śhāstras* also extends further to include the wide range of knowledge found throughout Vedic literature and sciences, including areas like *Jyotiṣha* (Vedic astrology), Yoga (a philosophy and practice for physical and mental control to achieve self-realization) and *Vāstu* (Vedic architecture, design and placement).

Each of these is a well-developed stream of knowledge and practice in its own right. Traditionally, Vedic scholars would be cross-functionally trained in these and additional disciplines to provide a complete, comprehensive foundation of knowledge in their professional practice.

Today, these Vedic sciences can still be utilized and applied along with the practice of Āyurveda. However, their utility and function would likely be more recognized and needed among people who include these related Vedic practices in their daily lives. The practice of cross-functional training in Vedic sciences seems to be more appropriate for actively practicing Hindus or Vedic scholars who can readily understand and apply these principles in an appropriate manner.

Because its principles are innately founded in natural law, Āyurveda can also be understood through streams of knowledge or sciences which are also based in the principles of nature. These include Western sciences such as astronomy, meteorology, environmental science, physics, chemistry, biology, anatomy and physiology.

Classical Āyurvedic laws can be seen in each of these when both perspectives are thoroughly understood and accurately applied. Āyurveda is capable of being applied in Western spheres and communities today. This allows scholars to communicate more effectively with their target audience in a language which is commonly known and well-accepted.

TEST YOURSELF

Learn, review and memorize key terms from this section.

Agada Tantra

Bhūtavidya

Charaka sampradāya

Jyotiṣha

Kaumāra-bhṛtya

Kāya-chikitsā

Rasāyana

Śhālākya-tantra

Śhalya-tantra

sampradāya

śhāstra

Suśhruta sampradāya

Vājīkaraṇa

Vāstu

Viṣha-gara

Yoga

EMERGING PRACTICE OF ĀYURVEDA

Looking at Āyurveda as a medical system today, it can be considered complete in its core principles and methodologies. The conspicuously missing component is a current collection of evidence and efficacy data recorded in an Āyurvedic scientific format which can be applied appropriately in localized communities and cultures.

The classical science contains a finite set of known, standard principles, or tenets upon which it operates. It divides itself nicely into two major areas for the purposes of prevention and cure. And within each of those areas, it contains a multitude of approaches, tools, procedures and processes for achieving specific goals.

To effectively prevent disease and maintain health, several frameworks are described in the classics that allow complete analysis of an individual covering 12 main categories of factors that directly influence the state of individual health.

To cure disease, methodologies determine the root cause, understand the disease manifestation and attempt to predict the likely outcome (curable, or otherwise) with varying degrees of confidence. Appropriate intervention is planned and enacted to create supportive mechanisms covering all aspects of life to support disease management and promote health. When managed properly, these personalized approaches stop the pathology, effectively reverse it, and restore an individual's health over time.

These principles and frameworks, along with the surviving body of applied knowledge are more than sufficient to practice Āyurveda in its original scope today. In fact, they can and should be developed to meet the ever increasing health demands of the rising population today.

Over the last few decades, a global resurgence of interest in Āyurveda has grown. This is being largely driven by the ever-increasing need for health care capable of effectively addressing today's most common issues. These including chronic disease, lifestyle disorders, and other non-emergency health pandemics. Āyurveda is uniquely positioned to offer effective, reliable and affordable solutions to manage and potentially cure many common health issues.

Chapter 4: Review

ADDITIONAL READING

Utilize these references to expand your understanding of the concepts in this chapter.

CLASSICS		1st read	2nd read
Charaka	Cha. Sū. 30/28 Cha. Sū. 30/32		
Suśhruta	Su. Sū. 1/7 Su. Sū. 4/7 Su. Sū. 34/14		

References

Cole, F. T. (2012) Science Of Light, Volume II. Nevada City, CA: Science of Light, LLC.

Śarmā, R. K., & Dāsa, B. Agniveśha's Charaka Saṃhitā. Varanasi: Chowkhamba Sanskrit Series Office; Reprint Edition. 2016. Cha. Sū. 30/.

Singhal, G.D., et al. Suśhruta Saṁhitā of Suśhruta. Chaukhamba Sanskrit Pratiśhthan, Reprint Edition. 2015. Sū. Sū.

Murthy, K. R. Srikantha. Vāgbhaṭa's Aṣhṭāṅga Hṛdayam. Chowkhamba Kṛṣhṇadas Academy, Varanasi. Reprint Edition. 2016. AH. Sū. 1/.

QUESTIONS & ANSWERS

Record your questions for this chapter here for further research and discussion.

Question:

Answer:

Question:

Answer:

Question:

Answer:

SELF-ASSESSMENT

1. When Suśhruta recommends studying additional *śhāstras* to improve one's practice of Āyurveda, which would provide the most benefit?
   a. *Jyotiṣha*
   b. *Kāyachikitsā*
   c. *Mānasaroga*
   d. *Śhalyatantra*
   e. the *Charaka sampradāya*

2. Classical *rasāyana* can be correlated today with
   a. Functional medicine
   b. Genomics
   c. Integrative medicine
   d. Precision medicine
   e. Regenerative medicine

3. Charaka includes the study of pathology under
   a. *hetu*
   b. *kāla*
   c. *kārya*
   d. *vidhi*
   e. *vyādhi*

4. The role of *kāla* in health is seen through
   a. normal progression of disease
   b. seasonal changes
   c. stages of life
   d. All of the above
   e. None of the above

5. *Śhālākya-tantra* most closely relates to which specialty today?
   a. HEENT
   b. Internal Medicine
   c. Obstetrics
   d. Pediatrics
   e. Surgery

6. Classically, *Śhalya-tantra* includes
   a. cauterization
   b. use of alkalis
   c. use of blunt instruments
   d. use of sharp instruments
   e. All of the above

7. Classically, Yoga's role in context of Āyurveda is
   a. as a secondary, allied *śhāstra*
   b. for deeper studies in HInduism
   c. to increase knowledge of Vedic sciences
   d. All of the above
   e. None of the above

8. Management of labor and delivery is practiced as
   a. *Kumāra-bhṛtya*
   b. Obstetrics
   c. Pediatrics
   d. Both A and B
   e. Both B and C

9. Consider a case of acute poisoning. Which classical specialty would be most apt for managing it?
   a. *Agada-tantra*
   b. *Bhūta-vidya*
   c. *Kāya-chikitsā*
   d. *Śhalya-tantra*
   e. None of the above

10. Consider a case of acute fever. Which classical specialty would be most apt for managing it?
   a. *Kāya-chikitsā*
   b. *Rasāyana*
   c. *Śhālākya-tantra*
   d. *Vājīkaraṇa*
   e. Any of the above

Chapter 5 : Models of Āyurvedic health care

The widest range of models of Āyurvedic health care can best be seen in practice in India today. The legal recognition of Āyurveda currently provides the most rigorous minimum standards for education, licensing and practice globally. While there are still many improvements that can be made, India is the leader in comprehensive Āyurvedic education and practice.

ĀYURVEDA IN INDIA

In India, Āyurveda has adapted itself over many centuries to continously meet the demands of the changing society. Today, Āyurveda can be found in almost every segment of society. Because it has evolved over millennia as an integrated component of daily living, a large portion of the Indian population could be considered to be using Āyurveda in some form on a daily basis, even if they do not directly recognize or admit to it.

On a professional level, Āyurveda is practiced in small, neighborhood clinics, nursing homes, rehabilitation centers, *Pañchakarma* centers, hospitals, retreat centers and through other specialty providers. A wide range of care is available which meets the needs of basic, common ailments and extends to delivery, surgery and other complex medical management in hospital settings.

With the increase in popularity of Āyurveda over the last decade, commercial interest in spa service, beauty treatments, natural cosmetics, nutraceuticals and medical tourism has mushroomed.

Maintaining high-quality services in these growing sectors has been a challenge. To improve standards, the Quality Council of India (QCI) developed and promoted current guidelines for AYUSH hospitals, including Āyurveda, through the National Accreditation Board for Hospitals & Health care Providers, or NABH (Accreditation of Ayurveda Hospitals, 2018).

Notably, the first Āyurvedic hospital to be formally accredited with NABH standards was AyurVAID Hospitals in 2010 (About Us, 2016). This chain of Āyurvedic hospitals is demonstrating effective practice of classical Āyurveda to meet the needs of the middle class in India today. It is an important example of Āyurveda's potential to impact and considerably improve health care now.

Traditional centers of Āyurveda include two significant establishments of South India which are currently the oldest, continuously operating centers - the Keraleeya Ayurveda Samajam ("About Us." Keraleeya Ayurveda Samajam, 2017) and the Kottakkal Arya Vaidya Sala ("About Us." Arya Vaidya Sala, Kottakkal, 2017), both established in 1902.

These two centers embody the traditional practices of Kerala-style Āyurveda in large establishments that combine education, classical medicine production, treatment and all other functional aspects. They are designed to handle a wide range of complex medical cases and patients seeking all forms of Āyurvedic health care. These institutions provide a window into effective methods and practices of traditional Āyurveda which continue to work today.

The public sector has recently begun advancing the scope and practice of Āyurveda as global interest has increased. Āyurvedic health care services are supplied through a multi-level approach of primary, secondary and tertiary levels. Each meets specific needs for the public in terms of hospital and clinic services, professional education and collaboration with other systems of medicine.

ĀYURVEDA GLOBALLY

Āyurveda is in its nascent stages of development outside of India. The historically recent popularization of Āyurveda primarily targets its easily marketable aspects and largely ignores the extensive health care potential.

Legal, social, environmental and educational obstacles have contributed to many of the misconceptions of Āyurveda today. Lack of advanced health care and medical infrastructure compounds these challenges.

In order for Āyurveda to become fully established outside of India, advanced education, legal practice and professional support must be available collectively. Until these components are accepted publicly and through necessary channels of regulation, Āyurveda will likely continue to exist in a reduced capacity.

EXAMPLES OF ĀYURVEDIC HEALTH CARE

The most complete, effective and diversified practice of Āyurveda is available in India today. A wide variety of hospitals, clinics, treatment centers, resorts and specialty centers serve the needs of urban and rural communities.

Outpatient facilities

For less complicated, outpatient care, Āyurvedic clinics are commonly available in most communities. These are typically staffed by at least one Āyurvedic Doctor and one or more assistants. Patients visit the clinic during the normal operating hours and at well-established clinics, there is almost always a wait to see the Āyurvedic Doctor.

The Āyurvedic Doctor performs an assessment of each patient using classical parameters and often times modern, Western diagnostic tools. Classically, this involves hearing the patient's main complaints and relevant history, asking the patient specific questions and observing any affected areas of the body.

Additionally, Western diagnostic methods are commonly utilized. These include laboratory work (blood, liver and kidney panels). diagnostic imaging (CT, MRI, Ultrasound), X-ray and other tools that may be available.

Inpatient facilities

For more serious, complicated cases, and especially with classical *Pañchakarma* , it is always preferable to have the patient remain in the hospital under supervision. Āyurvedic hospitals generally provide inpatient and outpatient services to support patients during each stage of management. At larger Āyurvedic hospitals, Āyurvedic Doctors are either on rotation 24 hours a day or on call.

Āyurvedic hospitals are often established in conjunction with Western medical hospitals in India. Āyurvedic services may be available as a wing in a Western hospital. This collaboration allows emergency medical care, life-saving drugs, tools and resources to be available to patients through practicing the full scope of both systems of health care. This is possible in India because of the acceptance and practice of medical pluralism.

Other forms of inpatient care exist in resort settings and provide similar, but generally less extensive services for Western medicine and emergency medical care. These traditional Āyurvedic hospitals mainly focus on *Pañchakarma* and *rasāyana*. Patients often prefer the natural setting for receiving long-term treatments and therapies.

In these environments, the traditional Āyurvedic hospital is structured quite differently from modern, Western medical facilities. Here, Āyurvedic Doctors and support staff are also present 24 hours a day, but they function somewhat differently.

The Āyurvedic hospital setting generally consists of either a large building with inpatient and outpatient facilities, treatment rooms, a kitchen and eating area, and a formulary with medicine dispensary. In more resort-like settings, inpatient facilities may be small, one or two bedroom cottages with individually attached treatment rooms.

For long-term, inpatient stays, the resort settings are often preferred for those who have the means to support themselves financially and completely disconnect themselves from regular commitments.

The complete Āyurvedic health care team functions in a cross-disciplinary format to provide all necessary steps in the patients' management plan. Āyurvedic Doctors assess patients typically twice each day to confirm results. Support staff perform a wide range of tasks including performing hands-on therapeutic treatments, medicine preparation, food preparation and maintenance. Many traditional Āyurvedic hospitals schedule support staff to work on rotating schedules in all areas of the facility.

These formats have worked well in India for centuries and they offer excellent insight and guidance for establishing Āyurvedic centers outside of India.

Rehabilitative care

In India, nursing homes and rehabilitation centers offer long-term care and support to patients who are chronically ill. The use of Āyurveda at these centers provides a more holistic approach by considering dietary needs, rehabilitative activities, treatments and strengthening Āyurvedic medicines.

Āyurveda also plays an important role in end of life care. This is most easily seen in it's cultural influences and ties to Hinduism. The process of dying and death due to natural causes is an expected stage of life in most Indian cultures. Families play the primary role of caregivers for ageing and dying relatives. As an anticipated life event, death is planned for and families are often prepared to follow specific cultural formalities.

Preventive care

Preventive care through Āyurveda is also largely found in cultural and religious habits, particularly in Hinduism. Preventive care is often considered related to "home remedies" and includes aspects of diet and lifestyle which are passed down through generations in families and communities.

Classically, this method of preventive care is very effective because it develops a strong tolerance and normalcy for the individual towards specific remedies.

Having personal, direct knowledge of effective remedies also highlights the importance of individual responsibility for health maintenance.

Emergency management

Prior to the widespread use of Western medicine in India, Āyurveda was regularly used for emergency management. Common, acute situations included trauma, fractures, poisoning from food, insects, snakes and other animals.

Classical literature, especially the Suśhruta Saṁhitā and later, consolidated works, provide detailed descriptions, instructions and management protocols for the complex management of emergency procedures, surgeries, complicated deliveries, plastic surgery, and surgeries for the eyes, ears, nose, throat and oral cavity. Management of wounds due to trauma, battle injuries and other blunt and sharp forces is also described in detail.

Today, Āyurveda is mostly relegated to secondary support in surgical and emergency management. Modern, Western tools like anesthesia, surgical instruments, catheters, injections and other methods take precedence over traditional management. When applied properly within this format, Āyurveda is capable of providing improved methods for patient preparation (when possible), and recovery.

Chapter 5: Review

ADDITIONAL READING

Utilize these references to expand your understanding of the concepts in this chapter.

REQUIRED READING	Chapters
Modern and Global Ayurveda	12, 13, 14

OPTIONAL READING	Format
AyurVaid Hospitals, https://ayurvaid.com/	online
Keraleeya Ayurveda Samajam, http://samajam.org/	online
Kottakkal Arya Vaidya Sala, https://www.aryavaidyasala.com/	online

References

"Accreditation of Ayurveda Hospitals." National Accreditation Board for Hospitals & Health care Providers, 2018. http://www.nabh.co/documents_Ayurveda.aspx

"About Us." AyurVAID Hospitals, 2016. https://ayurvaid.com/about-us

"About Us." Keraleeya Ayurveda Samajam, 2017. http://samajam.org/about

"About Us." Arya Vaidya Sala, Kottakkal, (AVS), 2017. http://www.aryavaidyasala.com/about-us.php

Wujastyk, D., Smith, F. (2008). (Eds.). Modern and Global Ayurveda: pluralism and paradigms. Albany, NY: State University of New York Press.

QUESTIONS & ANSWERS

Record your questions for this chapter here for further research and discussion.

Question:

Answer:

Question:

Answer:

Question:

Answer:

SELF-ASSESSMENT

1. The practice of *Śhalya-tantra* in India can be regularly seen today in
   a. Āyurvedic hospitals
   b. Āyurvedic retreat centers
   c. Āyurvedic spas and beauty parlors
   d. nursing homes
   e. neighborhood clinics

2. The widest range of Āyurvedic health care models in practice is available in
   a. Germany
   b. Great Britain
   c. India
   d. Malaysia
   e. United States

3. Western medicine and Āyurveda are readily available in India due to
   a. active business
   b. advanced education
   c. medical pluralism
   d. tradition
   e. None of the above

4. In India, Āyurveda is available at
   a. neighborhood clinics
   b. nursing homes
   c. *Pañchakarma* centers
   d. rehabilitation centers
   e. All of the above

5. Why is Āyurveda challenging to practice outside of India?
   a. Lack of advanced education
   b. Legal issues
   c. Professional support
   d. All of the above
   e. None of the above

6. What is NABH?
   a. National Accreditation Board for Homecare
   b. National Accreditation Board for Homeopathy
   c. National Accreditation Board of Hospitals
   d. National Accreditation Board for Hospitals & Health care Providers
   e. National Accreditation Board of Hospitals & Homecare

7. Āyurveda is particularly beneficial in rehabilitative care because of its
   a. holistic approach
   b. medicines without side effects
   c. relaxing spa treatments
   d. slow, gentle response time
   e. All of the above

8. Āyurvedic resorts generally focus on providing
   a. outpatient care
   b. *Pañchakarma*
   c. *Rasāyana*
   d. Both A and B
   e. Both B and C

9. In India, preventive care using Āyurveda over many generations has encouraged individuals to
   a. enter the Āyurvedic profession
   b. learn how to make complex Āyurvedic medicines
   c. recognize their personal responsibility for health maintenance
   d. All of the above
   e. None of the above

10. Emergency management in Āyurveda is originally a specialty of
    a. Charaka
    b. Integrative Medicine with Āyurveda
    c. lineage-based practice
    d. Suśhruta
    e. Vedic sciences

Chapter 6 : Āyurveda and holistic, sustainable health care

KEY TERMS

Āyurvedic health care	individual responsibility	macrocosm-microcosm	sustainability
ethical practice	interconnected factors	resource management	variable outcome
holism			

Āyurveda provides a robust framework for health care that encompasses health maintenance, disease management, root cause resolution, radical treatment and regeneration. It has the potential to provide a health care system that can support a wide range of basic and complex needs today.

With a recent resurgence of interest, Āyurveda has the opportunity to establish itself in many cultures on a global scale through a variety of languages and presentations. It can become a leader in 21st century primary health care through its inherent principles of holism, sustainability and personalization.

The concepts of holism and sustainability have always served as core principles and practices of Āyurveda. They can be found embedded in classical literature throughout its history and development.

These concepts are not new to Āyurveda but they were likely prioritized over periods of development due to many of the same mistakes that are being realized today in large scale societies. Issues that affect the human population on local, national and global scales are directly connected to health on individual and social levels. Āyurveda's ability to adapt itself to constantly changing needs and environments is one of its key features that has supported its continued practice and success.

HOLISM

The concept of holism is a well-established tenet in classical Āyurveda which has been recognized as a core principle of the science since its earliest records.

The Merriam-Webster Dictionary defines holism as (Holism, 2018):

1. a theory that the universe and especially living nature is correctly seen in terms of interacting wholes (as of living organisms) that are more than the mere sum of elementary particles

2. a study or method of treatment that is concerned with wholes or with complete systems

The New World Encyclopedia provides a more detailed definition of holism with additional descriptions of its use in specific fields of study and practice (Holism, 2018, January 12):

"Holism (from ὅλος *holos*, a Greek word meaning all, entire, total) is the idea that all the properties of a given system (biological, chemical, social, economic, mental, linguistic, etc.) cannot be determined or explained by the sum of its component parts alone. Instead, the system as a whole determines in an important way how the parts behave."

In the Western sphere, Aristotle is credited

with identifying this principle. He recorded it in his work *Metaphysics* by stating that "The whole is more than the sum of its parts." (Holism, 2018, January 12) It is possible that holism and several other principles were adapted from streams of knowledge shared through Vedic sciences. Historical records indicate strong ties between the Indian subcontinent, Europe and Central Asia that were prevalent during these time periods. Trade routes provided networks for sharing a wide range of knowledge, tools, products and other goods.

As the theory and philosophy of holism developed in Europe over Medieval periods, scholars associated its workings more closely with religion. Complexities of holistic approaches that could not be explained through the functions of individual components were eventually determined to be due to "God's design." Scientists of the time speculated that if this were the determining factor in complex, holistic scenarios, then these should not be considered scientific. This resulted in a sharp rejection of the principle of holism within developing and modernizing scientific communities.

Today, scholars and scientists are beginning to accept the complexities of holism and unpredictable outcomes as an inherent quality of the natural world. Āyurveda remains an unparalleled, foundational system to understand and investigate holism as a function of human health. Deeper study of the science and its frameworks along with appropriate research and analysis with current tools and technologies holds many possibilites to advance knowledge in human health and the natural world.

TEST YOURSELF

Learn, review and memorize key terms from this section.

holism

HOLISM IN ĀYURVEDA

Classical Āyurvedic works offer many examples of holism through functions of nature and the human body. Traditional scholars and practitioners explored, analyzed and documented these principles and their effects over large periods of time. Their work greatly advanced the understanding of connections between the external world and the inner workings of the human body.

As these principles were established and developed, traditional scholars also created very specific terminology for each concept. A thorough understanding of these concepts today will provide the means for current scientists to learn a framework for holistic health care and apply it effectively.

The following review of holism in Āyurveda discusses several key principles of the science.

Interconnected factors

The science of Āyurveda is built on a web of interconnected factors which traverse all life on earth. In the human body, Āyurveda classifies the main components into three factors called *doṣhas* which govern all physical manifestations and functions.

The *doṣhas* connect every aspect of structure and function within the human body and can be manipulated through Āyurveda to produce specific alterations in states of health as well as clinical interventions. The characteristics and functions used to describe the *doṣhas* provide the means to access and manipulate related factors within the system of the human body.

Vāgbhaṭa introduces the interconnected nature of the *doṣhas* through direct connections in the physical body and external world.

ते व्यापिनोऽपि हृन्नभ्योरधोमध्योर्ध्वसंश्रयाः ॥ ७
वयोहोरात्रिभुक्तानां तेऽन्तमध्यादिगाः क्रमात ।

अ. हृ. सू. १।७.५

Te vyāpino ' pi hṛnnabhyoradhomadhordhva saṁśhrayāḥ || 7
Vyohorātribhuktānāṁ te ' ntamadhādigāḥ kramāt |

AH Sū. 1/7.5

Te (They [the *doṣhas*]) *vyāpino* (spread throughout [the body]) *api* (and additionally) *hṛn* (the heart), *nabhi* (the umbilicus), *uru* (and the thighs) *adho* ([act as the markers for] the lower third [of the body]), *madha* (the middle), *urdhva* (and the upper) *saṁśhrayāḥ* (which are each the specific locations [where a *doṣha*, ie kapha, pitta and vāta] are localized). *Vyoho* ([Likewise] during the day) *rātri* (and the night), *bhuktānāṁ* (and during the [three] stages of digestion) *te* (they [the *doṣhas*] are found) *anta* (before), *madhādi* (during the middle) *gāḥ* (and afterwards) *kramāt* (in varying degrees).

In a short verse, Vāgbhaṭa conveys extensive depth that covers several principles of the *doṣhas*. He recognizes their interconnectedness between the human body and external world through circadian rhythyms. The details of these principles and their implications in practice will be discussed in depth in subsequent volumes.

In advanced studies of Āyurveda, these interconnected principles continue to expand. As they become more complex, they function in a multifactorial manner to provide a framework for highly personlized and highly specified individual assessment, diagnosis and treatment. Charaka provides detailed explanations and instructions through the text of the Charaka Saṁhitā.

On the level of the individual human body, interconnected factors can also be seen through the relationship between the physical body and the mind. While these are both stated to reside within the physical body itself, they are not one and the same. Specific channels allow them to connect and transfer certain effects, including disease, between them.

Chakrapāṇi specifically comments on the ability for disease to move between the mind and body especially in chronic conditions (Cha. Ni. 1/4).

Variable outcome

The sciences of complexity and chaos theory now recognize variability and unpredictability in closed systems given the same inputs. Scientific holism holds that the behavior of a system cannot be perfectly predicted, no matter how much data is available. Natural systems can produce surprisingly unexpected behavior, and it is suspected that behavior of such systems might be computationally irreducible, which means it would not be possible to even approximate the system state without a full simulation of all the events occurring in the system (Holism, 2018, January 12).

Complex, chaotic results are often seen in all health care disciplines. No intervention or treatment is capable of a 100% positive outcome because of myriad variations in each individual. This variability inherently leads to a certain degree of unpredictability in every system.

As a complex framework of health care, Āyurveda has developed and refined a systemmatic approach to identifying variables and measuring them with a high level of precision. Systemmatic practice of classical Āyurveda would be more likely to reveal higher quality outcomes than a disjointed, fractured or integrative approach.

Examples of variable outcomes appear frequently in classical literature. Charaka clearly states that the same *doṣhas* present within a single individual have the potential to produce health or disease depending on their input factors (Cha. Śhā. 6/18). The variable outcome is strongly influenced by the functions of the *doṣhas* at any given point in time. Their functioning is highly dependent upon every other possible factor in the framework.

Macrocosm-microcosm

The internal and external dimensions of the physical world are represented by the human body and the external world in the context of Āyurveda. This is a principle popularly known as the theory of macrocosm-microcosm.

Charaka mentions this principle in many instances throughout the text (Cha. Sū. 12/, Cha. Śhā. 4/13, Cha. Śhā. 5/3-8). He correlates the internal *doṣhas* with specific external functions of nature. Using this methodology, he is able to understand the functions of the *doṣhas* and predict their behavior.

TEST YOURSELF

Learn, review and memorize key terms from this section.

interconnected factors

macrocosm-microcosm

variable outcome

SUSTAINABILITY

The concept of sustainability has only arisen recently to be recognized in Western spheres. In traditional cultures around the globe however, it has been a well-known, common component of individual life and society for millennia or more.

The use of the term sustainability has grown since it was first coined in 1980 by the International Union for the Conservation of Nature as the phrase "sustainable development" (Sustainable development, 2015). Its primary intention is that economic and social growth "meets the needs of the present without compromising the ability of future generations to meet their own needs" (United Nations Department of Economic and Social Affairs 1987).

Sustainability is defined as (Sustainability, 2018):

1. capable of being sustained
2. of, relating to, or being a method of harvesting or using a resource so that the resource is not depleted or permanently damaged; sustainable techniques, sustainable agriculture
3. of or relating to a lifestyle involving the use of sustainable methods; sustainable society

The concept of sustainability in every aspect of life is not new. As sustainability becomes an increasing priority over the coming years and decades on a global scale, it will be obvious that its application must extend to all aspects in all societies.

Within the scope of health care, the Alliance for Natural Health defines sustainable health care as ("What is sustainable healthcare?" 2019):

"A complex system of interacting approaches to the restoration, management and optimisation of human health that has an ecological base, that is environmentally, economically and socially viable indefinitely, that functions harmoniously both with the human body and the non-human environment, and which does not result in unfair or disproportionate impacts on any significant contributory element of the healthcare system."

TEST YOURSELF

Learn, review and memorize key terms from this section.

sustainability

SUSTAINABILITY IN ĀYURVEDA

The concept of sustainability has been engrained into the practice of Āyurveda likely since its inception. However, several key references exist indicating that sustainability was not always adhered to over various periods in history.

The most prominant example of disregard for sustainability in the records of the classical texts is the extinction of many species of medicinal plants over the course of time. In earlier works, references to medicinal plants cannot be found or correlated to an existing species today. And in later works, the extinction of highly prized species is diretly mentioned by stating their non-availability and providing replacements.

Sustainability in Āyurveda, any health care system or aspect of life must be prioritized among individuals and entire societies. Dozens of examples exist today that demonstrate the negative outcomes of human behavior and habits when sustainability is ignored.

There is likely a continuous shift between priotization and disregard towards the issue that occurs over several generations. The negative consequences are often easy to ignore until the problem becomes significant.

Just as the scholars and practitioners of Āyurveda recognized and documented over time the imiportance of prioritizing and maintaining sustainability, professionals today must do the same.

The following key examples from the Āyurvedic classics demonstrate sustainability in action.

Resource management

As previously mentioned, resource management is one of the most critical factors to consider for sustainability in Āyurveda. Charaka recommends that specific medicinal plants and their appropriate parts be harvested during certain seasons to maximize their potency and efficacy (Cha. Ka. 1/10). This effective strategy allowed for reduced consumption of precious natural resources.

Similary, in *Bhāva Prakāśha*, specific replacements for non-existant medicinal plants have been provided with recognition that the original medicinal plants are likely unavailable (ie, extinct). This practice probably developed as a direct outcome of prior overharvesting.

In clinical practice, Charaka additionally states that rare medicaments and supplies should be reserved for those who could afford them. Practitioners were acutely aware of resource limitations especially with medicinal formulations, source ingredients and the requirements for compounding. In order to sustain their availability, they would need to be compensated appropriately. This compensation was not restricted to financial means only but could be any form that supported the process required to procure the final medicine (Cha. Sū. 15/19-21).

Individual responsibility

As a complete, primary health care system, Āyurveda provides specific expectations for everyone and everything involved in the health care management team. Patients who come to Āyurveda are expected to adhere to certain guidelines to improve their outcomes.

In clinical scenarios, guidelines are structured to support the targeted therapeutic interventions that are required to remove a disorder and re-establish a normal state of health. These include (Cha. Sū. 9/9):

1. Attention and focus to the treatment; prioritization of treatment over other life commitments and activities
2. Compliance and discipline to adhere to protocols appropriately
3. Trust in the Āyurvedic professional along with fortitude and bravery to follow through with all required aspects of management
4. Sufficient knowledge about themselves to recognize responses and changes, and the ability to convey those accurately and meaningfully

Additionally, for ongoing health maintenance, individuals are expected to adhere to daily and seasonal routines that promote health and reduce the opportunity for disease. These routines are well-developed for populations in the Indian subcontinent and are often applied as part of family or cultural tradition.

By following these routines of *dina cārya* (daily routines) and *ṛtu cārya* (seasonal routines), entire communities support each other in positive ways to produce healthy individuals, families and groups.

Included in these routines are recommendations for diet, activities, sleep schedules and many other aspects of life. The classics provide detailed references for all in the context of the Indian subcontinent and population.

Ethical practice

A final major component of sustainability in Āyurveda is demonstrated through its adherence to ethical professional practice.

All classical authors describe the extensive level of education that is required before one could practice as a qualified *Vaidya* (Āyurvedic Doctor). This training lasted multiple years and was considered complete only after the student was capable of reciting the science through classical references, demonstrating competence in practice and receiving final recognition from the teacher that they were prepared to begin their career.

Vaidyas were then held to minimum standards of practice and in earlier times were highly respected members of society. Proper behavior towards patients, especially those of the opposite sex, was one of many strict rules for ethical practice.

Today, a similar and appropriate approach must be implemented for the profession. In India and globally, Āyurveda has succumbed to many compromises of its most basic standards. Professional education, clinical practice, research and development have all been depressed and negatively affected over several centuries. These require a comprehensive approach and actionable plan to restore the practice and image of the profession.

TEST YOURSELF

Learn, review and memorize key terms from this section.

ethical practice

---

individual responsibility

---

resource management

ĀYURVEDIC HEALTH CARE

Āyurveda can be applied and practiced today in ways that further enhance its focus on holism and sustainability. With the judicious use of available tools and technology, Āyurveda can provide a means and pathway to long-term, sustainable health for individuals, communities and societies that are ready to take responsibility and actively participate to improve their personal health.

A model of primary Āyurvedic health care would ideally include minimum standards that expect active participation from everyone involved. These standards should emphasize:

1. Individual responsibility
2. Affordable, accessible, reliable and timely care
3. Individual health education
4. Actionable steps to improve individual health, and prevent abnormalities and dysfunction
5. Providing the simplest treatment required to effect a proper, positive clinical outcome and restoration of normal health
6. Identification of root cause along with its resolution
7. Clear plans for annual health maintenance through multiple formats of daily, seasonal and annual therapeutics
8. Maintain a goal to stabilize patients and end treatment at the appropriate time
9. Promote an adaptable, flexible and personalized approach to health care

Most of these standards are immediate needs today for societies around the globe. Āyurveda has the capacity to provide primary health care right now to meet these needs and more.

TEST YOURSELF

Learn, review and memorize key terms from this section.

Āyurvedic health care

Chapter 6: Review

ADDITIONAL READING

Utilize these references to expand your understanding of the concepts in this chapter.

REQUIRED READING	Chapters
Holism, https://www.newworldencyclopedia.org/entry/Holism	online
Sustainable development, https://www.newworldencyclopedia.org/entry/Sustainable_development	online

OPTIONAL READING	Format
Sustainable health care, https://www.resilience.org/stories/2012-08-03/sustainable-health care/	online

References

"Holism." Merriam-Webster, 2018, https://www.merriam-webster.com/dictionary/holism

"Holism." (2018, January 12). New World Encyclopedia, Retrieved April 26, 2019 from https://www.newworldencyclopedia.org/entry/Holism

"Sustainability." Merriam-Webster, 2018, https://www.merriam-webster.com/dictionary/sustainability

"Sustainable development." (2015, November 6). New World Encyclopedia, Retrieved April 26, 2019 from https://www.newworldencyclopedia.org/entry/Sustainable_development.

United Nations Department of Social and Economic Affairs. 1987. Report of the World Commission on Environment and Development United Nations. Retrieved December 23, 2007.

"What is sustainable healthcare?" Alliance for Natural Health, Retrieved April 26, 2019 from https://anh-usa.org/position-papers/sustainable-healthcare/

QUESTIONS & ANSWERS

Record your questions for this chapter here for further research and discussion.

Question: ______________________________

Answer: ______________________________

Question: ______________________________

Answer: ______________________________

Question: ______________________________

Answer: ______________________________

SELF-ASSESSMENT

1. Complexity theory and its related modes of thought are the opposite of
   a. adaptive systems
   b. Āyurveda
   c. biology
   d. reductionism
   e. scientific holism

2. Holism between the individual human being and the natural world is described by
   a. interconnected factors
   b. macrocosm-microcosm
   c. sustainability
   d. All of the above
   e. None of the above

3. "The whole is more than the sum of its parts," is the definition of holism stated by
   a. Aristotle
   b. Charaka
   c. Euclid
   d. Plato
   e. Socrates

4. During the Medieval period and until the 20th century holism was considered
   a. a law of biology
   b. a law of physics
   c. the God particle
   d. unscientific
   e. None of the above

5. Holism in Āyurveda is seen through the functions of
   a. *doṣhas*
   b. ethical practice
   c. external environment
   d. spirituality
   e. sustainability

6. Within the context of health care, sustainability focuses on
   a. dietary requirements
   b. economics
   c. environmental needs
   d. human health
   e. social growth

7. Resource management in Āyurveda is likely a direct outcome of
   a. harvesting medicinal plants only at specific times of the year
   b. high demand for medicines
   c. judicious use of medicines
   d. overharvesting
   e. poor soil quality

8. Prioritization of individual responsibility in Āyurvedic health care empowers the
   a. Āyurvedic doctor
   b. Āyurvedic medicine
   c. nurse
   d. patient
   e. Western doctor

9. Lack of ethical practice in Āyurveda today can be seen in
   a. common adulteration of Āyurvedic medicines in India
   b. lack of professional adherence to practicing within scope
   c. low quality professional Āyurvedic education
   d. All of the above
   e. None of the above

10. Instead of masking symptoms, Āyurvedic health care works to
    a. adhere only to classical *dina cārya* and *ṛtu cārya*
    b. educate patients and expect immediate changes
    c. prioritize dietary recommendations
    d. resolve the root cause
    e. utilize complex medicinal formulations for all disorders

Chapter 7 : Western health care, biomedicine and Āyurveda

KEY TERMS

Complementary and Alternative medicine (CAM)	health care	Western health care	Western medicine

Traditional health care in the United States has been dominated by Western medicine or biomedicine for over 100 years. While these services have met certain needs well through emergency care, surgeries and life saving methods, they have not adequately addressed more simple, common ailments or chronic lifestyle disorders. Many, including Western health care professionals, recognize these deficiencies and are seeking viable solutions or alternatives.

The National Center for Complementary and Integrative Health, part of the National Institutes of Health, recognizes the need and practices of Complementary, Alternative and Integrative Medicine practices as they support traditional Western medicine (Complementary, Alternative, or Integrative Health, 2016). According to the definitions provided by the NCCIH, Āyurveda may contribute to an individual's health care and wellbeing as a complementary, alternative or integrative practice. While this recognition is laudable, it unfortunately overlooks Āyurveda's potential to provide primary health care services, which is presently does for millions globally.

The Merriam-Webster Dictionary defines health care as (Health care, 2018):

1. efforts made to maintain or restore physical, mental, or emotional well-being especially by trained and licensed professionals
2. the maintaining and restoration of health by the treatment and prevention of disease especially by trained and licensed professionals (as in medicine, dentistry, clinical psychology, and public health)

Āyurveda currently stands at a critical juncture in its development and scope in the United States. Because it is largely misunderstood and misrepresented, it is outrightly ignored on many key positions that it has held and sustained for centuries.

Numerous concepts, disciplines and practices are being claimed as "discoveries" through Western medicine yet they have clear, documented evidence with active practice today in India. Examples include the practices of Functional Medicine, Precision or Personalized Medicine, Regenerative Medicine and Integrative Medicine which strongly echo key components of long-standing Āyurvedic practices.

For Āyurveda to advance in comprehensive form over the next decade, professionals representing the science and practice will be required to demonstrate the value, efficacy and outcomes to scientific communities.

WESTERN HEALTH CARE

The National Cancer Institute defines Western medicine as (NCI Dictionary of Cancer Terms, 2019):

"A system in which medical doctors and other healthcare professionals (such as nurses, pharmacists, and therapists) treat symptoms and diseases using drugs, radiation, or surgery. Also called allopathic medicine, biomedicine, conventional medicine, mainstream medicine, and orthodox medicine."

The Western health care system is the administrative structure that provides access to Western medicine, its facilities and professionals in the United States. Facilities include general hospitals, specialty hospitals, emergency centers, urgent care centers, diagnostic centers, laboratories, outpatient clinics, home health care and more.

Western medicine recognizes a large number of professionals today who contribute to the functions of this system. The system's development over the last century using the reductionist approach has lead to a highly specialized infrastructure. This presents many challenges today for patients who are unable to access the specific professional for required care.

Over the last few decades, the rise of Complementary and Alternative Medicine (CAM) has brought traditional systems of medicine including Āyurveda into the outer spheres of Western medicine. This is largely due to patient demand for choice in health care and access to modalities that produce results.

As this demand continues to rise, Western medicine appears to be willing to subsume practices and methods of management which are capable of proving themselves through Western standards of Evidence-based Medicine. This approach, however, is inherently biased and unscientific in its structure as it selectively chooses components and attempts to structure them into a Western framework.

Āyurveda has its own complete framework of theory and practice. The scientific approach to testing Āyurvedic protocols and interventions is to do so within its structure of practice.

TEST YOURSELF

Learn, review and memorize key terms from this section.

Complementary and Alternative medicine (CAM)

____

health care

____

Western health care

____

Western medicine

____

Chapter 7: Review

ADDITIONAL READING

Utilize these references to expand your understanding of the concepts in this chapter.

REQUIRED READING	Chapters
Modern and Global Ayurveda	2
Overview of the American Healthcare System, http://sphweb.bumc.bu.edu/otlt/MPH-Modules/HPM/AmericanHealthCare_Overview/AmericanHealthCare_Overview_print.html	Module
"Complementary, Alternative, or Integrative Health: What's In a Name?" https://nccih.nih.gov/health/integrative-health	General article
Whole Medical Systems versus the System of Conventional Biomedicine, https://www.ncbi.nlm.nih.gov/pmc/articles/PMC5530407/	Journal article

OPTIONAL READING	Format
WHO: Traditional Medicine Strategy 2014-2023, http://apps.who.int/medicinedocs/en/m/abstract/Js21201en/	Report
Conceptual framework for new models of integrative medicine, https://www.ncbi.nlm.nih.gov/pmc/articles/PMC3149389/	Journal article
The Flexner Report of 1910 and Its Impact on CAM, https://www.ncbi.nlm.nih.gov/pubmed/23346209	Journal article

References

"Complementary, Alternative, or Integrative Health: What's In a Name?" National Center for Complementary and Integrative Health (NCCIH), 2016, https://nccih.nih.gov/health/integrative-health

"Health care." Merriam-Webster, 2018, https://www.merriam-webster.com/dictionary/health%20care

"NCI Dictionary of Cancer Terms" National Cancer Institute (NCI), 2019, https://www.cancer.gov/publications/dictionaries/cancer-terms/def/western-medicine

Wujastyk, D., Smith, F. (2008). (Eds.). Modern and Global Ayurveda: pluralism and paradigms. Albany, NY: State University of New York Press.

QUESTIONS & ANSWERS

Record your questions for this chapter here for further research and discussion.

Question:

Answer:

Question:

Answer:

Question:

Answer:

SELF-ASSESSMENT

1. A main barrier to access of care in the American health care system is
   a. age
   b. pre-existing conditions
   c. quality of care
   d. sexual orientation
   e. socio-economic status

2. The US spends more than any other country on health care and compared to other countries it ranks
   a. average
   b. average in all causes
   c. high in life expectancy
   d. highest
   e. poorly

3. Examples of whole medical systems include
   a. Anthroposophic Medicine (AM)
   b. Āyurveda
   c. Traditional Chinese Medicine (TCM)
   d. Unani Medicine
   e. All of the above

4. Integration of CAM into Western Medicine is most reliable for specific indications using
   a. complex interventions
   b. multimodal CAM treatments
   c. personalized combinations of CAM interventions
   d. single component CAM interventions
   e. whole medical systems

5. The current scientific empirical model (Evidence-based medicine) causes
   a. a negative image of whole medical systems
   b. higher incidence of “false-negative results” in Western-structured clinical trials
   c. insufficient or inappropriate testing of whole medical systems
   d. rejection of whole medical systems by the Western scientific community
   e. All of the above

6. Whole medical systems view reality as
   a. holistic
   b. nonatomistic
   c. ontological
   d. All of the above
   e. None of the above

7. An important, positive example of integration between whole medical systems and Western medicine is found in
   a. Canada, through CAM
   b. India, through AYUSH
   c. India, through CCIM
   d. India, through Indian Council for Cultural Relations
   e. the United States, through CAM

8. The increasing dominance of evidence-based medicine
   a. discourages whole medical systems
   b. encourages whole medical systems
   c. promotes medical pluralism
   d. recognizes the efficacy of holistic medicine
   e. All of the above

9. The goal of Western medicine is to
   a. develop advanced treatment for cancer
   b. manage chronic illness with lifelong drug prescriptions
   c. treat symptoms and disease using drugs, radiation or surgery
   d. All of the above
   e. None of the above

10. Combining diverse single component CAM interventions into a Western medical structure is inherently unscientific because
    a. it cannot be tested with RCTs
    b. it demonstrates efficacy through outcomes only
    c. it does not require sufficient clinical trials
    d. it lacks a uniform conceptual understanding
    e. it is a personalized approach

Unit Review

ORAL EXAM QUESTIONS

Use these questions to prepare answers for the oral examination. You may create written statements or cue cards to memorize the key points that should be included in your response. Scoring is based on your accuracy, brevity, clarity (ABC), use of Sanskrit terms and concepts, and confidence.

1. What is the professional definition of Āyurveda?
2. How can Āyurveda be defined and explained to the general public?
3. Define the term *'āyu.'*
4. Define the term '*veda*.'
5. What is the meaning of the word Āyurveda based on its Sanskrit root terms?
6. Explain each of the terms in Charaka's definition of Āyurveda, and translate the *śhloka* completely: "*Sukha-asukhato hita-ahitataḥ pramāṇa-apramāṇataśhcha; yat-śhcha-āyuṣhyāṇya-na-āyuṣhyāṇi cha dravya-guṇa-karmāṇi vedayat-yato-apy-āyurvedah* |" Cha. Sū. 30/23
7. Explain each of the terms in Charaka's definition of Āyurveda, and translate the *śhloka* completely: "*Hita-ahitam sukham duhkham-āyustasya hita-ahitam* | *Mānam cha tachchha yatr-oktam āyurvedah sa uchyate* ||" Cha. Sū. 1/41
8. Explain each of the terms in Susruta's definition of Āyurveda, and translate the *śhloka* completely: "*Āyur-asmin vidyate, anena vā ' ' yurvindanti ityāyurvedaḥ* |" Su. Sū. 1/15
9. Name and explain two synonyms of Āyurveda with their classical reference.
10. Explain Charaka's statement of purpose of Āyurveda: "*Prayojanaṁ chāsya svasthasya svāsthya-rakṣhaṇam-āturasya vikāra-praśhamanaṁ cha* |" Cha. Sū. 30/26
11. Explain Susruta's statement of purpose of Āyurveda: "*Iha khalv-āyurveda-prayojanaṁ - vyādhy-upasṛṣhṭānāṁ vyādhi-parimokṣhaḥ, svasthasya rakṣhaṇaṁ cha* ||" Su. Sū. 1/14
12. List the four *puruṣhārthas* mentioned by Charaka in order, and transliterate their names correctly. Explain their meanings.
13. What are the main goals of Āyurveda according to the classical texts?
14. Why are the *puruṣhārthas* significant to the purpose of Āyurveda?
15. Describe any one branch of Āyurvedic medicine and explain its use in detail.
16. What are the eight branches of Āyurvedic medicine?
17. Which aspects of Āyurveda can be seen in emerging fields of medicine today?

MODERN AND GLOBAL AYURVEDA

1. Explain the term "Global Ayurveda."
2. Explain the term "Modern Ayurveda."
3. Explain the term "New Age Ayurveda."
4. What are the benefits and shortcomings of New Age Ayurveda?
5. Discuss Āyurveda's position in CAM, and explain the benefits and drawbacks of this classification.

UNIT II

Philosophy and Science Prerequisites for Āyurveda

Chapter 8 : Traditional medicine: the intersection of philosophy and science

KEY TERMS			
holism	reductionism	science	Veda vid

The debate about whether alternative, complementary or traditional medicines are scientific is long-standing. Many factors complicate our understanding of the power of traditional systems of medicine today because of political influence, bias, colonialism and other controlling factors.

> "There is no alternative medicine. There is only scientifically proven, evidence-based medicine supported by solid data or unproven medicine, for which scientific evidence is lacking. Whether a therapeutic practice is "Eastern" or "Western," is unconventional or mainstream, or involves mind-body techniques or molecular genetics is largely irrelevant except for historical purposes and cultural interest. We recognize that there are vastly different types of practitioners and proponents of the various forms of alternative medicine and conventional medicine, and that there are vast differences in the skills, capabilities, and beliefs of individuals within them and the nature of their actual practices. Moreover, the economic and political forces in these fields are large and increasingly complex and have the capability for being highly contentious. Nonetheless, as believers in science and evidence, we must focus on fundamental issues—namely, the patient, the target disease or condition, the proposed or practiced treatment, and the need for convincing data on safety and therapeutic efficacy."
>
> - Fontanarosa and Lundberg, "Alternative Medicine Meets Science," JAMA, November 11, 1998

As these practices continue to grow in popularity globally, the traditional western medical fraternity recognizes the need to acknowledge them and respond. In some circles, western professionals themselves are eager to explore and adopt practices which they find clinically effective, while others completely admonish that which does not fit their understanding of science.

One of the major obstacles to establishing common ground among professionals from various health care modalities is correcting the perception that "Many advocates of alternative medicine...believe the scientific method is simply not applicable to their remedies," (Angell, M. and Kassirer, J., 1998). It is unfortunately too easy for non-western practitioners to portray this image which creates a negative impression for the larger group.

The World Health Organization created definitions for these important phrases (WHO Traditional Medicine Strategy: 2014-2023, 2013).

"Traditional medicine (TM) has a long history. It is the sum total of the knowledge, skill, and practices based on the theories, beliefs, and experiences indigenous to different cultures, whether explicable or not, used in the maintenance of health as well as in the prevention, diagnosis, improvement or treatment of physical and mental illness."

"The terms 'complementary medicine' (CM) or 'alternative medicine' refer to a broad set of health care practices that are not part of that country's own tradition or conventional medicine and are not fully integrated into the dominant health-care system. They are used interchangeably with traditional medicine in some countries."

"Traditional and complementary medicine (T&CM) merges the terms TM and CM, encompassing products, practices and practitioners."

The ability to understand the workings of traditional medicine by those unfamiliar with their frameworks, systems and practices is a prime issue. Is it the responsibility of the traditional practitioners to explain their systems in a new or different manner for others to understand? Or is it the responsibility of those who want to understand to learn the traditional systems through their existing methods?

IS ĀYURVEDA TRULY A SCIENCE?

This question must be answered from two perspectives in order to understand the full implications. Today, in many modern, Western-based societies and cultures, the general understanding of science implies reductionism, or a procedure or theory that reduces complex data and phenomena to simple terms. More specifically, reductionism attempts an explanation of complex life-science processes and phenomena in terms of the laws of physics and chemistry, (Reductionism, 2018). The classical foundations of Āyurveda and its train of thought, however, do not operate solely based on reductionism. Nor do they rely only on the current standing laws and views of nature. The Āyurvedic train of thought encompasses both expansionism and reductionism to produce a broader mindset which tends to produce a circular pattern of thought rather than a linear one.

The word Āyurveda itself indicates that it is a body of knowledge which is held to laws of its own scientific foundations by the inclusion of the term *Veda* in its name. *Veda* originates from the Sanskrit root √ *vid* meaning "to exist, know or achieve." While this root meaning is short and simple, its full explanation in classical Āyurvedic literature is greatly expanded and many examples can be cited to demonstrate that it meets today's definition and specific criteria of science. Ḍalhaṇa, one of the most important commentators on the Suśhruta Saṁhitā mentions the connection of Āyurveda to the Vedas in Suśhruta *sūtrasthāna* 1/15.

आयुरस्मिन् विद्यते, अनेन वाऽऽयुर्विन्दन्ति इत्यायुर्वेदः । १५

सु. सू. १।१५

Āyurasmin vidyate, anena vā ' ' yurvindanti ityāyurvedaḥ | 15

Su. Sū. 1/15

Āyur-asmin vidyate (As it allows one to become proficient with the knowledge of life) *anena vā* (and) *āyurvindanti* (it creates and achieves a full, complete life or lifespan), *Iti-āyurvedaḥ* (it is called Āyurveda.)

While this single definition may not directly state science in terms that are familiar today, it application be seen throughout the classical treatises and in the current practice of Āyurveda in well-developed institutions in India. The challenge in seeing the scientific practices occurs for those who have not been fully trained in Āyurveda. The scientific framework of Āyurveda is quite complex and it provides mechanisms for overcoming many medical challenges today to fully integrate factors and aspects of life to measure health and disease.

The currently accepted definition of science is (Science, 2018):

1. the state of knowing : knowledge as distinguished from ignorance or misunderstanding
2.
    a. a department of systematized knowledge as an object of study
    b. something (such as a sport or technique) that may be studied or learned like systematized knowledge
3.
    a. knowledge or a system of knowledge covering general truths or the operation of general laws especially as obtained and tested through scientific method
    b. such knowledge or such a system of knowledge concerned with the physical world and its phenomena
4. a system or method reconciling practical ends with scientific laws

Āyurveda meets the definition of science with its core principles, applications, and knowledge body. Examples of these can be seen throughout professional study and practice.

MAINTAINING OBJECTIVITY IN STUDY AND PRACTICE

Considering the current perspectives and opinions towards traditional medicine, it is imperative that qualified professionals in these modalities uphold high levels of objectivity in study and practice. In the recent development of Āyurveda in particular, a significant interest stemmed from communities of western cultures that emphasize belief over science. This has created widespread confusion has even further discredited Āyurveda as formidable science even in India. The advancement of Āyurveda in the 21st century requires that its representative professional body strive for higher standards and objectivity in all areas of study and practice.

TEST YOURSELF

Learn, review and memorize key terms from this section.

Veda

vid

CURRENT SCIENTIFIC JOURNALS

A generally reliable measure for the health and viability of any scientific discipline is the existence of an active body of knowledge including research and development within its practicing community. In India, Āyurveda has seen a wide range of literature over the past few decades as the science establishes itself in the context of changing perceptions from society.

A few notable scientific journals have been consistently publishing and delivering high-quality, original articles. These include:

1. AYU (An International Quarterly Journal of Research in Ayurveda), the official publication of Institute For Post Graduate Teaching & Research in Ayurveda, Jamnagar. Published by Wolters Kluwer - Medknow. http://www.ayujournal.org/

2. Journal of Ayurveda and Integrative Medicine. Transdisciplinary University, Bangalore and World Ayurveda Foundation. Publishing Services by Elsevier B.V. https://www.journals.elsevier.com/journal-of-ayurveda-and-integrative-medicine
3. Ancient Science of Life. Published by Wolters Kluwer - Medknow. http://www.ancientscienceoflife.org/

During the early part of the 21st century, a number of factors caused a sudden demand in advanced Āyurvedic education in India resulting in the mushrooming of journals and literature with substandard publication policies. Known as predatory journals, many of these publications appeared and disappeared quickly with the sole intent of producing income from authors' fees. The professional Āyurvedic community in India has made efforts to stop these practices. Generally, articles that can be found through stringent indexes like PubMed are reliable and trustworthy (Patwardhan, 2017).

The professional Āyurvedic community in India has made strong efforts to resolve this issue. The University Grants Commission Consortium for Academic and Research Ethics (UGC-CARE) provides extensive information on the issue, and search tools for valid information.

https://ugccare.unipune.ac.in/apps1/home/index

Chapter 8: Review

ADDITIONAL READING

Utilize these references to expand your understanding of the concepts in this chapter.

CLASSICS	1st read	2nd read

REQUIRED READING	Chapters
Need of new research methodology for Ayurveda, https://www.ncbi.nlm.nih.gov/pmc/articles/PMC3215413/	

OPTIONAL READING	Format

References

WHO Traditional Medicine Strategy: 2014-2023. (2013). Geneva, Switzerland: World Health Organization.

Fontanarosa PB, Lundberg GD. Alternative Medicine Meets Science. JAMA. 1998;280(18):1618–1619. doi:10.1001/jama.280.18.1618

Walker, L. “Can science and alternative medicine shake hands?” 21stC Vol. 3, Issue 4. http://www.columbia.edu/cu/21stC/issue-3.4/walker.html

Angell, M. and Kassirer, J. (1998, September 17). “Alternative Medicine — The Risks of Untested and Unregulated Remedies.” NEJM. https://www.ncbi.nlm.nih.gov/pubmed/9738094

“Reductionism.” Merriam-Webster, 2018, https://www.merriam-webster.com/dictionary/reductionism

“Science.” Merriam-Webster, 2018, https://www.merriam-webster.com/dictionary/science

University Grants Commission Consortium for Academic and Research Ethics (UGC-CARE). (n.d.). Retrieved from https://ugccare.unipune.ac.in/apps1/home/index

QUESTIONS & ANSWERS

Record your questions for this chapter here for further research and discussion.

Question:

Answer:

Question:

Answer:

Question:

Answer:

SELF-ASSESSMENT

1. Āyurveda's scientific framework is
   a. incomplete
   b. inherent
   c. missing
   d. All of the above
   e. None of the above

2. Āyurveda meets the current definition of science with its
   a. applications
   b. core principles
   c. knowledge body
   d. All of the above
   e. None of the above

3. The World Health Organization considers Āyurveda to be
   a. Alternative medicine
   b. Complementary medicine
   c. Traditional medicine
   d. All of the above
   e. None of the above

4. The currently accepted definition of sciences states that science is
   a. a state of knowing, knowledge
   b. a system or method reconciling practical ends with scientific laws
   c. something learned
   d. All of the above
   e. None of the above

5. The Sanskrit root √ vid means
   a. Āyurveda
   b. to be
   c. to experiment
   d. to know
   e. to move

6. A major foundation of scientific thought in Western spheres is
   a. expansionism
   b. holism
   c. reductionism
   d. the scientific method
   e. None of the above

7. Understanding the scientific framework of Āyurveda is challenging because
   a. Āyurvedic professionals explain concepts in Sanskrit
   b. it originates from Eastern philosophy
   c. it requires extensive study of the science
   d. All of the above
   e. None of the above

8. Predatory journals are scientific publications that
   a. allow substandard publication policies
   b. detrimental to the entire scientific community
   c. operate solely to generate income from author's fees
   d. All of the above
   e. None of the above

9. Regular research and discovery in any field of science indicates
   a. an active professional community
   b. development of knowledge
   c. high level of competitiveness
   d. Both A and B
   e. Both B and C

10. AYU Journal is the official publication of
    a. Banaras Hindu University, Varanasi
    b. Chaukhambha Publications
    c. Institute For Post Graduate Teaching & Research in Ayurveda, Jamnagar
    d. Transdisciplinary University, Bangalore and World Ayurveda Foundation
    e. Wolters Kluwer - Medknow

Chapter 9 : The scientific method

KEY TERMS			
āgama	darśhana	Occam's razor	scientific method
āptopadeśha	good science	pratyakṣha	yukti

SCIENTIFIC METHOD

The fundamental principles and body of scientific knowledge in Āyurveda are intended to be applied in practice. Because of the complexity of the system, this application truly is a "practice" in the sense that no case presentation will ever be the same when all factors are considered. This results in every case and every patient encounter being unique and requires complex application of logical thought processes.

Because of this, the Āyurvedic professional must be fully prepared to apply the knowledge of Āyurveda in an appropriate manner. Professional application and practice can be greatly supported by understanding and utilizing the Western scientific method to guide the process.

The scientific method practiced today provides an excellent framework for Āyurveda. At its most basic, the traditional scientific method is a five step process (Malachowski, 1999):

1. Definition of the problem
2. Gathering of relevant data
3. Formulation of a hypothesis
4. Observation or experimentation to test hypothesis
5. Acceptance, modification, or rejection of the hypothesis

Start with a basic review of the process by reading through the article on the following website: https://fog.ccsf.edu/~mmalacho/ScientificMethod.html

The scientific method strives to adhere specifically to "good science" which is defined based upon the following factors:

1. Not based on authority
2. Testable
3. Repeatable
4. Universal
5. Measurable (Tangible)
6. Observable
7. Narrow (Occam's razor or Ockham's razor)/Simple

Once you have read online article, "The Scientific Method," written by M.J. Malachowski Ph.D., review how each of these requirements is fulfilled in the framework of classical, scientific Āyurvedic practice.

Not based on authority

This can be understood through several classical concepts. First, *āgama* is a standing body of applied knowledge recorded in the classical treatises that is the collective result of effective practice. This information is similar to the working body of scientific knowledge and evidence found today in advanced disciplines. *Āptopadeśha* are experts who provide reliable knowledge tested over time and found to be valid or invalid. Applying knowledge from these sources after appropriate study and comprehension of the science allows one to utilize *yukti*, the application of logical thought process. Today, one of the ways that *yukti* can be demonstrated is through application of the scientific method.

Testable

When the complete framework of Āyurveda is applied, it allows for controls and variables making testing possible. Each factor (control or variable) can also be measured using classical principles. This provides a clear picture of the scenario, its components, inputs, actions and outcomes.

Repeatable

With the Āyurvedic framework, scenarios can also be repeated assuming the controls and variables are properly established and a proper, reliable baseline has been determined.

Universal

The principles of Āyurveda can be applied and demonstrated universally. This also requires a complete understanding of the scenarios and their controls and variables.

Measurable (Tangible)

Measurement of factors is based on classical Āyurvedic principles. Traditionally, measurements are approximated in general levels of relativity (ie, low, medium, high) rather than numerically. While some may consider this unscientific today, it should be given deeper analysis for its ability to allow the science to be practiced in a very personalized, customized format. Measurable, subjective levels of relativity actually allow the individual and Āyurvedic healthcare professional to determine levels of health and disease which are directly applicable to the person affected.

Observable

This can be understood through several classical concepts. First, *āgama* is a standing body of applied knowledge recorded in the classical treatises that is the collective result of effective practice. This information is similar to the working body of scientific knowledge and evidence found today in advanced disciplines. Second, *pratyakṣha* is knowledge gained from individual direct perception through the sense organs and is utilized to assess the expression of health and disease in the health care setting similar to the way a scientist would observe a scientific study through utilizing the sense organs and aggregating the observed data for analysis. With direct perception the Āyurvedic health care professional is able to directly assess the person affected and is then able to apply and compare the knowledge gained through *āgama*. Within the classical Āyurvedic principles there is another concept utilized during *rogi parīkṣhā*, assessment of the diseased person, called *darśhana* or observation. Āyurvedic health care professionals are trained to observe the minute changes and shifts occurring for an individual or a population given one simple variable.

Narrow (Occam's razor)/Simple

Occam's razor is a problem-solving principle used in various branches of science to determine the simplest solution to a problem. The principle, *Essentia non sunt multiplicanda praeter necessitatem*, stated by William of Occam, a 14th century philosopher, means that "Entities should not be multiplied beyond necessity." This principle can be readily applied in the practice of Āyurveda by positing and testing multiple hypotheses to identify the most efficient solution to a specific health issue that has been well-defined within an individual or known group. It is very likely that throughout Āyurveda's development in the Indian subcontinent, this principle was commonly applied with relative ease due to the normalcy in ethnicity, environment, diet, habits and other influential factors.

When practicing Āyurveda using the scientific method, the specifics of the science become clear when the controls and variables are properly understood and measurable. A general principle for successful practice is well-summarized in "The Scientific Method" (Malachowski, 1999):

"A good experiment is difficult to design. It is best to keep experiments simple, to pare them down to the least number of elements possible, and to design it to produce definitive results, which can be unequivocally interpreted. In reality, it is frequently better to run a series of tests, experiments, rather than performing only one. The reason is we are frequently seeking to identify what happens when we do something; we want to know what will happen if we make a single change, all other factors held constant.

That change we are making is called a variable; the constant portion is called the control. We would prefer to only change one variable at a time; because, if we make a whole bunch of changes, it is difficult to determine a direct cause and effect. We are frequently better off making a small change, observing the result, making a little bigger change, observing the result, and then evaluating this sequence of events."

The Scientific Method as an Ongoing Process

By ArchonMagnus [CC BY-SA 4.0 (https://creativecommons.org/licenses/by-sa/4.0)], from Wikimedia Commons

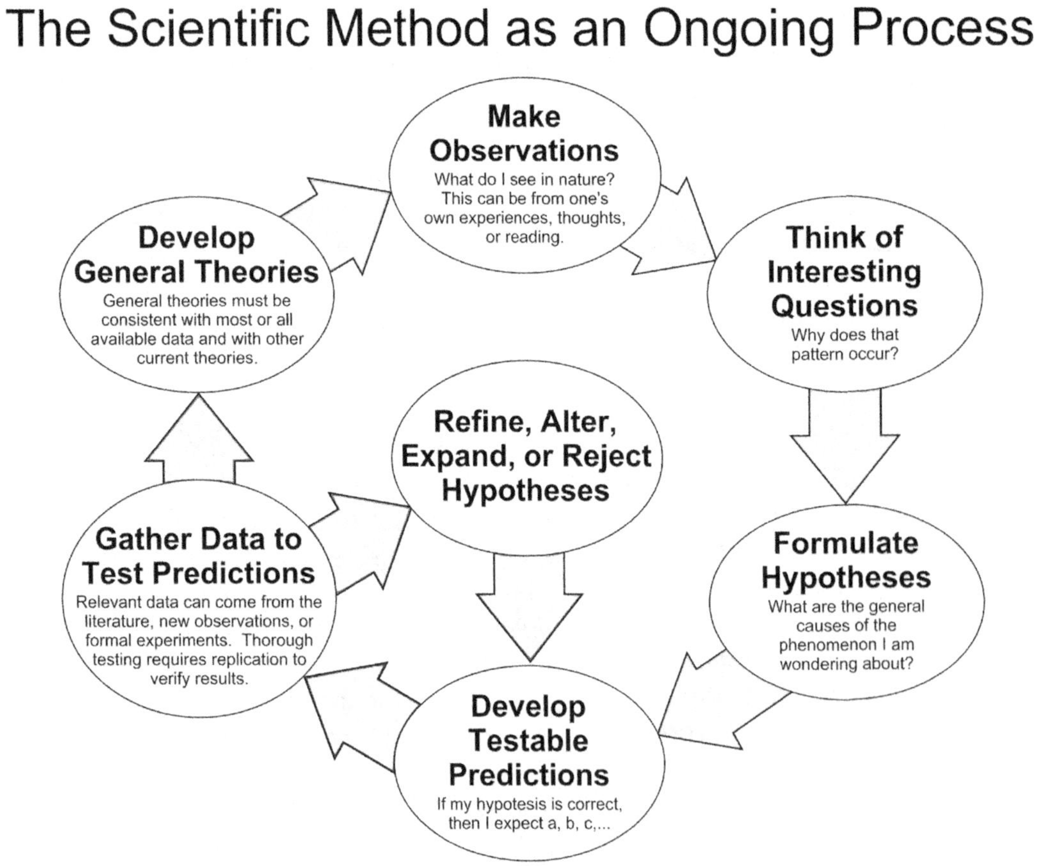

TEST YOURSELF

Learn, review and memorize key terms from this section.

āgama

āptopadeśha

darśhana

good science

Occam's razor

pratyakṣha

scientific method

yukti

Chapter 9: Review

ADDITIONAL READING

Utilize these references to expand your understanding of the concepts in this chapter.

REQUIRED READING	Chapters
The Scientific Method, https://fog.ccsf.edu/~mmalacho/ScientificMethod.html	
The Scientific Method, https://www.youtube.com/watch?v=tYGiCDZ7B6k	
Scientific Method, example, https://www.youtube.com/watch?v=lOerfJcBWI0	
The Scientific Process, https://www.windows2universe.org/people/scientific_process.html	

OPTIONAL READING	Format
Indian Science and Predatory Journals, https://www.ncbi.nlm.nih.gov/pmc/articles/PMC5377474/	
Predatory Conferences in the Field of Ayurveda and Alternative Medicine: Need for Quality Checks, https://www.ncbi.nlm.nih.gov/pmc/articles/PMC5566821/	
"Writing a Scientific Research Paper"	
William of Ockham, https://www.iep.utm.edu/ockham/	

References

ArchonMagnus [CC BY-SA 4.0 (https://creativecommons.org/licenses/by-sa/4.0)]. "The Scientific Method as an Ongoing Process.svg" (2015, 7 August) Wikimedia Commons, https://commons.wikimedia.org/wiki/File:The_Scientific_Method_as_an_Ongoing_Process.svg

Malachowski, M. (1999). "The Scientific Method." https://fog.ccsf.edu/~mmalacho/ScientificMethod.html

Manohar, P. R. (2017). Predatory Conferences in the Field of Ayurveda and Alternative Medicine: Need for Quality Checks. Ancient Science of Life, 36(3), 115–116. http://doi.org/10.4103/asl.ASL_128_17

Patwardhan, B. (2017). Indian Science and Predatory Journals. Journal of Ayurveda and Integrative Medicine, 8(1), 1–2. http://doi.org/10.1016/j.jaim.2017.02.004

QUESTIONS & ANSWERS

Record your questions for this chapter here for further research and discussion.

Question:

Answer:

Question:

Answer:

Question:

Answer:

SELF-ASSESSMENT

1. What are the steps of the Scientific Method?
   a. accept, modify, or reject the hypothesis
   b. defining the problem and gathering relevant data
   c. formulate a hypothesis
   d. observe or experiment to test a hypothesis
   e. All of the above

2. Āyurveda be considered "good science" because it is
   a. ancient
   b. follows the scientific method when practiced classically
   c. life science
   d. testable
   e. None of the above

3. The first step of the scientific method is to
   a. analyze outcome data
   b. formulate hypotheses
   c. make observations
   d. refine hypotheses
   e. test predictions

4. The principle of Occam's razor is based on
   a. entities should be multiplied necessarily
   b. entities should not be multiplied beyond necessity
   c. testing multiple hypotheses
   d. Western philosophy
   e. None of the above

5. The scientific method requires that components of the experiment be
   a. common
   b. measurable
   c. practical
   d. realistic
   e. All of the above

6. Not basing knowledge on authority is evident in Āyurveda through
   a. classical texts
   b. observation
   c. pratyakṣha
   d. theoretical principles
   e. yukti

7. What is *āgama*?
   a. Classical treatise of the working body of Āyurvedic knowledge
   b. Textbook
   c. Medical reference
   d. Knowledge gained through direct perception
   e. None of the above

8. What is *Āptopadeśha*?
   a. A student dedicated to learning the complete science of Āyurveda
   b. An instructor
   c. Experts who provide reliable knowledge that has been tested over time
   d. Apprentice who studies with an expert
   e. None of the above

9. What is *yukti*?
   a. The ability to derive an understanding, answer or conclusion based on logical thought
   b. One of the four *pramānas*, or sources of knowledge
   c. Logical thinking
   d. All of the above
   e. None of the above

10. What do classical Āyurvedic measurements allow that standard numerical measurements exclude?
    a. Personalization to the individual
    b. Customizable analysis to the individual
    c. Clear statistical values
    d. Data that can be applied to large populations
    e. Both A and B

Chapter 10 : Scientific thought and logic

The study and development of philosophy in western spheres has traditionally been intertwined with science and mathematics. Early philosophers like Pythagoras, Aristotle and Plato were very possibly influenced by eastern philosophies including the Vedas. Discourse, debates and developments of philosophical tenets over centuries have played key roles in producing current perspectives and applications of reasoning and logic.

According to the Encyclopædia Britannica, "Reason [is], in philosophy, the faculty or process of drawing logical inferences. The term 'reason' is also used in several other, narrower senses. Reason is in opposition to sensation, perception, feeling, desire, as the faculty (the existence of which is denied by empiricists) by which fundamental truths are intuitively apprehended. These fundamental truths are the causes or 'reasons' of all derivative facts. According to the German philosopher Immanuel Kant, reason is the power of synthesizing into unity, by means of comprehensive principles, the concepts that are provided by the intellect." (The Editors of Encyclopaedia Britannica, 2018)

While similar, reasoning and logic have developed distinct meanings. Logic is the study of correct reasoning, especially as it involves the drawing of inferences (Hintikka, 2018). The philosophical field of logic studies the ways of formal reasoning through argument (Hintikka, 2018). Ultimately, both require the process of thinking, which is "the action of using one's mind to produce thoughts." (Thinking, 2018).

Primary methods of reasoning and logic are based on deduction and inference. Deduction is "the deriving of a conclusion by reasoning; a conclusion reached by logical deduction" (Deduction, 2018). Inference is similar but possibly less reliable. To infer means "to derive as a conclusion from facts or premises; to guess or surmise; to involve as a normal outcome of thought" (Infer, 2018).

BASIC PRINCIPLES OF LOGIC

Read the "Basic concepts of logic" for a comprehensive overview of this field of study.

DEFINITION OF STATISTICS

"Statistics is the science concerned with developing and studying methods for collecting, analyzing, interpreting and presenting empirical data. Statistics is a highly interdisciplinary field; research in statistics finds applicability in virtually all scientific fields and research questions in the various scientific fields motivate the development of new statistical methods and theory. In developing methods and studying the theory that underlies the methods statisticians draw on a variety of mathematical and computational tools.

Two fundamental ideas in the field of statistics are uncertainty and variation. There are many situations that we encounter in science (or more generally in life) in which the outcome is uncertain. In some cases the uncertainty is because the outcome in question is not determined yet (e.g., we may not know whether it will rain tomorrow) while in other cases the uncertainty is because although the outcome has been determined already we are not aware of it (e.g., we may not know whether we passed a particular exam).

Probability is a mathematical language used

to discuss uncertain events and probability plays a key role in statistics. Any measurement or data collection effort is subject to a number of sources of variation. By this we mean that if the same measurement were repeated, then the answer would likely change. Statisticians attempt to understand and control (where possible) the sources of variation in any situation. (UC Regents, 2018)"

Chapter 10: Review

ADDITIONAL READING

Utilize these references to expand your understanding of the concepts in this chapter.

REQUIRED READING	Chapters
Venn diagram: Logic and Mathematics, https://www.britannica.com/topic/Venn-diagram	
Venn Diagrams Logic, https://www.youtube.com/watch?v=5XbCoyvByBo	
Chapter 1: Basic concepts of logic http://courses.umass.edu/phil110-gmh/MAIN/IHome-5.htm	

OPTIONAL READING	Format
Introduction to medical statistics Part 1, 2 and 3	

References

The Editors of Encyclopaedia Britannica. (2018). “Reason.” Encyclopædia Britannica. https://www.britannica.com/topic/reason

Hintikka, J. (2018). “Logic.” Encyclopædia Britannica. https://www.britannica.com/topic/logic

Hintikka, J. (2018). "Philosophy of logic". Encyclopædia Britannica. https://www.britannica.com/topic/philosophy-of-logic

“Thinking.” Merriam-Webster, 2018, https://www.merriam-webster.com/dictionary/thinking

“Deduction.” Merriam-Webster, 2018, https://www.merriam-webster.com/dictionary/deduction

“Infer.” Merriam-Webster, 2018, https://www.merriam-webster.com/dictionary/infer

Buckner, E.D. 2005. “Principles of logic.” http://www.logicmuseum.com/joyce/LOGIC-Chapter-I.HTM

UC Regents, 2018. “What is Statistics?” https://www.stat.uci.edu/what-is-statistics/

Fischer, Ismor. (2012, May 29). “The Classical Scientific Method and Statistical Inference.” http://pages.stat.wisc.edu/~ifischer/Intro_Stat/Lecture_Notes/1_-_Introduction/1.2_-_Classical_Scientific_Method.pdf

Fischer, Ismor. (2013, May 17). “Definitions and examples.” http://pages.stat.wisc.edu/~ifischer/Intro_Stat/Lecture_Notes/1_-_Introduction/1.3_-_Definitions_and_Examples.pdf

QUESTIONS & ANSWERS

Record your questions for this chapter here for further research and discussion.

Question:

Answer:

Question:

Answer:

Question:

Answer:

SELF-ASSESSMENT

1. What does the Venn Diagram introduced by English logician and philosopher John Venn represent within the study and field of logic?
   a. Relations of inclusion or exclusion between classes or sets
   b. Existence and non-existence between classes or sets.
   c. Categorical propositions within the field of logic.
   d. All of the above
   e. None of the above
2. What is a syllogism in relation to the field of logic?
   a. The study of venn diagrams.
   b. A valid deductive argument having two premises and a conclusion.
   c. A non valid argument having two premises and a conclusion.
   d. All of the above
   e. None of the above
3. Which statement is an example of a valid syllogism form?
   a. All X are Y, some Y are Z, All X are Z.
   b. All X are Y, All Y are Z, All X are Z.
   c. All X are Z, No Y are Z, No X are Y.
   d. All of the above
   e. None of the above
4. What is the definition of logic?
   a. The study of correct reasoning, especially as it involves the drawing of inferences.
   b. The study of making informed decisions based on facts.
   c. The study of utilizing statistical data to come to a conclusion.
   d. The study of utilizing the scientific method to determine a hypothesis.
   e. None of the above
5. What is the definition of reason according to the *Encyclopedia Britannica*?
   a. The faculty or process of drawing logical inferences.
   b. The faculty by which fundamental truths are intuitively apprehended.
   c. The faculty by which fundamental truths are intuitively apprehended.
   d. All of the above
   e. None of the above
6. What factors make an argument a *sound* argument?
   a. All of its premises are true.
   b. Its conclusion follows from its premises.
   c. It is both factually correct and valid.
   d. All of the above
   e. None of the above
7. What makes an argument invalid?
   a. An argument with false premises and a false conclusion is invalid.
   b. An argument with true premises but a false conclusion is invalid.
   c. An argument with true premises and a true conclusion is invalid.
   d. All of the above
   e. None of the above
8. What are statistics?
   a. The science concerned with developing and studying methods for collecting empirical data.
   b. The science concerned with developing and studying methods for analyzing empirical data.
   c. The science concerned with developing and studying methods for interpreting empirical data.
   d. The science concerned with developing and studying methods for presenting empirical data.
   e. All of the above
9. What is the most appropriate definition of deduction within the study of logic?
   a. It is the act of taking away.
   b. It is something that is or may be subtracted.
   c. It is the deriving of a conclusion by reasoning.
   d. All of the above
   e. None of the above
10. What is the most appropriate definition of inference within the study of logic?
    a. To guess
    b. To surmise
    c. To indicate
    d. To derive as a conclusion from facts or premises
    e. None of the above

Chapter 11 : Pramāṇa

KEY TERMS

āgama	āptopadeśha	pramāṇa	sat
anumāna	asat	pratyakṣha	upamāna
āpta	epistemology	Ṣhaḍ Darśhana	yukti

Classically, the *pramāṇa* consisted of the means to attain knowledge, understanding or information. Today, *pramāṇa* can be correlated to the study of epistemology, which is defined as (Epistemology, 2018):

1. the study or a theory of the nature and grounds of knowledge especially with reference to its limits and validity

PRAMĀṆA

The classics had clear, specific methodologies for obtaining and validating knowledge. Classically, the methods were grouped under the term *pramāṇa* and recognized by major authors. An affinity towards a certain methodology was often influenced by the philosophical system (one or more of the *Ṣhaḍ Darśhanas*) which served as the foundation for the learning and practice methodologies within that *sampradāya*, or school of thought.

Knowledge was considered to be either *sat* or *asat* (true or false) by Caraka in Sūtrasthāna 11/17. The purpose of *pramāṇa* was to allow an individual to examine and assess any given information to determine its truthfulness or otherwise. To do this, four methods of *pramāṇa* could be applied to make the determination.

The major classifications of *pramāṇa* include:

Caraka Sūtrasthāna 11/20	Suśhruta Sūtrasthāna 1/16
Āptopadeśha Authoritative knowledge	*Pratyakṣha* Direct perception
Pratyakṣha Direct perception	*Āgama* Authoritative knowledge
Anumāna Inferred knowledge	*Anumāna* Inferred knowledge
Yukti Logical knowledge	*Upamāna* Analogical reasoning

Caraka explains *pramāṇa* through its component methods in Ca. Sū. 11/17.

द्विविधमेव खलु सर्वं सच्चासच्च; तस्य चतुर्विधा परीक्षा - आप्तोपदेशः, प्रत्यक्षम्, अनुमानं, युक्तिश्चेति || च. सू. ११।१७

Dvividhameva khalu sarvaṁ saccāsacca; tasya caturvidhā parīkṣhā - āptopadeśhaḥ, pratyakṣham, anumānaṁ, yuktiśhcēti || Ca. Sū. 11/17

The order of presentation varies slightly among authors and that can be interpreted according to the situation in which the methodologies are applied. This variance indicates that the individual student or practitioner must determine the correct order of application and usage that is appropriate to each unique event and its requirements.

Āptopadeśha and *Āgama* include the knowledge which comes from highly reliable sources. Classically, these sources were *āptas*, or experts in their field who had a combination of factual, accurate core knowledge, a clear understanding of practical experience reinforced by strong, reliable mental stability. The information and knowledge garnered from these sources could always then be applied, tested, and determined to be true or false through reasoning in any specific instance. Because of limitations with storing information in written format during classical times, transmission of valid knowledge through *āptas* was key to maintaining an ongoing body of applied principles.

Pratyakṣha refers to that knowledge which can be ascertained directly through the sense organs, as direct perception. The ability to discern truthful versus invalid knowledge can be directly related to the individual's base level of accurate knowledge and their ability to recognize and interpret reality. These both depend heavily on education and training which can be accomplished through study of accurate information from reliable sources. This typically includes knowledge gained through *Āptopadeśha*, and can include authoritative, classical texts as a valid source.

Anumāna is valid, inferred knowledge from any of the three time periods, past, present and future, which is generated out of the application of *yukti*, or logical reasoning. This relies on the previous existence of *Pratyakṣha* and is one of the most important aspects of applied knowledge in the practice of Āyurveda. The fact that knowledge can be accurately inferred from the past and confidently predicted demonstrates the scientific nature of Āyurveda in practical terms.

Yukti is defined by Caraka in Sūtrasthāna 11/25 as the logical process which is capable of taking multiple inputs of various factors and predicting or determining their outcome. This can also help produce the knowledge of *Anumāna* which may be applicable to the past, present or future.

Each *pramāṇa* is a required component for successful education, training and practice of Āyurveda. In various stages of education and training, certain *pramāṇas* may be used more frequently than others. In practice, all four are typically applied in a single case encounter. The ability to recognize the source of knowledge in practice is a key component to determining accuracy and confidence levels which can directly influence clinical decisions.

TEST YOURSELF

Learn, review and memorize key terms from this section.

āgama

anumāna

āpta

āptopadeśha

asat

pramāṇa

pratyakṣha

Ṣhaḍ Darśhana

sat

upamāna

yukti

Chapter 11: Review

ADDITIONAL READING

Utilize these references to expand your understanding of the concepts in this chapter.

CLASSICS	1st read	2nd read
Ca. Sū. 11/		
Ca. Vi. 4/		
Su. Sū. 2/ – 4/		

REQUIRED READING	Chapters
Patil, S., Baghel, A., Dwivedi, R. (2014). Methods of Examination and Investigation in Ayurveda : A review in reference to Pramana Vijnana (Epistemology). Annals of Ayurvedic Medicine, 3(1-2), 42-47, http://www.scopemed.org/?mno=170945	

References

"Epistemology." Merriam-Webster, 2018, https://www.merriam-webster.com/dictionary/epistemology

Śarmā, R. K., & Dāsa, B. Agniveśa's Caraka Saṃhitā. Varanasi: Chowkhamba Sanskrit Series Office; Reprint Edition. 2016. Ca. Sū. 11/, Ca. Vi. 4/.

Singhal, G.D., et al. Suśhruta Saṁhitā of Suśhruta. Chaukhamba Sanskrit Pratiśhthan, Reprint Edition. 2015. Sū. Sū. 2/-4/.

.

QUESTIONS & ANSWERS

Record your questions for this chapter here for further research and discussion.

Question:

Answer:

Question:

Answer:

Question:

Answer:

SELF-ASSESSMENT

1. What is *pramāṇa*?
   a. It is a measurement.
   b. It is a means of obtaining knowledge about measurement.
   c. It is any proof, testament, or knowledge gained through the four classical classifications.
   d. All of the above
   e. None of the above

2. According to *Caraka* in *Sūtrasthāna* 11/17, which of the following are included in the named *pramāṇa?*
   a. *āptopadeśha*
   b. *pratyakṣha*
   c. *anumāna*
   d. *yukti*
   e. All of the above

3. Which *pramāṇa* does *Suśhruta* include that *Caraka* does not include in the four major classifications?
   a. *āptopadeśha*
   b. *āgama*
   c. *upamāna*
   d. *yukti*
   e. Answers b and c

4. Which of the following terms are synonyms?
   a. āptopadeśha and āgama
   b. *yukti* and *upamāna*
   c. *Āptopadeśha* and *yukti*
   d. All of the above
   e. None of the above

5. In present day, which of the following could best be considered knowledge gained through *āptopadeśha?*
   a. Reading articles from a trusted source from the internet.
   b. Reading the classical texts with the guidance of a new teacher.
   c. Listening to a lecture given by an expert in the field who has studied the classical texts and who has had ample experience working in the field.
   d. All of the above
   e. None of the above

6. Which sense organs can be utilized to learn through *pratyakṣha*?
   a. Eyes
   b. Ears
   c. Nose
   d. Tongue
   e. All of the above

7. What are the limitations of relying on *pratyakṣha* as one's sole way of gaining knowledge?
   a. The individual's base level of accurate knowledge can be a limitation.
   b. Education and training can be a limitation.
   c. One's ability to accurately recognize and interpret reality.
   d. All of the above
   e. None of the above

8. What classification of *pramāṇa* would best be correlated to the study of logic?
   a. *āptopadeśha*
   b. *pratyakṣha*
   c. *anumāna*
   d. *yukti*
   e. None of the above

9. *Anumāna* is valid inferred knowledge and is generated out of the application of what other *pramāṇa?*
   a. *āptopadeśha*
   b. *pratyakṣha*
   c. *anumāna*
   d. *yukti*
   e. None of the above

10. Which *pramāṇa* is required for successful education, training, and practice in Āyurveda?
    a. *āptopadeśha*
    b. *pratyakṣha*
    c. *anumāna*
    d. *yukti*
    e. All of the above

Chapter 12 : Astronomy and time

KEY TERMS

astronomy	declination	latitude	poles
axis	equator	longitutde	precession
celestial equator	equinox	lunar calendar	solar calendar
celestial poles	Gregorian calendar	moon	solar system
celestial sphere	heliocentricity	obliquity	soli-lunar calendar
		planet	solstice

Astronomy is the scientific study of the universe and the objects in it. To fully understand Āyurveda, comprehension of certain basic principles in astronomy is required. These principles explain the physical mechanics of changes that occur in the human body due to the environment, geographical location, climate and seasons.

Astronomy is defined as (American Heritage Student Science Dictionary, 2014):

The scientific study of the universe and the objects in it, including stars, planets, and nebulae. Astronomy deals with the position, size, motion, composition, energy, and evolution of celestial objects. Astronomers analyze not only visible light but also radio waves, x-rays, and other ranges of radiation that come from sources outside the Earth's atmosphere.

BASIC MECHANICS OF THE SOLAR SYSTEM

Heliocentricity

Heliocentricity is defined as (American Heritage Student Science Dictionary, 2014):

1. In relation to the sun as seen from the sun's center: the heliocentric position of a planet
2. Relating to a model of the solar system or universe having the sun as the center

Heliocentrism is a cosmological model in which the Sun is assumed to lie at or near a central point (ie, of the solar system or of the universe) while the Earth and other bodies revolve around it.

The solar system

The solar system is the collection of eight planets and their moons in orbit around the sun, together with smaller bodies in the form of asteroids, meteoroids, and comets.

The solar system is named for its main and central feature, the Sun. The first four planets are terrestrial, or rocky, and include Mercury, Venus, Earth and Mars. A large asteroid belt lies beyond Mars and is likely held in place by the strong gravity of Jupiter. The final four planets are jovian or gaseous, and include Jupiter, Saturn, Uranus and Neptune. The dwarf planet, Pluto, is no longer considered a true planet.

The solar system is also home to comets, Kuiper Belt Object, Trans-Neptunian Object and the Oort cloud (Solar System Basics, 2013).

Planets

A planet is a celestial body moving in an elliptical orbit around a star. The earth is a planet.

To be considered a planet, the object must:

1. orbit a star (like the sun)
2. be large enough to create its own gravitational force to produce a spherical shape
3. be large enough so that its gravity can clear away any other objects of a similar size near its orbit around the sun.

The International Astronomical Union, or IAU, has created three distinct categories for planets which includes the description in the previous paragraph. It now accepts dwarf planets which meets the first two criteria but not the third. The third category includes all other objects except satellites orbiting the sun which are called "Small Solar System Bodies" (Planets, 2018).

Celestial sphere

The Merriam-Webster Dictionary defines the celestial sphere as (Celestial sphere, 2018):

An imaginary sphere of infinite radius against which the celestial bodies appear to be projected and of which the apparent dome of the visible sky forms half.

The celestial sphere includes the portion of the sky which can be seen from an individual's perspective on earth. This perspective changes depending on the individual's location on the planet and their vantage point.

The celestial sphere is an imaginary sphere of which the observer is the center and on which all celestial objects are considered to lie.

Celestial poles are the two imaginary points in the sky where the Earth's axis of rotation, indefinitely extended, intersects the celestial sphere. The north celestial pole is the point in the sky about which all the stars seen from the Northern Hemisphere rotate. The south celestial pole is the point in the sky about which all the stars seen from the Southern Hemisphere rotate.

The celestial equator is the projection into space of the earth's equator; an imaginary circle equidistant from the celestial poles. The ecliptic is a great circle on the celestial sphere representing the sun's apparent path during the year, so called because lunar and solar eclipses can occur only when the moon crosses it.

The celestial sphere is the view of the sky from earth. The path of the sun on the ecliptic appears to move or change throughout the year as the earth rotates on its own axis and revolves around the sun. These apparent motions are expressed as seasons on earth.

Motion of the planets

Orbits of planets around the sun are elliptical. In a given period of time, objects are going to move and sweep out an equal area over time. As a planet moves around the sun it appears to move faster as it gets closer to the sun and slower when it's further away.

The motion of the earth and all planets around the sun produce the following effects:

- Motions of the earth around the sun and the moon around the earth create night and day every 24 hours.
- Motions explain why seasons occur.
- Motions explain the phases of moon.
- Motions cause tides due to the gravitational forces between the moon and earth.
- Motions cause solar and lunar eclipses based on the tilt of the earth's axis.
- Planetary motion causes some planets to appear to move backwards (retrograde) or forwards in the night

sky.

- Venus is only visible in the early morning or just after sunset because of its location between the earth and the sun.

The laws of planetary motion have been explained in detail by scientists over the last few hundred years, including Johannes Kepler. Sir Isaac Newton is credited with explaining the laws of motion and gravity.

THE EARTH

The earth is 13,000 kilometers in diameter by approximately 11 kilometers high. It is surrounded by a magnetic field that protects from the onslaught of subatomic particles from the sun 150 million kilometers away. It is considered an oblate spheroid or ellipsoid. The Poles (the top and bottom) are squished, creating a bulge at the equator. Gravity causes the contraction to make the sphere shape. Earth is slowing down over time.

Earth is not straight up and down in relation to the sun, but slightly tilted. As this tilt or angle changes over time, it wobbles producing variations in its elliptical orbit called precession. All these variations can lead to changes in climate and weather patterns on earth. This occurred during the Ice Ages due to changes in the orbit of the earth and its tilt over time.

Axis

The Earth's axis is positioned at an angle of 23.5 degrees away from the plane of the ecliptic. An objects axis, or axial tilt, also referred to as obliquity, is the angle between an objects' orbital axis and rotational axis, or regularly, the angle between its orbital plane and equatorial plane.

Obliquity

Obliquity is an astronomical term describing the angle of tilt of the Earth's axis of rotation. In technical jargon, it is the angle between the plane of the Earth's equator and the plane of the Earth's orbit around the Sun.

The axial tilt or obliquity is the angle between the axis of rotation of the Earth and its orbital plane, it remains confined between 21.8° and 24.4°. Currently, it is 23°26'14" but the axis is recovering about 0.46" per year or ≈1 degree every 7800 years.

Precession

Precession is caused by the gravitational pull of the Sun and the Moon on the Earth.

Precession refers to a change in the direction of the axis of a rotating object.

In certain contexts, "precession" may refer to the precession that the Earth experiences, the effects of this type of precession on astronomical observation, or to the precession of orbital objects.

The revolution of a planet in its orbit around the Sun is also a form of rotary motion. (In this case, the combined system of Earth and Sun is rotating.) So the axis of a planet's orbital plane will also precess over time.

The major axis of each planet's elliptical orbit also precesses within its orbital plane, in response to perturbations in the form of the changing gravitational forces exerted by other planets.

Precession is a change in the orientation of the rotational axis of a rotating body.

If the axis of rotation of a body is itself rotating about a second axis, that body is said to be precessing about the second axis.

Poles

Earth has two geographic poles: the North Pole and the South Pole. They are the places on Earth's surface that Earth's imaginary spin axis passes through. Our planet also has two magnetic poles: the North Magnetic Pole and the South Magnetic Pole. The magnetic poles are near, but not quite in the same places as the geographic poles. The needle in a compass points towards a magnetic pole.

Interestingly, the magnetic poles actually move around. Remember, swirling motions of molten metal in Earth's outer core make our planet's magnetic field. Those swirling motions are changing all the time. That means the magnetic field is changing, so the magnetic poles move.

Equator

The Equator is an imaginary line around the middle of the Earth. It is halfway between the North and South Poles, and divides the Earth into the Northern and Southern Hemispheres.

MOTION OF THE EARTH AND MOON

The sun rises due east and sets due west on only two days of every year. Sunrises and sunsets happen because earth spins counterclockwise on its axis aligned to the north pole. The sun rises and sets exactly due east and west only when the circular path of the turn on earth's surface splits into two equal parts, half in the light and half in the dark. As the planet's rotation axis tilts by 23.5° with respect to its orbital plane, this alignment happens only at the spring and fall equinoxes. During an equinox, the plane separating earth's day and night sides contains both the north and south poles. On any days other than the equinoxes, this plane is askew and the circular path of rotation passes unequally through earth's lit and dark sides. Therefore, the lengths of night and day vary, as do the position of the sun's rise and set on the horizon.

Moon

The moon's orbit around earth forms an angle of about 5° with respect to earth's orbital plane. Earth's rotation axis tilts by about 28.5° with respect to the moon's orbital plane. The moonrise shifts north or south of due east as the moon completes its orbit. In this case, though, the changes occur over the period of roughly a month instead of a year. Earth must complete a full orbit around the sun to go through its extremes, rising the furthest north of east during summer solstice and the furthest south of east during winter solstice. The same occurs with the moon which must also complete a full orbit around earth to go through the extremes of its rising and setting locations.

As both the earth and moon are moving in their orbits, moonrise occurs later every day. Just as earth spins counterclockwise when viewed from the north pole, the moon also orbits earth counterclockwise. Therefore, every time the earth spins 360° with respect to the stars completing a sidereal day (23 hours and 56 minutes), the moon has moved a little in its orbit around earth. The moon orbits earth every 27.32 days with respect to the stars, marking a sidereal month. The amount it moves in one sidereal day is (360/27.32) degrees is approximately 13°. Earth turns 360° every sidereal day and takes about 13*(23.9/360) hours to make up the remaining 13° and 52 minutes. Each moonrise occurs roughly 52 minutes later than the one before it.

Moon phases are determined by the relative positions of the moon, earth and sun. Common misconceptions are that earth's shadow on the moon causes these phases or that the moon changes shape due to clouds. Actually, the moon's phase depends only on its position relative to earth and the sun.

The moon does not create its own light. It reflects the sun's light as all planets do. The sun always illuminates one half of the moon. Since the moon is tidally locked, the same side is always visible from Earth. There is no permanent "dark side of the Moon." The sun lights up different sides of the moon as it orbits around earth. It is the fraction of the moon from which reflected sunlight is visible that determines the lunar phase (Vecchiato, 2018).

Tides

Most locations around the earth experience two high tides and two low tides each day. The difference in height between high and low tides varies as the moon waxes and wanes from new to full and full to new. The moon and sun are primarily responsible for the rising and falling of ocean tides.

If the moon is primarily responsible for the tides, why are there two high tides and two low tides each day in most places, for example, the U.S. eastern seaboard? It seems as if there should just be one. When picturing the part of Earth closest to the moon, it's easy to see that the ocean is drawn toward the moon. Gravity depends in part on how close two objects are.

But then on the opposite side of Earth another tidal bulge occurs in the direction opposite of the moon. This second bulge happens at the part of Earth where the moon's gravity is pulling the least. Earth spins once every 24 hours. So a given location on earth will pass through both bulges of water each day. The bulges do not stay fixed in time, however. They move at the slow rate of about 13.1 degrees per day which is the same rate as the monthly motion of the moon relative to the stars. Other factors, including the shape of coastlines also influence the time of the tides (Byrd, 2018).

HOW SEASONS WORK

The tilt of earth's axis determines the seasons. With the north pole tilted towards the sun, summer occurs in the northern hemisphere. And with the north pole tilted away from the sun, winter occurs in the northern hemisphere. During the northern hemisphere's winter, the earth is closer to the sun than during the summer but the tilt determines the direct light and the seasons. The southern hemisphere experiences seasons at opposite times of the year because of these same phenomena.

By observing seasonal characteristics, sunrise and sunset times, it is possible to learn and better understand the patterns of the earth's movement and their direct effects on life. This chart demonstrates how sunrise and sunset times do not directly correspond to the equinoxes. These variations may be found at many locations around earth (American Āyurvedic Journal of Health, Vol 1, Issue 1).

Path of the Sun

The intense gravitational force of the sun led to the formation of the solar system. Current theories propose that it used to be a massive disc made up of dust. Gravity pulled those dust particles together allowing them to grow bigger and bigger and eventually creating the sun and planets. The gravitational effects continue to produce the paths of movement for these celestial bodies. Galileo, Brahe, Kepler proved that the movement of the planets occurs around the sun.

Declination. The Declination of a celestial body is its angular distance North or South of the Celestial Equator. The declination of the Sun changes from 23.5 degrees North to 23.5 degrees South and back again during the course of a year. Declination can be summarized as the celestial equivalent of Latitude since it is the angular distance of a celestial body North or South of the Celestial Equator.

The Equinoxes

The Sun crosses the celestial equator on two occasions during the course of a year and these occasions are known as the equinoxes. At the equinoxes, at all places on Earth, the nights and days are of equal duration (i.e. 12 hours) hence the term equinoxes (equal nights). Because the Sun is on the celestial equator at the equinoxes, its declination is of course 0 degrees.

The Autumnal Equinox occurs on or about the 22nd of September when the Sun crosses the celestial equator as it moves southwards from 23.5 degrees North, the northernmost limit of its declination.

The Vernal Equinox occurs on or about the 21st of March when the Sun crosses the celestial equator as it moves northwards from 23.5 degrees South, the southernmost limit of its declination.

The Solstices

The times when the Sun reaches the limits of its path of declination are known as the solstices. The word solstice is taken from 'solstitium', the latin for 'sun stands still'. This is because the apparent movement of the Sun seems to stop before it changes direction.

The Summer Solstice (mid-summer in the northern hemisphere) occurs on about the 21st of June when the Sun's declination reaches 23.5 degrees North (the tropic of Cancer).

The Winter Solstice (mid-winter in the northern hemisphere) occurs on about the 21st of December when the Sun's declination is 23.5 degrees South (the tropic of Capricorn).

Note. The latitude of the tropic of Cancer is currently drifting south at approximately 0.5" per year while the latitude of the tropic of Capricorn is drifting north at the same rate.

The dates of the equinoxes and the solstices will vary slightly during the four-year cycle between leap years for the following reason: Each year is approximately 365.25 days in length. However; for the sake of convenience, the Gregorian calendar divides three years of the cycle into 365 days and the fourth (the leap year) into 366. So, the Vernal Equinox sometimes falls on the 20th of March and sometimes on the 21st of March. The Autumnal Equinox sometimes falls on the 22nd of September and sometimes on the 23rd of September. Similarly, the Summer Solstice usually falls on the 21st of June but sometimes falls on the 20th of June. The Winter Solstice usually falls on the 21st of December but sometimes falls on the 22nd of December.

LATITUDE AND LONGITUDE

The development of cartography, or map-making, provides a system to identify locations on earth using latitude and longitude lines that are equally divided horizontally and vertically. Latitude is represented by horizontal lines called parallels and they measure distance north or south of the equator. They range from from 0 degrees at the equator to 90 degrees at the poles. Longitude is represented by vertical lines called meridians and they measure distance east or west of the Prime Meridian. They range from from 0 degrees to 180 degrees. The 180 degree line is called the International Date Line.

Latitude is divided into (Units of Longitude and Latitude, 2018):

- Arctic Circle 66°33' N
- Tropic of Cancer 23°27' N
- Equator 0°

- Tropic of Capricorn 23°27' S
- Antarctic Circle 66°33' S

The variations in direct sunlight, heat and wind currents affect the climate patterns seen at different latitudes around the earth. Generally, it is tropical and rainy at the equator, desert-like around 30° north or south of the equator, and temperate with boreal forests beyond 30°.

SOLAR TIME, LUNAR TIME, CLOCK TIME

It would make sense for the summer solstice to also be the date at which sunrise is earliest and sunset is latest; and for the winter solstice to be the date when sunrise is latest and sunset is earliest. However, that is not what happens! Nature sometimes defies our expectations. Our clock time and the Sun do not keep the same kind of time.

We don't tell time using the solar day, because we want all days to have exactly the same length. So we use clocks that run at a constant rate independent of the sun, ticking off exactly 24 hours each day. These clocks average out the variations in the solar day, making all days the same length, and so don't agree with the solar day. But when we ask about "earliest" sunset, of course we mean earliest according to the constantly-running clocks.

There are two factors that change the time of sunset. The first is the change in the number of hours of daylight—we get fewer hours of daylight as we move towards December, which is reflected in earlier sunsets. The second factor is the difference between solar time and clock time. The first factor is the dominating factor through most of the year. Near the summer and winter solstices, though, the amount of daylight in the day is essentially constant, changing only a tiny amount from day to day, and then the second factor comes into play.

We can apply the same reasoning to the summer solstice to conclude that the latest sunset must follow the summer solstice, and the earliest sunrise must precede the summer solstice.

The length of the solar day is determined mostly by the rotation of the earth on its axis but is also affected a little bit by the revolution of the earth around the sun. The rotation by itself would create a solar day of constant length whether the axis was tilted or not. The slight change caused by the revolution would be a constant if the earth were not tilted, but because of the tilt it is not constant; this effect varies through the year and makes the solar day longer near the solstices and shorter near the equinoxes. Therefore, we effectively have two kinds of time. Nature sometimes defies our expectations.

SOLAR & LUNAR CALENDARS AND THE SUN & THE MOON

Throughout history, people have used different types of calendars to help them know when to plant crops, choose the best hunting times, plan meetings and observe religious holidays. All calendars work by making it possible for you to organize time units by observing astronomical cycles. Months are based on the moon's orbit around the Earth, years are based on Earth's orbit around the sun and days measure the time as the Earth revolves once around its axis.

The principal astronomical cycles are the day (based on the rotation of the Earth on its axis), the year (based on the revolution of the Earth around the Sun), and the month (based on the revolution of the Moon around the Earth). The complexity of calendars arises because the year does not comprise an integral number of days or an integral number of lunar months.

Scientists define a solar year based on the movements of the sun, but use the movements of the moon to define a lunar year. Most places across the globe use the solar calendar to track the passage of the year. The difference between the lunar calendar and the solar calendar is of course, the celestial body used to measure the passage of time. The lunar calendar measures the time from new moon to new moon as one month. The time required for the Earth to rotate around the Sun is one solar year. The solar calendar typically measures the time between vernal equinoxes.

Solar calendars, such as the Gregorian calendar, track time using tropical years. A tropical year, also called a solar year, measures the length of time between two vernal equinoxes. That time period is 365 days, five hours, 48 minutes and 46 seconds. Many people refer to a vernal equinox as the first day of spring. While most people use the Gregorian calendar, no U.S. law forces people to observe Gregorian solar calendar dates. The use of that calendar dates back to 1751 when the United Kingdom told its colonies to use the Gregorian calendar.

A new moon is the opposite of a full moon. As the moon orbits the Earth, its position relative to the Earth and sun changes, and the moon appears to go through phases. When the Earth sits between the moon and sun, people on Earth see a full moon at night. A new moon occurs when the moon sits between the sun and the Earth. New moons occur during the day, so you can't see them because of the sun's brightness. A quarter moon, on the other hand, occurs when the moon completes 25 percent of its orbit around this planet.

Because the moon circles the Earth in the same time it takes to rotate once, the moon always shows the same face to the Earth. That's why you never see its far side. A new moon occurs every 29.5 days. Astronomers call the time between new moons a synodic month. All lunar calendars that people create base their months on the synodic month rather than the months you find on a solar calendar.

The civil calendar in use around the world (Gregorian calendar) is a solar calendar. Solar calendars are based on the progression through the seasons as the Earth revolves around the Sun, but neglect any attempt to keep the months synchronous with the lunar phases. A lunar calendar bases each month on a full cycle of the Moon’s phases (called a lunation or synodic month) without regard to the solar year. Lunar calendars usually start each month with a New Moon or the first visible crescent moon after New Moon. Luni-solar calendars try to remain synchronous with both the solar year and the moon phases. However, a solar year does not contain an integral number of days or an integral number of lunar months. To compensate for this, many luni-solar calendars adjust the length of their years and months. Without such an adjustment the seasons will steadily drift through the months.

TEST YOURSELF

Learn, review and memorize key terms from this section.

astronomy

axis

celestial equator

celestial poles

celestial sphere

declination

equator

equinox

Gregorian calendar

heliocentricity

latitude

longitutde

lunar calendar

moon

obliquity

planet

poles

precession

solar calendar

solar system

soli-lunar calendar

solstice

Chapter 12: Review

ADDITIONAL READING

Utilize these references to expand your understanding of the concepts in this chapter.

REQUIRED READING	Chapters
Crash Course Introduction to Astronomy: Crash Course Astronomy #1 Phil Plait, 1/15/2015, https://www.youtube.com/watch?v=0rHUDWjR5gg	
Sunrise and sunset times near the solstices, http://aa.usno.navy.mil/faq/docs/rs_solstices.php	
How earth moves, https://www.youtube.com/watch?v=IJhgZBn-LHg	
How to start with the basics of (theoretical) Astronomy?, http://www.backyard-astro.com/beginner/basicastronomy.html	
Bozeman Science - ESS1B Earth and the Solar System, https://www.youtube.com/watch?v=mxl7vRv8HT0	

References

The American Heritage Student Science Dictionary, Second Edition. (2014). Houghton Mifflin Harcourt Publishing Company.

"Celestial sphere." Merriam-Webster, 2018, https://www.merriam-webster.com/dictionary/celestial%20sphere

"Solar System Basics." Astronomy Online, 2013. http://astronomyonline.org/SolarSystem/Introduction.asp?Cate=SolarSystem&SubCate=Introduction&SubCate2=SS00

"Units of Longitude and Latitude." Astronomy Education at the University of Nebraska-Lincoln, 2018. http://astro.unl.edu/naap/motion1/tc_units.html

American Āyurvedic Journal of Health (Vol 1, Issue 1). http://www.aachealth.us/journal/issues/

Temming, M. (2014, July 15). "What Is a Star?" Sky and Telescope. http://www.skyandtelescope.com/astronomy-resources/what-is-a-star/

"Planets." NASA Science Solar System Exploration, 2018, https://solarsystem.nasa.gov/planets/in-depth/

"Mercator projection." Encyclopædia Britannica, 2018, https://www.britannica.com/science/Mercator-projection

Vecchiato, A. (2018, January 2). "Do the Sun and Moon Really Rise in the East?" Sky and Telescope. http://www.skyandtelescope.com/astronomy-resources/sunrise-moonrise-east/

Byrd, D. (2018, January 31). "Tides, and the pull of the moon and sun." EarthSky. http://earthsky.org/earth/tides-and-the-pull-of-the-moon-and-sun#two-tides

QUESTIONS & ANSWERS

Record your questions for this chapter here for further research and discussion.

Question:

Answer:

Question:

Answer:

Question:

Answer:

SELF-ASSESSMENT

1. Astronomy relates to Āyurveda through ____?
   a. understanding the seasons
   b. Astrology
   c. the sun, moon and wind
   d. Both A and C
   e. All of the above

2. Latitude is represented by the ___.
   a. vertical lines
   b. meridians
   c. parallels
   d. B and C
   e. None of the above

3. Variations produced within the elliptical orbit of the Earth is called ___.
   a. precession
   b. axis tilt
   c. an anomaly
   d. All of the above
   e. None of the above

4. Our clock time ___ the variations in the solar day.
   a. is in sync with
   b. is opposite from
   c. averages out
   d. equals
   e. None of the above

5. The length of a day and night vary due to ____.
   a. the stars
   b. the Sun
   c. the Moon
   d. Mars
   e. Venus

6. The Celestial sphere is ___.
   a. an actual sphere
   b. a dome shaped projection
   c. perspective of sky from space
   d. a projected circular shape
   e. an imaginary sphere

7. What determines the seasons?
   a. The tilt of the Earths' axis
   b. Precession
   c. The tides
   d. The Moon
   e. None of the above

8. Motion is a cause for ___.
   a. the phases of the Moon
   b. solar and lunar eclipses
   c. night and day
   d. planets appearing to move backwards
   e. All of the above

9. The length of a solar day is determined by ___ and ___.
   a. the Sun and tides
   b. the Earth and Moon
   c. rotation and revolution
   d. the sun and motion
   e. None of the above

10. Moon phases are determined by which planets?
    a. The Moon.
    b. The Sun.
    c. The Earth.
    d. All of the above
    e. None of the above

Chapter 13 : Meteorology and earth science

The Merriam-Webster Dictionary defines meteorology as (Meteorology, 2018):

1. a science that deals with the atmosphere and its phenomena and especially with weather and weather forecasting
2. the atmospheric phenomena and weather of a region

While it may not seem as if Astronomy and Meteorology have anything to do with Āyurveda, they do indeed. There is a great deal of reflection of the macrocosm in the microcosm and vice versa.

KEY CONCEPTS AND DEFINITIONS

Review these key concepts and memorize their definitions (Weather for dummies cheat sheet, 2018).

Atmosphere - The envelope of gases that compose the air surrounding Earth

Low Pressure - An area of rising air usually marked by cloudiness, often referred to as a storm

Chaos - A state of a system in which disturbances large and small grow and decay; considered chaotic as it is unpredictable beyond a few days

Climate - The average, long term weather of a place

Precipitation - Water vapor that condenses in the atmosphere, falling to the surface as rain, snow or ice

Coriolis Effect - The bending effect of the Earth's rotation on the path of things in motion in the atmosphere and the ocean. The bending of deflection of its course is to the right in the Northern Hemisphere and to the left in Southern Hemisphere.

Pressure - The weight of the air overhead, exerted in all directions on everything air touches. Horizontal differences in pressure cause winds. Vertical differences in air pressure influence cloud formation and storm development.

Dew point - The temperature to which air must be cooled in order for it to become saturated with water vapor

Relative Humidity - The percentage of the air that is saturated with water vapor at the current temperature. A value that changes with temperature. Air that is saturated at 50 degrees - 100% relative humidity - falls to about 50% when its temperature rises to 70 degrees.

Solstice - The point reached on or about June 21 and December 21 when the seasonal track of sunlight over the Earth reaches its northernmost and southernmost progress

Equinox - Latin for "equal nights." The time in spring and autumn when the sun shines directly over the equator and hours of daylight and darkness are equal everywhere.

Stratosphere - The layer of much thinner gases in the atmosphere above the troposphere, between 7 miles and 30 miles in height. It included the ozone layer. It is called the stratosphere because the temperatures are usually stratified and uniform at this level.

Troposphere - The lowest part of the atmosphere, where all the weather takes place. Its height averages about 7 miles, ranging from 5 miles at the poles to about 10 miles at the equator.

High pressure system - An area where more air has been added overhead compared to surrounding areas creating higher barometric pressure. Typically, the air enters at high altitudes, sinks, and exits at ground level. The sinking motion causes warming and drying, leaving the clear sky often found in high pressure areas.

Wind Chill - The additional cooling effect of wind blowing on bare skin

AIR MASSES

Air masses are created by different landmasses modifying the air above them to have the same properties as the ground. There are four primary groups of air masses:

- Those formed over cold water maritime polar or mP
- Those formed over warm water called maritime tropical or mT
- Those formed over cold land called continental polar or cP
- Those formed over warm land and is called continental tropical or cT

The creation process of an air mass requires low wind to allow the air to sit over the ground for long periods of time of at least a week typically. Eventually these air masses drift into areas of stronger winds and are moved with them into other areas (Grey, 2018).

CLIMATE AND WEATHER

Climate is known as the general or average weather conditions of a certain region that includes temperature, rainfall and wind. For example, Seattle has a rainy, wet climate for much of the year. Weather is the state of the atmosphere at any particular time and place. It is described by variable conditions like temperature, humidity, wind velocity, precipitation and barometric pressure. The key difference is time. Climate covers years and decades where weather is day to day to short term. Climate information is made up of statistical weather, weather that is normal as well as the range from one extreme to another (American Heritage Dictionary of Student Science, 2014).

RELATED FIELDS OF SCIENCE

Review these key concepts and memorize their definitions (American Heritage Dictionary of Student Science, 2014).

Earth Science is any of several sciences, such as geology, oceanography, or meteorology, that specialize in the origin, composition, and physical features of the Earth.

Geology

1. The scientific study of the origin of the earth along with its rocks, minerals, and landforms, and of the history of the changes these have undergone.

2. The structure of a specific region of the earth, including its rocks, soils, mountains, fossils, and other features.

Geography

The scientific study of the earth's surface and its various climates, countries, peoples and natural resources.

Climate

The general or average weather conditions of a certain region, including temperature, rainfall, and wind: Caribbean islands have a year-round climate of warm breezes and sunshine.

Weather

The state of the atmosphere at a particular time and place. Weather is described by variable conditions such as temperature, humidity, wind velocity, precipitation, and barometric pressure.

Geography and its relationship to climate

What is the relationship between the distance from the equator, sea elevation, distance from water, topography or the layout of the landscape and climate (basic patterns of temperature and precipitation)? All of these in the form of: higher latitudes, water bodies, mountains and higher elevations can all impact climate. They can create air currents, precipitation patterns and prolong colder seasons.

Environmental science

An interdisciplinary field that integrates all the sciences, such as biology, ecology, physics, geology, meteorology, chemistry. It also includes the social sciences as there is a direct relationship between humans and the environment.

Chapter 13: Review

ADDITIONAL READING

Utilize these references to expand your understanding of the concepts in this chapter.

REQUIRED READING	Chapters
Basic Meteorology: A Short Course, http://www.fortunearchive.com/Physics/Meteorology.pdf	
Basic Meteorology Concepts, https://www.vatsim.net/pilot-resource-centre/general-lessons/basic-meteorology-concepts	
Meteorology: An Educator's Resource, https://www.nasa.gov/pdf/288978main_Meteorology_Guide.pdf	

OPTIONAL READING	Format
Handbook of Meteorology, https://www.pssurvival.com/PS/Weather/Handbook_Of_Meteorology_1921.pdf	
Physical Geography: Weather and the Factors that Influence Climate, Mr. Naumann, University of Missouri, St. Louis	

References

"Meteorology." Merriam-Webster, 2018, https://www.merriam-webster.com/dictionary/meteorology

"Weather for dummies cheat sheet." Dummies, 2018. http://www.dummies.com/education/science/weather-for-dummies-cheat-sheet/

Grey, P. (2018). "Basic Meteorology Concepts." https://www.vatsim.net/pilot-resource-centre/general-lessons/basic-meteorology-concepts

QUESTIONS & ANSWERS

Record your questions for this chapter here for further research and discussion.

Question:

Answer:

Question:

Answer:

Question:

Answer:

SELF-ASSESSMENT

1. What is the definition of Meteorology according to Merriam-Webster?
   a. A science that deals with Geology, with special focus on how ecology affects the weather.
   b. A science that deals with the atmosphere and its phenomena and especially with weather and weather forecasting.
   c. The weight of the air overhead, exerted in all directions on everything air touches.
   d. The number of meteors that appear to radiate from one point in the sky at a particular date each year, due to the earth's regularly passing through a field of particles at that position in its orbit.
   e. All of the above

2. What's the definition of atmosphere?
   a. The envelope of gases that compose the air surrounding Earth.
   b. A combination of 80% nitrogen, 10% oxygen, 10% other trace gasses.
   c. The celestial body surrounding any object in the universe.
   d. Water vapor and carbon dioxide that surrounds the earth.
   e. None of the Above

3. What's the definition of precipitation?
   a. It is rain, snow, sleet, hail and lightning.
   b. Water vapor that condenses in the atmosphere, falling to the surface as rain, snow or ice.
   c. Spherical or irregular pellets of ice larger than 5 millimeters (0.2 inch) in diameter, usually associated with thunderstorms.
   d. Precipitation includes fog and mist.
   e. None of the above

4. What's the definition of Solstice?
   a. The day which marks the onset of Summer.
   b. The day which marks the onset of Fall.
   c. The point reached on or about June 21 and December 21 when the seasonal track of sunlight over the Earth reaches its northernmost and southernmost progress.
   d. Both A and B
   e. None of the above

5. What's the definition of "equinox"?
   a. It's Latin for "equal nights."
   b. The time in spring and autumn when the sun shines directly over the equator and hours of daylight and darkness are equal everywhere.
   c. It relates to or affects horses or other members of the horse family.
   d. Both A and B
   e. None of the above

6. Which of the following make up some of the earth sciences mentioned in Chapter 32?
   a. Geology, Geography, Oceanography and Meteorology
   b. Astronomy, Geology and Meteorology
   c. Geography and Meteorology
   d. All of the above
   e. None of the above

7. Which of the following is NOT one of the four primary groups of air masses?
   a. Those formed over hot land and is called subtropical or sT.
   b. Those formed over warm water called maritime tropical or mT.
   c. Those formed over cold water maritime polar or mP.
   d. Those formed over cold land called continental polar or cP.
   e. None of the above

8. Which of the following factors are included in what is known as climate?
   a. Temperature, rainfall and wind
   b. Humidity, precipitation and barometric pressure
   c. Carbon dioxide levels and water pollution
   d. A and B
   e. None of the above

9. What's the primary difference between climate and weather?
   a. Climate covers years and decades of weather patterns, where weather covers the day to day, short term state of the atmosphere of a particular place.
   b. There is no difference, they are the same thing.
   c. Weather only includes the average range of barometric pressure at any given place.
   d. Weather can only be described in terms of temperature.
   e. None of the above

10. What's the definition of Geography?
    a. The scientific study of the water bodies and how they relate to climate.
    b. The study of the relationship between the distance of the equator and the landscape.
    c. The study of the different land masses and the air above them in relation to temperature.
    d. The scientific study of the earth's surface and its various climates, countries, peoples and natural resources.
    e. None of the above

Chapter 14 : Physics

The Merriam-Webster Dictionary defines Physics as:

1. a science that deals with matter and energy and their interactions
2. the physical processes and phenomena of a particular system
3. the physical properties and composition of something (physics, 2018)

This chapter is meant to be a review as well as learning new ways to apply the concepts and Laws of physics to the study of Āyurveda. A student of Āyurveda needs to be able to move in and out of "multiple perspectives". These Laws and concepts can also be approached from the perspective of everyday application. It's much easier to apply the laws of physics through an everyday example.

LAW OF UNIVERSAL GRAVITATION

Sir Isaac Newton's groundbreaking work in physics was first published in 1687 in his book "The Mathematical Principles of Natural Philosophy," commonly known as the Principia. In it, he outlined theories about gravity and of motion. His physical law of gravity states that an object attracts another object in direct proportion to their combined mass and inversely related to the square of the distance between them. Newton understood that objects pull on each other - the earth pulls the apple to the ground, but the apple also pulls back on the Earth.

The most important part about this is not only that objects pull on each other, but that two objects attract each other with a force that is proportional to the product of their masses and inversely proportional to the square of the distance between them. This is known as Newton's law of universal gravitation. What this means is that for any two objects in the universe, the gravity between these two objects depends only on their mass and distance.

A more recent understanding of gravity explains it not as a force, but an effect of the way space rolls through itself. Imagine two entities aware of each other but not aware they are moving sideways toward a common convergence point. They would imagine there is a mysterious force drawing them together. Everything is on a convergence path, that is what we call gravity. It has to do with the way space moves.

Here are two common examples of the Law of Universal Gravitation:

- an apple falling towards the ground
- the moon orbiting around the earth

It was Newton's insight that a single physical law could describe these two, apparently different, sorts of motion that kick-started modern physics.

NEWTON'S THREE LAWS OF MOTION AND THEIR APPLICATION

Newton's three laws of motion, also found in the Principia, govern how the motion of physical objects change. They define the fundamental relationship between the acceleration of an object and the forces acting upon it.

Newtons First Law

Isaac Newton states that an object maintains a constant velocity unless acted upon by another force.

Examples:

A truck collides with another truck and the truck stops, but the driver keeps going. A rock won't move unless someone moves it.

Newtons Second Law

Acceleration increases with force and decreases with mass.

Example 1: Two objects of different weights are thrown off of a roof, you may assume that the heavier object will hit the ground first, but according to Newtons Second Law, the heavier objects acceleration decreases because it has more mass. The truth is, both objects will hit the ground at the same time.

Example 2: It is easier to push an empty shopping cart than a full one. If pushed with the same amount of force, the empty one will go farther while the full one will be harder to stop.

Newtons Third Law

For every action there is an equal and opposite reaction.

Example 1: When a rocket blasts off, the thrust produced pushes against the ground, forcing the rocket up.

Example 2: When walking, you are actually pushing on the earth and the earth pushes back, causing you to move.

Example 3: In yoga, it's referred to as "root and rise". Take a moment right now wherever you are sitting, draw your abdominal muscles in and press your sits bones downward into your seat and notice if you have a sense of lengthening or rising of your spine/torso.

The same applies to cars, bicycles, and boats.

There is no such thing as an unpaired force in the universe.

The table rests on the floor just as the book rests on it, and the floor pushes up on the table with a force equal in magnitude to that with which the table presses down on the floor. The same is true for the floor and the supporting beams that hold it up, and for the supporting beams and the foundation of the building, and the building and the ground, and so on.

These pairs of forces exist everywhere. When you walk, you move forward by pushing backward on the ground with a force equal to your mass multiplied by your rate of downward gravitational acceleration. (This force, in other words, is the same as weight.) At the same time, the ground actually pushes back with an equal force. You do not perceive the fact that Earth is pushing you upward, simply because its enormous mass makes this motion negligible—but it does push.

If you were stepping off of a small unmoored boat and onto a dock, however, something quite different would happen. The force of your leap to the dock would exert an equal force against the boat, pushing it further out into the water, and as a result, you would likely end up in the water as well. Again, the reaction is equal and opposite; the problem is that the boat in this illustration is not fixed in place like the ground beneath your feet.

Read more:

http://www.scienceclarified.com/everyday/Real-Life-Chemistry-Vol-3-Physics-Vol-1/Laws-of-Motion-Real-life-applications.html#ixzz5KQpqziWC

THREE LAWS OF THERMODYNAMICS

The laws of thermodynamics dictate energy behavior, for example, how and why heat, which is a form of energy, transfers between different objects. The laws of thermodynamics are actually specific manifestations of the law of conservation of mass-energy as it relates to thermodynamic processes. The field was first explored in the 1650s by Otto von Guericke in Germany and Robert Boyle and Robert Hooke in Britain. All three scientists used vacuum pumps, which von Guericke pioneered, to study the principles of pressure, temperature, and volume.

The zeroth law of thermodynamics makes the notion of temperature possible.

The first law of thermodynamics demonstrates the relationship between internal energy, added heat, and work within a system.

The second law of thermodynamics relates to the natural flow of heat within a closed system.

The third law of thermodynamics states that it is impossible to create a thermodynamic process that is perfectly efficient

1st Law - The Law of Conservation of Energy

This law states that energy can neither be created nor destroyed. It can only change from one form to another or transferred from one object to another.

Everyday examples of the Law of Conservation of Energy in action include:

Walking quickly and accidently bumping into someone so that they get knocked off their course.

Playing pool - when the cue ball is hit, it carries energy with it and if it hits another ball, that energy will be transferred.

The potential energy of oil or gas is turned into energy to heat a room.

When an electric heater is turned on, the electrical energy is converted into heat energy. If the amount of electricity supplied to the heater is measured, it equals the amount of heat produced by the heater.

The Law of Conservation of Mass is similar to that of the Law of Conservation of Energy.

Example: the combustion of a piece of paper to form ash, water vapor and carbon dioxide. In this process, the mass of the paper is not actually destroyed; instead, it is transformed into other forms. This best demonstrates the law that states matter cannot be created or destroyed. However, the form of matter can be changed.

2nd Law - The Second Law of Thermodynamics

This law states that in any energy conversion, some energy is wasted as heat; moreover, the entropy (lack of order or predictability) of any closed system always increases. Another way to understand this is to say that "things wear out". One expression of the 2nd law of thermodynamics is that heat cannot flow from a cold object to a hotter object of its own volition.

Example 1: One way we can see the Second Law at work is in our daily diet. We eat food each day, without gaining that same amount of body weight! The food we eat is largely expended as carbon dioxide and heat energy, plus some work done in repairing and rebuilding bodily cells and tissues, physical movement, and neuronal activity

Example 2: Place an ice cube in a cup of warm water, and the ice melts as heat flows into it from the water, ending up with a cup of slightly cooler water than you had before. You never see ice cubes spontaneously forming in cups of water, as heat drains out of the cold ice in to the hotter liquid. Ice cubes can only be made by using energy to pump heat out. (e.g.in a freezer.)

Example 3: If a house is left unattended for a

long time, it will crumble away by the influence of wind and weather but a pile of bricks will not spontaneously form itself into a house.

Other examples include:

- a smell diffusing in a room
- ice melting in lukewarm water
- salt dissolving in water
- iron rusting

3rd Law - The Third Law of Thermodynamics

The third law of thermodynamics has very few practical applications in day-to-day life, as opposed to the first and the second laws. The third law essentially tells us that it is impossible, by any procedure, to reach the absolute zero of temperature in a finite number of steps. Study of the Third Law of Thermodynamics mainly supports the implications of the first two laws.

More common examples where we see the Laws of Thermodynamics in our everyday life.

Melting Ice Cube

Every day, ice needs to be maintained at a temperature below the freezing point of water to remain solid. On hot summer days, however, people often take out a tray of ice to cool beverages. In the process, they witness the first and second laws of thermodynamics. For example, someone might put an ice cube into a glass of warm lemonade and then forget to drink the beverage. An hour or two later, they will notice that the ice has melted but the temperature of the lemonade has cooled. This is because the total amount of heat in the system has remained the same, but has just gravitated towards equilibrium, where both the former ice cube (now water) and the lemonade are the same temperature. This is, of course, not a completely closed system. The lemonade will eventually become warm again, as heat from the environment is transferred to the glass and its contents.

Sweating in a Crowded Room

The human body obeys the laws of thermodynamics. Consider the experience of being in a small crowded room with lots of other people. In all likelihood, you'll start to feel very warm and will start sweating. This is the process your body uses to cool itself off. Heat from your body is transferred to the sweat. As the sweat absorbs more and more heat, it evaporates from your body, becoming more disordered and transferring heat to the air, which heats up the air temperature of the room. Many sweating people in a crowded room, "closed system," will quickly heat things up. This is both the first and second laws of thermodynamics in action: No heat is lost; it is merely transferred, and approaches equilibrium with maximum entropy.

Taking a Bath

Consider a situation where a person takes a very long bath. Immediately during and after filling up the bathtub, the water is very hot -- as high as 120 degrees Fahrenheit. The person will then turn off the water and submerge his body into it. Initially, the water feels comfortably warm, because the water's temperature is higher than the person's body temperature. After some time, however, some heat from the water will have transferred to the individual, and the two temperatures will meet. After a bit more time has passed, because this is not a closed system, the bath water will cool as heat is lost to the atmosphere. The person will cool as well, but not as much since his internal homeostatic mechanisms help keep his temperature adequately elevated.

Flipping a Light Switch

We rely on electricity to turn on our lights. Electricity is a form of energy; it is, however, a secondary source. A primary source of energy must be converted into electricity before we can flip on the lights. For example, water energy can be harnessed by building a dam to hold back the water of a large lake. If we slowly release water through a small opening in the dam, we can use the driving pressure of the water to turn a turbine. The work of the turbine can be used to generate electricity with the help of a generator. The electricity is sent to our homes via power lines. The electricity was not created out of nothing; it is the result of transforming water energy from the lake into another energy form.

ELECTROSTATIC LAWS

Two laws of physics govern the relationship between electrically charged particles and their ability to create electrostatic force and electrostatic fields. These laws look at the forces between particles that are caused by their electric charges.

Coulomb's law is named for Charles-Augustin Coulomb, a French researcher working in the 1700s. The force between two-point charges is directly proportional to the magnitude of each charge and inversely proportional to the square of the distance between their centers. More simply put, when you have two charged particles, an electric force is created. If you have larger charges, the forces will be larger. As distance increases, the forces and electric fields decrease. If the objects have the same charge, positive or negative, they will repel each other. If they have opposite charges, they will attract each other.

Gauss's law is named for Carl Friedrich Gauss, a German mathematician who worked in the early 19th century. This law states that net flow of an electric field through a closed surface is proportional to the enclosed electric charge. Gauss proposed similar laws relating to magnetism and electromagnetism as a whole.

Electrostatics and Everyday Life Examples

1. When you take off a pullover over a nylon shirt there is a crackling sound.

2. A pen rubbed with a piece of cloth will pick up small pieces of paper.

3. A television screen collects dust easily.

4. If you roll over in bed you can sometimes see small sparks between the sheets.

5. Cling wrap sticking to everything.

6. Getting a small electric shock from a cat that has rolled on a synthetic carpet.

7. In a thunder storm there are huge flashes of lightning.

8. An electrostatic dust collector in a chimney.

9. Paint sprays can be charged and the object they are spraying earthed to attract the paint towards it.

10. Photocopiers use a charged sheet to attract fine carbon powder.

11. Charge build up when emptying oil tankers or re-fueling planes.

FOUR FUNDAMENTAL FORCES

Gravity

Of the fundamental forces, gravity has the farthest reach but it's the weakest in actual magnitude. It is a purely attractive force which reaches through even the "empty" void of space to draw two masses toward each other. It keeps the planets in orbit around the sun and the moon in orbit around the Earth.

Gravitation is described under the theory of general relativity, which defines it as the curvature of spacetime around an object of mass. This curvature, in turn, creates a situation where the path of least energy is toward the other object of mass.

Example

The first force that you ever became aware of was probably gravity. As a toddler, you had to learn to rise up against it and walk. When you stumbled, you immediately felt gravity bring you back down to the floor. Besides giving toddlers trouble, gravity holds the moon, planets, sun, stars and galaxies together in the universe in their respective orbits. It can work over immense distances and has an infinite range.

Electromagnetism

Electromagnetism is the interaction of particles with an electrical charge. Charged particles at rest interact through electrostatic forces, while in motion they interact through both electrical and magnetic forces.

For a long time, the electric and magnetic forces were considered to be different forces, but they were finally unified by James Clerk Maxwell in 1864, under Maxwell's equations.

In the 1940s, quantum electrodynamics consolidated electromagnetism with quantum physics. Electromagnetism is perhaps the most obviously prevalent force in the world as it can affect things at a reasonable distance and with a fair amount of force.

Examples

If you brush your hair several times, your hair may stand on end and be attracted to the brush. Why? The movement of the brush imparts electrical charges to each hair and the identically charged individual hairs repel each other. Similarly, if you place identical poles of two bar magnets together, they will repel each other. But set the opposite poles of the magnets near one another, and the magnets will attract each other. These are familiar examples of electromagnetic forces where opposite charges attract, while like charges repel.

Weak Interaction

The weak interaction is a very powerful force that acts on the scale of the atomic nucleus.

It has been consolidated with electromagnetism as a single interaction called the "electroweak interaction." Weak interaction is responsible for certain kinds of radioactive decay. For example, the kind of decay measured by archaeologists when they perform radiocarbon dating.

Strong Interaction

The strongest of the forces is the aptly-named strong interaction, which is the force that, among other things, keeps nucleons (protons and neutrons) bound together. In the helium atom, for example, it is strong enough to bind two protons together despite the fact that their positive electrical charges cause them to repulse each other.

Interesting Note

Which force is the mightiest of them all? That would be the strong nuclear force. However, it acts only over a short range, approximately the size of a nucleus. The weak nuclear force is one-millionth as strong as the strong nuclear force and has an even shorter range, less than a proton's diameter. The electromagnetic force is about 0.7 percent as strong as the strong nuclear force, but has an infinite range because photons carrying the electromagnetic force travel at the speed of light. Finally, gravity is the weakest force at about 6 x 10-29 times that of the strong nuclear force. Gravity, however, has an infinite range.

Physicists are currently pursuing the ideas

that the four fundamental forces may be related and that they sprang from one force early in the universe. The idea isn't unprecedented. We once thought of electricity and magnetism as separate entities, but the work of Oersted, Faraday, Maxwell and others showed that they were related.

Unifying the Fundamental Forces

Many physicists believe that all four of the fundamental forces are, in fact, the manifestations of a single underlying (or unified) force which has yet to be discovered. Just as electricity, magnetism, and the weak force were unified into the electroweak interaction, they work to unify all of the fundamental forces.

The current quantum mechanical interpretation of these forces is that the particles do not interact directly, but rather manifest virtual particles that mediate the actual interactions. All of the forces except for gravity have been consolidated into this "Standard Model" of interaction.

The effort to unify gravity with the other three fundamental forces is called quantum gravity. It postulates the existence of a virtual particle called the graviton, which would be the mediating element in gravity interactions. To date, gravitons have not been detected and no theories of quantum gravity have been successful or universally adopted (Jones, 2018).

A major point to take away from these sciences is that while the laws are discussed separately, they are actually interwoven with each other. The familiar force of gravity pulls you down into your seat, toward the Earth's center. You feel it as your weight. How come you don't fall through your seat? Another force, electromagnetism, holds the atoms of your seat together, preventing your atoms from intruding on those of your seat. Electromagnetic interactions in your computer monitor are also responsible for generating light that allows you to read the screen.

Gravity and electromagnetism are just two of the four fundamental forces of nature, specifically two that you can observe every day. What are the other two, and how do they affect you if you can't see them?

The remaining two forces work at the atomic level, which we never feel, despite being made of atoms. The strong force holds the nucleus together. Lastly, the weak force is responsible for radioactive decay, specifically, beta decay where a neutron within the nucleus changes into a proton and an electron, which is ejected from the nucleus.

Without these fundamental forces, you and all the other matter in the universe would fall apart and float away. Let's look at each fundamental force, what each does, how it was discovered and how it relates to the others.

STATES OF MATTER

Solid

Solids have structural rigidity and a strong resistance to environmental changes. Solids have their own shape and will not take the shape of the container in which they are put. The tiny particles of a solid are compactly bound together.

Example

Ice is a solid but when it melts it becomes a liquid. Other examples of solids are cars, books and clothes. Solids can be different colors and textures, and they can be turned into different shapes, such as clay.

Liquid

Liquids have a definite volume but take the shape of the container in which they occupy.

This means liquids do not have shape. They are made up of vibrating particles that are held together by intermolecular bonds.

Examples

Tea, water and blood. They can be different colors and thickness; for example, custard is a thicker liquid than tea and doesn't flow as quickly as tea. You can measure a liquid in a cup or a spoon.

Gas

Gases have no shape and will assume the shape of the container in which they are placed. They are made up of tiny particles that are vastly separated and are in constant vibration. When liquids are heated, they tend to change into gases.

Example

We are surrounded by different gases in the air we breathe.

Plasma

Similar to liquids and gases, plasma does not have a definite shape. It is created when energy is added to a gas

PHASE CHANGES IN STATES OF MATTER

These include evaporation, condensation, melting, freezing, sublimation, and deposition.

Melting and Freezing

If solid matters gain enough heat they change state from a solid to a liquid. Heat is a form of energy and in this situation, it is used to break the bonds of the atoms and molecules. Heated atoms and molecules vibrate more quickly and break their bonds. We call this process melting as it changes the state from solid to liquid. Inverse of melting is called freezing, changing state from a liquid to solid, in which atoms and molecules lost heat and come together, their motion slows down and distance between them decreases.

Melting occurs when a solid is heated until its particles reach a high enough energy to reach its melting point, changing it into the liquid state. An example of melting is an ice cube turning into liquid water when you set it on a surface or hold it in your hand.

Freezing occurs when a liquid is cooled until its particles reach a low enough energy to reach its freezing point, changing it into the solid state. This occurs to liquid water when it is placed in a freezer.

Boiling, Evaporation and Condensation

Evaporation, a type of vaporization, occurs when particles of a liquid reach a high enough energy to leave the surface of the liquid and change into the gas state. An example of evaporation is a puddle of water drying out. It dries out because the molecules of water evaporate into the atmosphere.

Boiling is a type of rapid vaporization that occurs when the particles of a liquid are heated to its boiling point. Large bubbles of gas form throughout the liquid and move to the surface, leaving the liquid. Steam is the gaseous water molecules that form above boiling water.

Condensation occurs when the particles in a gas cool enough (lose energy) to change to the liquid state. An example of condensation is when a glass of ice water forms water droplets on the outside. The molecules of water vapor next to the glass cool and condense into liquid water.

Sublimation and Deposition

Sublimation occurs when a solid changes into the gas state without passing through the liquid state. Iodine is an example of a substance that sublimes, as well as solid carbon dioxide (dry ice), snow, and ice.

Deposition occurs when a gas changes into a solid without passing through the liquid state. Examples of deposition include the formation of snow in clouds, formation of frost on windows and the ground, and discharging a CO2 fire extinguisher.

CLOSED AND OPEN SYSTEMS

The basics of an Open/Closed System theory is that an open system interacts with its environment, taking in information and sending out information to the outside. A closed system does just the opposite. It does not incorporate new ideas or get involved with the environment. Examples can be found in the world of computers/operating technologies, large and small businesses and all the way to the physical and life sciences such as biology and chemistry.

The basic mechanics involved include the system which could be a cell or complex organism and its surrounding environment. The factors that require the life form to interact with the external environment determine whether it behaves as an open or closed system.

CONTROLLING THE ENVIRONMENT

The widespread use of heating and cooling systems affects a large majority of the modern, urban world today, especially in westernized countries. Heating and cooling systems proliferate in homes, offices, shopping centers, indoor recreation areas and almost every enclosed building. This insulates inhabitants from fully experiencing the effects of the more extreme external environment and may have direct impacts on human health.

Heating systems

Forced hot air- Air is heated directly then circulated through ventilation ducts.

Gas furnace

Oil furnace

Space heaters with blowers

Convection- Air is heated and circulated slowly by air movement based on temperature differences. Heating elements that heat up quickly also cool quickly.

Electric baseboards

Space heaters (ceramic)

Hydronic baseboards

Portable oil-filled radiators

Non-steam radiators

Steam radiators

Radiant- heats the cooler objects through direct contact.

Radiant floor heating with hot water tubes

Wood and pellet stoves

Infrared heaters

Cooling systems

Air conditioning- Air is cooled and dehumidified directly then circulated through ventilation ducts.

Evaporative water cooler

Single room a/c

Central a/c

MEASUREMENT SCALES: IMPERIAL AND METRIC SYSTEMS

The United States is one of only two countries in the world where the Imperial System is commonly used. It is the older of the two systems and is based on inches, feet, yards and miles for length. Fluid volume is measured in fluid ounces, cups, pints, quarts and gallons. Weight is measured in ounces, pounds and tons. In this system, it is difficult to compare measurements.

The Metric System is newer and simpler to use. It utilizes a basic unit of meter for distance, gram for mass and liter for volume. Prefixes are then added on making it much easier to work with measurements. Measurements increase and decrease by powers of ten making the system very easy to use.

Chapter 14: Review

ADDITIONAL READING

Utilize these references to expand your understanding of the concepts in this chapter.

REQUIRED READING	Chapters
Fundamental Physics, https://www.windows2universe.org/physical_science/physics/physics.html	
Introduction to the Major Laws of Physics, https://www.thoughtco.com/major-laws-of-physics-2699071	
The Basics of Physics in Scientific Study, https://www.thoughtco.com/physics-basics-4140295	

References

Jones, Andrew Zimmerman. (2017, July 10). "How Physics Works." ThoughtCo. https://www.thoughtco.com/what-is-physics-2699069

Jones, Andrew Zimmerman. (2018, February 19). "The 4 Fundamental Forces of Physics." ThoughtCo. https://www.thoughtco.com/what-are-fundamental-forces-of-physics-2699070

Helmenstine, Anne Marie. (2018, January 31). "What Are the States of Matter?" ThoughtCo. https://www.thoughtco.com/states-of-matter-p2-608184

QUESTIONS & ANSWERS

Record your questions for this chapter here for further research and discussion.

Question:

Answer:

Question:

Answer:

Question:

Answer:

SELF-ASSESSMENT

1. What is the definition of Physics?
   a. A science that deals with matter and energy and their interactions.
   b. A science that deals with that which relates to the body and all that is seen through the senses.
   c. The science of physical exertion, physical effort; that which causes the body to sweat.
   d. All of the above
   e. None of the above
2. Physics can describe the concepts of the following:
   a. inflammation and degeneration
   b. hydrogen and oxygen
   c. motion, forces and Thermodynamics
   d. weather patterns
   e. All of the above
3. What book by Sir Isaac Newton was groundbreaking in the field of Physics?
   a. *The Mathematical Principles of Natural Philosophy*
   b. *The Opticks*
   c. *Method of Fluxions*
   d. *The Unpublished Papers*
   e. None of the above
4. What is Newton's First Law of Motion?
   a. Every particle attracts every other particle in the universe with a force which is directly proportional to the product of their masses and inversely proportional to the square of the distance between their centers.
   b. An object maintains a constant velocity unless acted upon by another force.
   c. For every action in nature there is an equal and opposite reaction.
   d. All of the above
   e. None of the above
5. What is Newton's Second Law of Motion?
   a. For every action in nature there is an equal and opposite reaction.
   b. Acceleration increases with force and decreases with mass.
   c. The rate of change in momentum is not directly proportional to the amount of force applied.
   d. All of the above
   e. None of the above
6. The First Law of Thermodynamics demonstrates the relationship between internal energy, added heat, and ______.
   a. work within the system
   b. momentum
   c. gravity
   d. wind
   e. None of the above
7. The Second Law of Thermodynamics relates to the natural flow of____ within a closed system.
   a. wind
   b. heat
   c. cold
   d. A and C
   e. None of the above
8. The Third Law of Thermodynamics states that it is impossible to create a _______ that is perfectly efficient.
   a. state of inertia
   b. state of momentum
   c. thermodynamic process
   d. process in motion
   e. condition of stasis
9. Gravitation is described under the Theory of General Relativity, which defines it as _______.
   a. The curvature of spacetime around an object of mass.
   b. The tendency to do nothing or remain unchanged.
   c. The curvature of heat around an object or mass.
   d. All of the above
   e. None of the above
10. What are the states of matter?
    a. water, ice and humidity
    b. hydrogen, oxygen and sodium
    c. Solid, liquid and gas
    d. All of the above
    e. None of the above

Chapter 15 : Chemistry

The Merriam-Webster Dictionary defines chemistry as (Chemistry, 2018):

1. a science that deals with the composition, structure, and properties of substances and with the transformations that they undergo.
2. the composition and chemical properties of a substance.
3. chemical processes and phenomena (as of an organism).
4. a strong mutual attraction, attachment, or sympathy.
5. interaction between people working together.

BASIC CONCEPTS

Review the following concepts and memorize their definitions (Applegate, 2006).

Elements - The basic components of all matter; the simplest form of matter

Structure of Atoms - The smallest particle of an element that still retains the properties of that element. The atom is made up of still smaller subunits - protons, neutrons and electrons. The dense region of the nucleus holds the protons and neutrons. The electrons are outside the nucleus.

Protons - Have a positive charge and have a mass of one atomic unit. The number of protons in a nucleus is called the atomic number. This is the number on a periodic table for each element.

Neutrons - Have the same mass as protons but no charge. Together, protons and neutrons account for the mass of the atom and this number is called the mass number.

Electrons - Small, negatively charged particles. Their number and arrangement determine how an atom reacts. Electrons are located in the space surrounding the nucleus. The number of negatively charged electrons in an atom is always equal to the number of positively charged protons so that the atom is electrically neutral.

Chemical Bonds - An atom's chemical behavior is determined largely by the electrons in the outermost energy shell. Atoms have a tendency to transfer or share electrons to achieve a stable configuration in this shell. When electrons from the outer most energy level are transferred or shared, attractive forces called chemical bonds develop that hold the atoms together to form a molecule.

Molecule - When two or more atoms chemically bond together, a molecule is formed.

Compound - Formed when two or more different types of atoms chemically combine in a definite, or fixed, ratio to form a new substance that is different from any of the original atoms, ie, water.

MIXTURES, SOLUTIONS AND SUSPENSIONS

A mixture is a combination of two or more substances in varying proportions that can be separated by ordinary physical means. The substances retain their original properties after they have been combined in a mixture. The components of a mixture may be elements, compounds or elements and compounds.

Solutions are mixtures in which the component particles remain evenly distributed. All solutions consist of two parts - the solute and the solvent. The solute is the substance that is present in the smaller amount and that is being dissolved. It can be a gas, liquid, or solid. The solvent usually a gas or liquid is the component that is present in the larger amount and that does the dissolving. The universal solvent is water but alcohol and carbon tetrachloride are commonly used. When alcohol is used as the solvent, the solution is called a tincture.

A suspension is a mixture where settling occurs like sand mixed in water. The fluid in the body that fills the cells is the cytoplasm, a colloidal suspension. (Applegate, 2006)

Review the following concepts and memorize their definitions (Helmenstine, 2018):

Colloids are a type of homogeneous mixture where the dispersed particles do not settle out, such as butter or paint.

Simple chemical reactions are chemical reactions happen every day in our lives. A few common examples include:

- Photosynthesis - converts carbon dioxide and water into glucose and oxygen.
- Breathing - energy molecules are combined with the oxygen we breath to release energy needed by the cells. This energy is in the form ATP.
- Combustion - energetic molecules with oxygen produce carbon dioxide and water.
- Digestion - thousands of chemical reactions take place during digestion, all with specific jobs.
- Soap and Detergents - emulsifiers allow oily stains to bind with soap.
- Cooking - uses heat to cause chemical changes.

Concentration refers to the amount of a substance per defined space. It is the ratio of the solute to the solvent or the total solution. Two related terms are concentrated and dilute. Concentrated solutions have high concentrations of the solute. Dilute solutions contain a small amount of solvent compared with the amount of the solvent.

Extractions are separations of substances when they are mixed with others. Making tea is a simple example. Tea leaves are heated in water and the components come out of the tea and into the water.

Solubility is the maximum quantity of a substance that may be dissolved in another. It is the maximum amount of solute that may be dissolved in a solvent at equilibrium which produces a saturated solution.

Osmosis is the process where solvent molecules move through a semipermeable membrane from a dilute solution into a more concentrated solution. Osmosis acts to equalize concentration on both sides of a membrane.

Chapter 15: Review

ADDITIONAL READING

Utilize these references to expand your understanding of the concepts in this chapter.

REQUIRED READING	Chapters
Basic Chemistry Concepts Part I, https://www.youtube.com/watch?v=MYuh5yErdfA	
Atomic Bonds - Chemistry Basics Part II, https://www.youtube.com/watch?v=Juw7HBg0zZs	
Making Sense of Chemical Structures, https://www.youtube.com/watch?v=FbaXQ8u6IP8	

References

"Chemistry." Merriam-Webster, 2018, https://www.merriam-webster.com/dictionary/chemistry

Applegate, Edith J. (2006) The Anatomy and Physiology Learning System, 3e 3rd Edition. St. Louis, Missouri: Saunders.

Helmenstine, Anne Marie. (2018, May 8). "A to Z Chemistry Dictionary." ThoughtCo. https://www.thoughtco.com/a-to-z-chemistry-dictionary-4143188

QUESTIONS & ANSWERS

Record your questions for this chapter here for further research and discussion.

Question:

Answer:

Question:

Answer:

Question:

Answer:

SELF-ASSESSMENT

1. What's the definition of Chemistry?
   a. The composition and physical properties of a substance.
   b. A science that deals with the composition, structure, and properties of substances including the transformations that they undergo.
   c. The science of the elements and elemental structures.
   d. A and C
   e. None of the above

2. What are the basic components of all matter?
   a. chemical bonds
   b. electrons
   c. elements
   d. Atoms
   e. None of the above

3. The atom is made up of still smaller subunits of _______.
   a. protons, neutrons and electrons
   b. just protons
   c. neurons
   d. All of the above
   e. None of the above

4. What is the definition of an electron?
   a. The outermost energy level in a chemical bond.
   b. The simplest form of matter.
   c. It is a small, negative charged particle.
   d. All of the above
   e. None of the above

5. What is the definition of a molecule?
   a. The bond of two or more atoms chemically.
   b. A type of homogeneous mixture where the dispersed particles do not settle out.
   c. It is positively charged protons.
   d. B and C
   e. A and B

6. A mixture is a combination of two or more_____, in varying proportions that can be separated by ordinary physical means.
   a. protons
   b. liquids
   c. substances
   d. powders
   e. Molecules

7. ______ are a type of homogeneous mixture where the dispersed particles do not settle out, such as butter or paint.
   a. Fats
   b. Colloids
   c. Gasses
   d. Solvents
   e. All of the above

8. Which is an example of a chemical reaction?
   a. cooking
   b. digestion
   c. breathing
   d. All of the above
   e. None of the above

9. _________ is the ratio of the solute to the solvent or the total solution.
   a. A concentration
   b. Osmosis
   c. A solute
   d. Permeability
   e. None of the above

10. The process where solvent molecules move through a semipermeable membrane from a dilute solution into a more concentrated solution.
    a. Solubility
    b. Breathing
    c. Osmosis
    d. Concentrations
    e. Permeability

Chapter 16 : Biology

Biology is:

1. a branch of knowledge that deals with living organisms and vital processes.
2. the plant and animal life of a region or environment.
    a. the biology of the rain forest.
    b. the life processes especially of an organism or group.
    c. the biology of cancer cells.

AREAS OF STUDY

Life science is a branch of science (such as biology, medicine, and sometimes anthropology or sociology) that deals with living organisms and life processes. Life Sciences is a broad system with Biology as a type of life science.

Taxonomy is the branch of science concerned with classification, especially of organisms.

Developmental biology is the study of the process by which organisms grow and develop. Modern developmental biology studies the genetic control of cell growth, differentiation and "morphogenesis," which is the process that gives rise to tissues, organs and anatomy.

Embryology is a subfield, the study of organisms between the one-cell stage (generally, the zygote) and the end of the embryonic stage. Embryology and developmental biology today deal with the various steps necessary for the correct and complete formation of the body of a living organism.

Cellular biology is the study of cells. As a diagnostic discipline, cellular biology is better designated as cytology, a subspecialty of anatomic pathology. And, as a broadly defined field of natural science, the preferred term is cell biology, which often overlaps with molecular biology.

Molecular biology is the branch of biology that deals with the structure, function, and manipulation of nucleic acids and proteins.

Biochemistry is the branch of science concerned with the chemical and physical-chemical processes and substances that occur within living organisms.

Pathology is the science of the causes and effects of diseases, especially the branch of medicine that deals with the laboratory examination of samples of body tissue for diagnostic or forensic purposes.

Systems biology is an emerging approach applied to biomedical and biological scientific research. Systems biology is a biology-based inter-disciplinary field of study that focuses on complex interactions within biological systems, using a more holistic perspective approach to biological and biomedical research.

Chapter 16: Review

ADDITIONAL READING

Utilize these references to expand your understanding of the concepts in this chapter.

REQUIRED READING	Chapters
The Biology Corner, https://www.biologycorner.com/	

References

QUESTIONS & ANSWERS

Record your questions for this chapter here for further research and discussion.

Question:

Answer:

Question:

Answer:

Question:

Answer:

SELF-ASSESSMENT

1. Which of the following describes a cell?
   a. It is the basic unit of all life.
   b. A structure that shows certain characteristics of life such as organization, metabolism and homeostasis.
   c. A cell structure that contains a plasma membrane.
   d. All of the above
   e. None of the above
2. What's the definition of Biology?
   a. A branch of knowledge that deals with living organisms and vital processes.
   b. The science related to diagnosis and treatment of pathology.
   c. The study of rod shaped bodies near the nucleus of a cell.
   d. All of the above
   e. None of the above
3. What best describes the nucleus of the cell?
   a. It contains the chromosomes of the cell.
   b. It picks up and transmits electrical impulses.
   c. A large membrane-bound, dark staining organelle near the center of a cell.
   d. A and C
   e. All of the above
4. Which of the following are parts of a cell?
   a. Microvilli
   b. Cytosol
   c. Ribosomes
   d. All of the above
   e. None of the above
5. What's the definition of "metabolism"?
   a. One of the two stages of glucose catabolism.
   b. The breakdown of carbohydrates in normal digestion.
   c. All of the physical and chemical processes by which an organism is maintained.
   d. All of the above
   e. None of the above
6. What is the definition of tissues?
   a. They are layers of membranes.
   b. A group of similar cells that perform a specialized function.
   c. Small membrane-bound sacs in the cytoplasm
   d. All of the above
   e. None of the above
7. Molecular biology is the branch of biology that deals with the structure, function, and manipulation of ______ and proteins.
   a. protons
   b. nucleic acids
   c. vesicles
   d. All of the above
   e. None of the above
8. Biochemistry is the branch of science concerned with the chemical and physiochemical processes and substances that occur within _______.
   a. animals
   b. cell membranes
   c. non-living organisms
   d. living organisms
   e. All of the above
9. _____ is a type of life science.
   a. Botany
   b. Zoology
   c. Biology
   d. All of the above
   e. None of the above
10. Pathology is the science of the causes and effects of diseases, especially the branch of medicine that deals with the laboratory examination of body tissue samples for diagnostic or ______ purposes.
    a. psychological
    b. chemical
    c. academic
    d. All the above
    e. None of the above

Unit Review

ORAL EXAM QUESTIONS

Use these questions to prepare answers for the oral examination. You may create written statements or cue cards to memorize the key points that should be included in your response. Scoring is based on your accuracy, brevity, clarity (ABC), use of Sanskrit terms and concepts, and confidence.

1. Propose a method to bridge communication among professionals from various modalities to open dialog for improving health care outcomes.
2. Explain three reasons why it might be challenging for modern or Western people today to accept Āyurveda as "good science."
3. Describe the scientific method and Occam's razor through an example of a simple experiment.
4. Complete as many questions from "Basic concepts of logic" as possible.
5. Using the diagram from chapter 28, "The Scientific Method as an Ongoing Process," identify where each of the pramāṇa can be applied with examples.
6. Demonstrate one or more examples showing how each of the pramāṇa can be employed in typical situations today. How reliable is each type of pramāṇa in providing accurate, truthful knowledge with high confidence?
7. Explain the accuracy and confidence that can be generally expected from each pramāṇa when applied in the scientific method to test a hypothesis.
8. Explain a concept described by astronomy that is relevant to understanding Āyurveda.
9. How does declination influence the seasons?
10. Explain a concept or perspective that you learned in this chapter that can be applied to better understand Āyurveda.
11. Research moon phases and explain them through any model.
12. How might climate and weather impact an individual's health differently?
13. Describe at least three examples of everyday application or expression of any of the Laws explained in this unit.
14. Take any three concepts from this unit and explain how they are applied in regular, daily life.

UNIT III

A brief history of Traditional Āyurvedic Medicine (TAM) and Literature

Chapter 17 : Origins

KEY TERMS

anādi smṛti śhruti

PERSPECTIVES ON TRADITIONAL MEDICINE TODAY

The true historical origins of Āyurveda may never be fully known. The science is estimated to be at least several thousand years old based on surviving historical records. Proving a definitive start date should be considered nearly impossible since it is fairly certain that the oldest original records do not exist today.

The delicate, paper palm leaves on which the knowledge was originally transcribed have life spans of a few hundred years in the most optimal conditions. Additionally, the effort required to continuously maintain information is intense and requires a stable society capable of prioritizing and maintaining these types of activities.

Throughout its older periods of history, Āyurveda was said to be passed down through two main methods – *smṛti* and *śhruti*. According to its own account, Āyurveda claims to have been recalled or remembered through the process of *smṛti* because the nature of the knowledge is timeless, universal and has always been inherent in nature.

This knowledge was then passed down through *śhruti*, or the oral tradition. The body of knowledge would have to be recited and memorized completely before one could be considered competent in the subject.

More recently, in the last 2,000-3,000 years, Āyurveda has also been recorded in written manuscript form. The oldest surviving classical works, the Charaka Saṁhitā and Suśhruta Saṁhitā, provide records of a large part of the science.

Precise dates of origin for these manuscripts cannot be reliably determined. It is likely that many additional texts were also recorded around the same time periods but only a small portion of these are available in their complete forms today. The majority of works were either lost partially or completely, or destroyed over time.

Within some of the oldest existing texts of Āyurveda references state that the science is *anādi*, meaning it has "no beginning (and no end)." Charaka mentions this explicitly in Charaka Saṁhitā, *sūtrasthāna* 30/27. This indicates that the knowledge has always existed because they are fundamental laws that are inherent in the natural world. One of the most intriguing questions that strikes many during the study of this science is how did ancient people discover these principles and test them?

Āyurvedic origins and history are quite complicated, like any long-standing practice or culture is. Over the last two millennia, India has been a hotspot for political upheavals, major religious shifts, and social unrest. Through it all, the people of this geographical area have managed to adapt to new cultures, new rulers, and new ways of living while recognizing health as a priority at the levels of individual, family, community and society. The evolution of Āyurveda throughout history often echoes these events and reflects in the science as research, development and progression based on influential powers over time.

TEST YOURSELF

Learn, review and memorize key terms from this section.

anādi

smṛti

śhruti

Chapter 17: Review

ADDITIONAL READING

Utilize these references to expand your understanding of the concepts in this chapter.

CLASSICS	1st read	2nd read
Charaka Cha. Sū. 30/		

REQUIRED READING	Chapters
Origin and Development of Ayurveda (A Brief History), https://www.ncbi.nlm.nih.gov/pmc/articles/PMC3336651/	
A Myth of Aryan Invasions of India, Goel, ML	
History of Ayurveda, NV Krisnankutty: Introduction	

OPTIONAL READING	Format

References

Śarmā, R. K., & Dāsa, B. Agniveśa's Charaka Saṃhitā. Varanasi: Chowkhamba Sanskrit Series Office; Reprint Edition. 2016. Cha. Sū. 30/.

QUESTIONS & ANSWERS

Record your questions for this chapter here for further research and discussion.

Question:

Answer:

Question:

Answer:

Question:

Answer:

SELF-ASSESSMENT

1. In Charaka's historical account of Āyurveda, *anādi* refers to
   a. Āyurveda's start date
   b. no beginning or end of Āyurveda
   c. theoretical principles of Āyurveda
   d. All of the above
   e. None of the above

2. The oral traditional of Āyurvedic training is known as
   a. Charaka Saṁhitā
   b. *smṛti*
   c. *śhruti*
   d. *Suśhruta sampradāya*
   e. All of the above

3. Based on surviving historical records, Āyurveda is estimated to be at least
   a. 500 years old
   b. 3,000 years old
   c. 5,000 years old
   d. 10,000 years old
   e. None of the above

4. Traditionally, Āyurveda was recorded on
   a. birch paper
   b. palm leaves
   c. papyrus
   d. stone
   e. None of the above

5. The original manuscripts of Āyurveda include
   a. Charaka Saṁhitā
   b. *smṛti*
   c. *śhruti*
   d. *Suśhruta sampradāya*
   e. *sūtrasthāna*

6. Āyurveda's history has largely been influenced by
   a. long periods of peace
   b. major religious shifts
   c. political upheaval
   d. Both A and B
   e. Both B and C

7. Which commonly accepted, Western scientific law could today be considered as *smṛti*?
   a. heat transfer (first law of thermodynamics)
   b. Newton's law of gravity
   c. osmosis
   d. All of the above
   e. None of the above

8. Considering that written paper records generally do not survive well over several millennia, it is likely that Āyurveda is
   a. a good candidate for carbon dating
   b. eternal
   c. older than currently recognized
   d. younger than currently recognized
   e. None of the above

9. Throughout the history of Āyurveda, the science has demonstrated its
   a. adaptability
   b. ancient foundations
   c. bias for commodification
   d. irrefutable dogma
   e. orthodox, rigid nature

10. Āyurveda has always been prioritized for use among
    a. communities
    b. families
    c. individuals
    d. societies
    e. All of the above

Chapter 18 : Historical review

KEY TERMS

ahiṁsā
anādi
Aṣhṭa Vaidya
Aṣhṭāṅga Hṛdaya
Aṣhṭāṅga Saṅgraha
Atharva Veda
Bhaiṣhajya Ratnāvali
Bhāva Prakāśha
Bhela Saṁhitā
Bṛhat Trayī
Cakrapāṇi
Charaka
Charaka Saṁhitā
Charaka sampradāya
Dṛḍhabala
Hārīta Saṁhitā
hiṁsa
Kāśhyapa Saṁhitā
Laghu Trayī
Laghu Vāgbhaṭa
Mādhava Nidāna
nāḍī parīkṣha
Nāgārjuna
Nighaṇṭu
Punarvasu Ātreya
rasa
Rasa Śhāstra
Ṛg Veda
ṛṣhi
Sāma Veda
saṁhitā
sampradāya
Śhāraṅgadhāra Saṁhitā
siddhānta
smṛti
śhruti
Suśhruta
Suśhruta Saṁhitā
Suśhruta sampradāya
Vāgbhaṭa
Veda
Vṛddha Vāgbhaṭa
Yajur Veda
Yogaratnākara

"History will be kind to me for I intend to write it."

- Winston S. Churchill

Historical accounts are perspectives of past events. They can range from factually incomplete to ornately embellished, and they can lack an objective point of view. Belief systems that are influenced through recollection of historical information tend to have a strong influence on mainstream perspectives. These accounts can influence the generations that follow and their cultural, social and political trends for centuries.

Āyurvedic history is no different. Āyurveda is a comprehensive system of medicine that evolved in agitated environments and was regularly influenced by political, social and religious pressures. These pressures helped shape what currently remains of the present-day understanding and practice of this scientific medical system. They have also strongly influenced the system's current legal standing and public perception in its homeland of India.

This historical review of Āyurveda will focus on objective, factual events to the greatest extent possible and it will include popular theories to cover a wide range of perspectives. These events are most important wherever they influenced the classical Āyurvedic texts. The texts which remain today continue to serve as the basis for Āyurvedic medical education both in and outside India.

A HISTORY OF CONTROVERSY

The one commonality that can be found across all historical accounts is that human activity in and around the Indian subcontinent has been very active for a long time. Over millennia, there has been a constant influx of foreign invasions with changes in leadership and all the associated cultural, societal and religious adjustments that accompanied the ruling parties.

India as it is known today was historically not a single, unified country or kingdom. Internal disputes were constant along with continuous struggles for control within the subcontinent.

Assigning specific dates or even broad time ranges to many events is perhaps the most controversial part of documenting history in the Indian subcontinent. There are major differences proposed depending on the source of the historical account. Comparing Indian and European versions can often result in time period differences of 1,000 years or more. Because of this, associating specific dates to events is best reserved for historians. Here, approximate time ranges will be provided instead. The sequence of historical events that is particularly relevant to classical Āyurvedic literature will be reviewed in detail.

ORIGINS

There are three main sources that provide insight into the origins of Vedic culture, Sanskrit and Āyurveda:

1. Common historical theories
2. Evidence from Āyurvedic literature
3. Mythological accounts

The common driving force of Āyurveda has always been the preservation and promotion of human health. The two main theories that have dominated the Āyurvedic history books for decades are the Indo-Aryan and the Indian subcontinent origin theories.

Indo-Aryan origin

The Indo-Aryan origin theory postulates that Sanskrit originated in the areas currently known as Syria, Turkey and Iraq. They propose that Sanskrit is a Proto-Indo-European language. As the people of these regions migrated eastward somewhere between 2000 to 1000 BCE, the language evolved into Vedic Sanskrit which was used to record the Vedas.

As these people migrated further south, they entered the Indian subcontinent. During this period of migration and development, Vedic Sanskrit progressed into the Sanskrit known today.

This theory is often promoted by scholars who maintain a European-centric view of world history. Extensive analysis of language developments in the ancient and modern worlds have been performed to support this theory. And in 2018, a large study was published using genomic evidence to explain migration patterns in South and Central Asia.

Indian Subcontinent origin

The Indian Subcontinent origin theory proposes that Sanskrit was born in the Indian subcontinent. Supporters of this perspective contend that absence of written Sanskrit prior to the Vedas indicates that the language arose from the people of the Indian subcontinent.

This perspective is commonly supported by Indian historians who claim the language, culture and origins to have originated in the Indian subcontinent. With the rise of the Modi government in 2016, there has been a resurgence of Hindu nationalism in India which aligns with these beliefs. Scholars of the opposing Indo-Aryan origin theory believe that the Indian historians deny linguistic evidence that demonstrates otherwise.

There is strong genetic evidence now to support migration of peoples from the Near East to South and Central Asia. These migration patterns could provide stronger support for the Indo-Aryan origin theory.

Previously, genetic evidence had been used to support the Indian Subcontinent origin theory through matrilineal DNA testing. This demonstrated little change in the gene pool for 12,000 years.

However, the male-specific Y-DNA shows signs that 17% of Indian male DNA contains haplogroup R1a. This has been found across Central Asia, Europe and South Asia. This new discovery is likely because of the "sex bias in Bronze Age migrations."

It is possible that both of these theories will

continue to discover and demonstrate evidence to support each of their viewpoints. Like most historical accounts, a final, truthful determination may never be known.

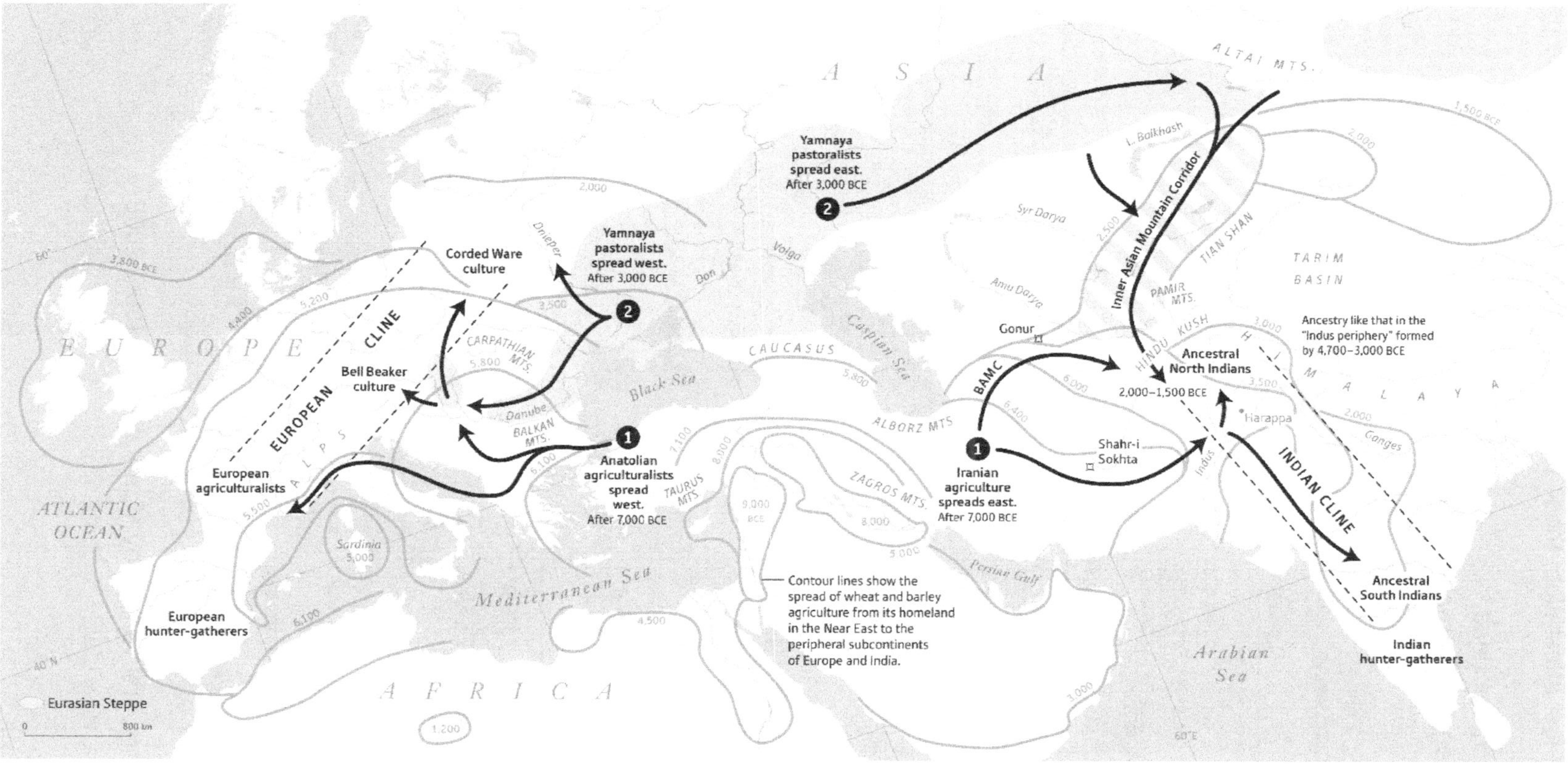

The prehistory of South Asia and Europe are parallel in both being impacted by two successive spreads, the first from the Near East after 7000 BCE bringing agriculturalists who mixed with local hunter-gatherers, and the second from the Steppe after 3000 BCE bringing people who spoke Indo-European languages and who mixed with those they encountered during their migratory movement. Mixtures of these mixed populations then produced the rough clines of ancestry present in both South Asia and in Europe today (albeit 63 with more variable proportions of local hunter-gatherer-related ancestry in Europe than in India), which are (imperfectly) correlated to geography. The plot shows in contour lines the time of the expansion of Near Eastern agriculture. Human movements and mixtures, which also plausibly contributed to the spread of languages, are shown with arrows.

The Genomic Formation of South and Central Asia, https://www.biorxiv.org/content/biorxiv/early/2018/03/31/292581.full.pdf

Partial tree of Indo-European languages

- Branches are in order of first attestation; those to the left are Centum, those to the right are Satem.
- Languages in red are extinct or dead.
- White labels indicate categories / un-attested proto-languages.

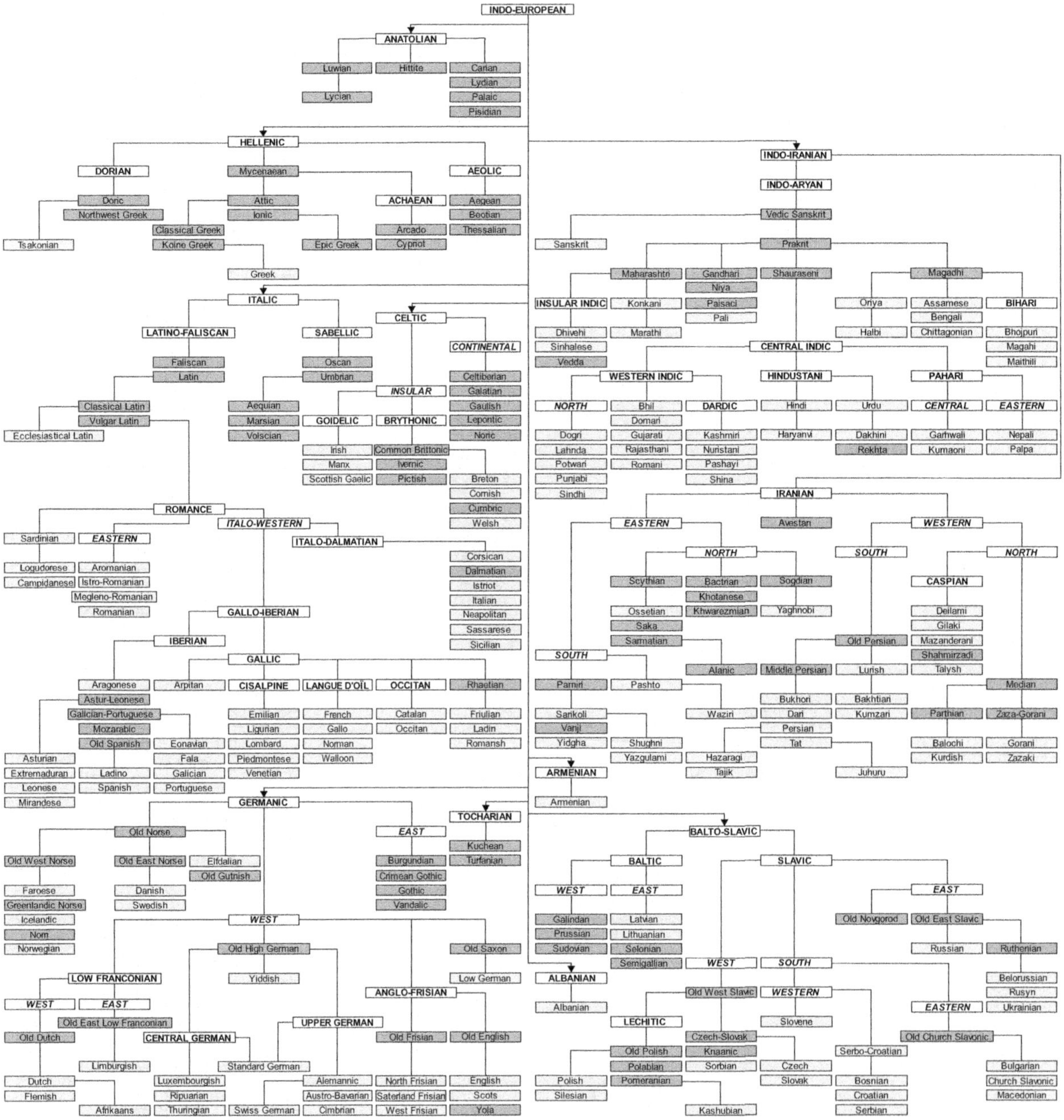

Multiple authors, first version by Mandrak, 18 October 2008

https://commons.wikimedia.org/wiki/File:IndoEuropeanTree.svg

Evidence from Āyurvedic literature

For the purposes of Āyurvedic professional education, knowledge of the historical evidence found directly in the classical texts takes priority. Generally, all authors attribute their work to a lineage, teacher, predecessor or currently accepted, standing body of knowledge.

Based on these references and by understanding the progression of the science over time through recorded research and developments found in various texts, an approximate timeline can be constructed. Although this timeline may not include exact dates, it shines an important light on the order in which the classics were written and popularized. Understanding this allows one to gain a better grasp of the progression of the science, its knowledge and applied aspects.

The knowledge of Āyurveda is considered in two ways from a historical perspective, according to references from Charaka. First, Āyurveda is a set of universal truths and natural laws, which Charaka calls *anādi* in *sūtrasthāna* 30/27.

The Monier-Williams dictionary defines *anādi* as "having no beginning, existing from eternity" and Charaka elaborates this by directly stating that the knowledge of Āyurveda has existed in nature since nature itself has existed.

Second, Āyurveda is an active body of applied knowledge and practice which has been passed down through various schools and teachers. To recognize the source of knowledge, each text includes respectful references to their appropriate teacher(s) or lineage usually at the very beginning of the work.

The classics also refer to groups of learned scholars, or *ṛṣhis*, who traditionally helped maintain the knowledge of Āyurveda. In Charaka *sūtrasthāna* 1/7-14, the author mentions many of these *ṛṣhis* by name and describes their characteristics and purpose. They directly witnessed the suffering of mankind and were aware that as long as man existed, so would his diseases. Since this would be an obstacle to pursuing life goals and being able to achieve them, these *ṛṣhis* wanted to find a way to allay suffering for the benefit of all creatures. This is the original goal of Āyurveda.

Later in the text, at the beginning of Charaka *cikitsāsthāna* 1/ (*pāda* 4), an important account is provided which describes how the *ṛṣhis* needed the knowledge of Āyurveda to maintain their own health to fulfill their goals. These types of accounts provide unique insight into nature of the science, its scholars and practical applications from the earliest times.

Mythological accounts

Throughout the classics, the origins of Āyurveda are linked to mythology at their initial incarnations. Authors typically attribute *smṛti*, the first "knowing" of the science to a higher source which serves as the original transmission of knowledge to allow the information to be passed down through a specific lineage into the form currently expounded in the text.

The recognition of a source of knowledge which is separate from the human realm is considered an important form of respect and modesty in many traditional cultures and belief systems. It is noticeably present in Vedic and present-day Hindu customs. Mythology can be viewed as one means to represent concepts experienced in human life in a personified way which makes them relatable and meaningful.

Each of the classics credits their knowledge to a specific mythological source and describes its progression through notable individuals who helped shape its present form. Names and statements about these individuals can be found in the texts in chapter contents typically at the heading and colophon (end line). Here, the two major schools of thought are reviewed, including the direct lineages through the *Charaka sampradāya* and *Suśhruta sampradāya*. A summary of the consolidations found in the *Aṣhṭāṅga Hṛdāya* and *Bhāva Prakāśha* is also provided to show the literary progression over time.

The Charaka Saṁhitā begins by recounting the origin of Āyurveda according to the *Charaka sampradāya* in *sūtrasthāna* 1/1-14. Following the traditional form of reverence and respect, the text immediately starts off by crediting the source of knowledge to the individual Bharadvāja, who obtained the knowledge directly from Indra, a mythological personification of the lord of the gods.

In this *sampradāya*, the transmission of Āyurveda originally descended through several key mythological figures. It came from Brahmā, the personification of creation, through Dakṣha, then to the twins, the Aśhvini Kumāras, and finally to Indra. Bharadvāja volunteered to represent the group of *ṛṣhis* who sought the complete knowledge and understanding of Āyurveda to help alleviate suffering of all creatures and aid mankind in achieving their *puruṣhārthas*. With the focus of the Charaka sampradāya being *Kāya cikitsā*, the knowledge received is tailored to achieving the goal of health through the specialized practice of internal medicine.

After obtaining the full knowledge of the science and applying it to himself for realizing his own state of maximum health, Bharadvāja then shared this knowledge with the group of *ṛṣhis* who he volunteered to represent. From this large group, Punarvasu Ātreya then began to teach the science to his six disciples, Agniveśha, Bhela, Jatūkarṇa, Parāśhara, Hārita, Kṣhārapāṇi. Each of the six recorded what they learned in their own work.

Out of the six, Agniveśha's treatise was notably superior and was compiled as the Agniveśha Tantra. Over time, however, the work was not maintained and parts of it were lost. Charaka salvaged what remained of the text and completed the missing portions so that *sūtrasthāna* through the 13th chapter of cikitsāsthāna became available.

Dṛḍhabala then supplemented the remaining chapters of the text, from *cikitsāsthāna* chapter 14 through the end of *siddhisthāna*. This rendered the text complete once again at 120 chapters. However, even to this day, the actual number of lines found in the text is still less than the total number quoted by about 2,000 verses.

Charaka sampradāya

Brahmā

↓

Dakṣha (Prajāpati)

↓

Aśhvini Kumāras

↓

Indra

↓

Bharadvāja

↓

Ṛṣhis including Punarvasu Ātreya

↓

6 disciples:

Agniveśha, Bhela, Jatūkarṇa, Parāśhara, Hārita, Kṣhārapāṇi

↓

Agniveśha Tantra by Agniveśha

↓

Redacted by Charaka as the Charaka Saṁhitā

↓

Charaka Saṁhitā supplemented by Dṛḍhabala

The Suśhruta Saṁhitā begins by recounting the origin of Āyurveda according to the *Suśhruta sampradāya* in *sūtrasthāna* 1/1-22. Following the traditional form of reverence and respect, the text immediately starts off by crediting the source of knowledge to the present incarnation of the god Bhagavān Divodāsa Dhanvantari, as the king of Kāśhī.

In this *sampradāya*, the transmission of Āyurveda originally descended through several key mythological figures. It came from Brahmā, the personification of creation, through Prajāpati, then to the twins, the Aśhvini Kumāras, and finally to Indra. It was then passed on to the god Divodāsa Dhanvantari, who incarnated as the king of Kāśhī, also name Dhanvantari.

One day Dhanvantari was approached by a group of disciples, including Aupadhenava, Vaitaraṇa, Aurabhra, Pauṣhkalāvata, Karavīrya, Gopurarakṣhita, and Suśhruta. Out of concern for the suffering of mankind and all creatures, the students asked Dhanvantari to teach Āyurveda. After introducing the subject and its specialties, Dhanvantari asked the students which area they would like to concentrate in and they chose *Śhalya-tantra*, surgery, because of its ability to provide quick and effective results, and for its utility across all branches of Āyurveda.

Out of all the students, Suśhruta's recordings of the teacher's instructions were compiled and deemed to be the best. His work was completed as the Suśhruta Saṁhitā, consisting of 120 chapters in 5 *sthānas*. Over time this original work was not maintained and parts of it were lost. It is likely that another individual, also named Suśhruta, recompiled the text, which was then redacted into its current form by Nāgārjuna. Additionally, it was supplemented by other authors to include the final, sixth section called *uttara-tantra*. This rendered the text complete according to the standards of the full science of Āyurveda so that it contained instructions for managing diseases in all branches, in addition to surgery.

Suśhruta sampradāya

Brahmā

↓

Prajāpati

↓

Aśhvini Kumāras

↓

Indra

↓

Divodāsa Dhanvantari

↓

6 disciples:

Aupadhenava, Vaitaraṇa, Aurabhra, Pauṣhkalāvata, Karavīrya, Gopurarakṣhita, Suśhruta, etc.

↓

Suśhruta Saṁhitā

↓

Redacted by Nāgārjuna

↓

Appended to include Uttara-tantra

In Aṣhṭāṅga Hṛdaya, a very concise narration of the mythological origins of Āyurveda is provided exactly from the *Charaka sampradāya*. This reference appears within the first few lines of the entire text, again indicating the importance of crediting the source of knowledge from the beginning of the work. The author, Vāgbhaṭa, immediately follows this narration with the key statement that this text is the streamlined version of knowledge compiled from the larger, more elaborate recorded sources.

Bhāva Prakāśha contains perhaps the most elaborate explanation of the mythological origins of Āyurveda. The author dedicates the entire first chapter of the text to describing the key figures throughout Āyurvedic history and their stories and contributions. The information provided here appears to match very closely to the same accounts of the *Charaka sampradāya* and *Suśhruta sampradāya*, however there are a few important name changes. Ultimately, these minor variations are not critical to Āyurvedic history and can be attributed to common differences found in cultural history.

VEDIC PERIOD

Approximate time range

2,000 (or earlier) to 500 BCE

The Vedic Period of history covers the wide range of time where the oldest texts of were recorded in written format. Prior to their codification, they had been passed down via oral tradition, known as *śhruti*, or *śhrauta* (oral, or that which is spoken and heard).

The four Vedic texts were composed in one of the oldest known forms of writing, Vedic Sanskrit, which differs significantly from the form seen and used today.

According to Charaka and Suśhruta, these four texts include:

1. Ṛg, or Ṛk Veda
2. Yajus or Yajur Veda
3. Sāma Veda
4. Atharva Veda

The contents of the Vedas is wide and large, and beyond the scope of required study for professional Āyurvedic practice. Charaka himself mentions in *sūtrasthāna* 30/20-21 that the Veda which Āyurvedic scholars should consider as primary is the Atharva Veda because it serves are the basis for treatment of diseases, although mostly in a religious manner.

During the Vedic period, Āyurvedic literature as it is known today was in its infancy. The precursors to the currently accepted treatises were being laid down in more of a cultural and religious fashion. It is likely that the religious-based practices of this time period served to promote the movement towards theoretical and scientific styles of practice developed in later centuries.

This can be demonstrated by the references available within the Vedas which provided the foundations for some of the Āyurvedic *siddhānta* (core principles) later found in Charaka and Suśhruta. For example, the Vedas propound the theory of *Ojas-Tejas-Prāṇa* which graduated into the full-fledged *Tridoṣha siddhānta* in classical Āyurvedic literature. Although the word Āyurveda is not actually found in the Vedas, references to developing concepts like *Tridhātu* are seen.

SAṀHITĀ PERIOD

Approximate time range

500 BCE - 700 CE

The Saṁhitā period can arguably be considered the "Golden Age" of classical Āyurvedic literature. The progress made during this period has stood the test of time and the two original classics continue to stand as the most authoritative works today. These are the Charaka Saṁhitā and Suśhruta Saṁhitā, and they serve as primary clinical references in hospitals throughout India. Their knowledge, including the *siddhānta* and applied aspects, is regularly applied in practice.

During the Saṁhitā period, many works were recorded yet very few survived. Out of these, the most significant are grouped into the *Bṛhat Trayī*, or the "Great Three." The name can be slightly misleading because it refers to the three great authors, rather than texts. Four works are actually included in this classification.

1. Charaka Saṁhitā
2. Suśhruta Saṁhitā
3. Aṣhṭāṅga Saṅgraha
4. Aṣhṭāṅga Hṛdaya

Because the last two are attributed to an author of the same name, Vāgbhaṭa, they are both considered under this classification in the Saṁhitā period.

A few additional works from the same time period have survived but are usually reserved for more advanced professional studies. These include:

1. Kāśhyapa Saṁhitā
2. Bhela Saṁhitā
3. Hārīta Saṁhitā

These works were written by contemporaries of Agniveśha under the guidance of Punarvasu Ātreya. The Bhela and Hārīta Saṁhitās echo much of what is found in today's Charaka Saṁhitā. English translations for these works are difficult to obtain and the advanced level of knowledge is only valuable after thoroughly completing basic studies. The Kāśhyapa Saṁhitā is a unique literary composition because it focuses on obstetrics and pediatrics. Unfortunately it is missing quite a few chapters and verses and is presently incomplete.

The Charaka Saṁhitā and Suśhruta Saṁhitā lead the way by establishing the primary schools and specializations within the science. Aṣhṭāṅga Saṅgraha and Aṣhṭāṅga Hṛdaya followed by attempting to consolidate and streamline the knowledge of both major schools into single works. Both of these texts are attributed to the author Vāgbhaṭa, although it is still unclear as to whether this is one or more individuals, and which of the two works was created first. In some references, we find the author's name mentioned as Vṛddha Vāgbhaṭa or Laghu Vāgbhaṭa, meaning the senior (or major), and the younger (or minor) Vāgbhaṭa.

In Aṣhṭāṅga Saṅgraha, the author states at the beginning of the text that the information included here has been collected from the vast ocean of existing Āyurvedic knowledge. The author is drawing knowledge from Charaka and Suśhruta, and likely from other texts and sources which are not available today. In Aṣhṭāṅga Hṛdaya, the author clearly states the purpose of the work from the beginning as well. Here the goal is to record the science in a way which is neither too succinct nor too elaborate, again drawing on all of the well-known and accepted works of the time.

The consolidation and streamlining of information in these two works is an invaluable addition to the classical literature. It is especially helpful for advanced students and practitioners as a review of the entire body of knowledge. The Aṣhṭāṅga Hṛdaya is especially useful in a way similar to "Cliff's Notes" and today is popular in South Indian practice, particularly in Kerala. In certain institutions, an annual recitation of the text is held for students.

RASA ŚHĀSTRA PERIOD

Approximate time range

700 - 1500 CE

At the end of Saṁhitā period, the cultural and political landscape of the Indian subcontinent changed considerably. At the beginning of this period, the strong influence of the Brahman class and the Vedas temporarily waned in favor of Buddhism. During the latter part of this period, *Śhaṅkarācārya*, the popular proponent of the philosophy Advaita Vedanta, revived what has become a main practice in Hinduism today.

This greatly affected the practice of Āyurveda and the influences of both of these major religions and their philosophies can still be seen in the science today. During the Saṁhitā period, scholars and practitioners developed the science to utilize all natural resources, including a judicious use of animal products. Under Buddhism however, these activities were considered *hiṁsa*, or harmful to other life forms. There was a marked shift away from the use of animal products in favor of following the principles of *ahiṁsa*, or nonviolence.

This lead to one of the most innovative periods in Āyurvedic history and the development of a new branch of medicine production, called *Rasa Śhāstra*. This specialization focuses on using mineral and metallic ingredients to create broad-spectrum, long-lasting, and highly effective formulations. The ingredients undergo extensive purification processes for days, weeks, or months and are compounded using very specific methods to produce safe and highly efficacious formulations. The name *Rasa Śhāstra* is used for this specialized branch of Āyurveda because a majority of the formulations utilize one of the most powerful ingredients, *Rasa*. This ingredient goes by many synonymous names, including *Pārada*, and it has several mythological stories to personify its origins, benefits and dangers. Today, this ingredient is called Mercury and is considered highly toxic in its raw state, just as it was classically.

The Āyurvedic alchemical processes were able to transform toxic mercury into a highly efficacious and potent medicine after 30 days of continuous purification plus additional formulary processing. It is used in many Āyurvedic practices in India today with excellent results but must be sourced carefully from specific pharmacies.

The development of *Rasa Śhāstra* came to include over 100 metallic and mineral ingredients and today the purification and manufacturing instructions continue to be followed with effective results. During the *Rasa Śhāstra* period, a significant amount of literature was generated with specific instructions for these alchemical processes as they were discovered and standardized in this unique branch of the science. Very few of these texts are available today in English.

The most popular texts that arose from the Rasa Śhāstra period include the *Laghu Trayī*, or the "Lesser Three." Each of the texts in this group took an approach of specialization, as opposed to their predecessors in the Saṁhitā period. They include:

1. Mādhava Nidāna
2. Śhāraṅgadhāra Saṁhitā
3. Bhāva Prakāśha

Mādhava Nidāna is the first surviving text to focus only on the framework of diagnosis and its methodologies. It is a very practical resource and intended as a quick reference in clinical environments. Śhāraṅgadhāra Saṁhitā specializes in compiling the standard rules for compounding medicines, and includes other popular topics of the time period like *nāḍī parīkṣha*. Bhāva Prakāśha makes a very notable contribution to Āyurveda by organizing the *siddhānta* in a clean and thorough manner. He also includes a new type of resource, the *Nighaṇṭu* section, Āyurveda's first surviving herbal encyclopedia. Here, records of newly-available herbal resources and diseases are first seen in documentation, including the appearance of Syphilis, of European origin. This helps demonstrate the ability of Āyurveda to grow its practical knowledge base over time and implies a constant process of research and development, indicating a high level of continuous activity within the science. Bhāva Prakāśha is often considered the last innovative and influential text to appear in the course of Āyurvedic history in the 15th-16th centuries.

FOREIGN INVASION PERIOD

Approximate time range

1500CE - 1947CE

The research, developments and advancements in Āyurveda came to a grinding halt at the end of the Rasa Śhāstra period. Foreign invaders made their way into the Indian subcontinent starting with the Moghuls around the 16th century. They were soon followed by the British who held India under their rule until independence in 1947.

British invasion and control resulted in a massive drain of resources from the Indian subcontinent. Valuables including tons of gold, precious metals and stones were stolen, along with art, furniture, and other goods. Literature and knowledge were not spared either and a huge, unknown number of manuscripts were taken to be sold in shops in Britain, France and other countries (Rosu, 1993).

Some European scholars realized the value of Āyurveda and other bodies of Indian knowledge and during the 1800's there were attempts to translate manuscripts and better understand Sanskrit and other specialties. These attempts, however did not materialize very well and for the most part any significant information that was obtained was ignored, forgotten or worse, ridiculed. For an account of one attempt to better catalogue Indian manuscripts, read the journal article *Two French Pioneer Historians of Indian Medicine* by Arion Rosu.

The rich, localized practices that had developed throughout the Indian subcontinent among a wide range of families and lineages was forcefully interrupted by the British invasion. Records of specialized practices and localized knowledge were stolen and lost. Attempts were made by a few families and groups to hide whatever they could and some of these valuables still surface today. One example of a lineage-based practice of Āyurveda that was successful to some degree is the *Aṣhṭa Vaidya* group of families. Their history is long and complex, and worthy of its own focused study. Read *Religious Beliefs and Medical Practices A Sociological Study of Ashtavaidyas of Kerala*, chapter 5, by Leela PU, which documents the families' histories and practices through personal interviews.

During this time, two major literary works were completed, *Yogaratnākara* and *Bhaiṣhajya Ratnāvali*. These both have a heavy emphasis on *Kāya-cikitsā* rather than *Śhalya-tantra*, and include a summarized review of *siddhānta* followed by detailed instructions on diagnosis and treatment. The most popular medicines and therapeutic measures of the time are included, and in *Bhaiṣhajya Ratnāvali*, the list of formulations is exhaustive.

INDEPENDENCE

When India officially gained independence from the British on August 15th, 1947, the country was perceived to be unified for perhaps the first time in its history. Prior to the British, internal disputes were constant and regional kings and rulers were always attempting to gain control over their neighbors. Transitioning from this type of political and cultural environment to an imposed democracy with national unity was perhaps even more foreign than being under the control of a forceful ruling group.

Being left to now fend for themselves, the newly appointed Government of India proceeded to implement the skeleton system of democracy left behind by the British. Government and regulatory bodies were established to manage the country, but the system was rife with corruption from the very beginning.

Perspectives towards medicine had shifted greatly under British rule, and the idea that English or Western medicine was superior was now well-rooted in the minds of the country's most elite. All other traditional practices were not only outdated but were considered poor and barbaric, including Āyurveda. The newly-appointed government immediately set its sights and objectives on establishing regulation for English medicine as the primary health care system, with management for Āyurveda following a decade later, purposely structured in a format as close to the English system as possible.

Since the inception of bodies like the Central Council for Indian Medicine (CCIM), and Ayurveda, Yoga & Naturopathy, Unani, Siddha and Homeopathy (AYUSH) in the 1960's, not too much has changed in regulation for Āyurvedic professional education and practice. Much of the syllabus still reflects what was set in a 1970 Act for educational requirements. The Āyurvedic professional community of India has been actively stating for decades that a complete overhaul is necessary but this, like many other things in India, tends to continue as is.

TEST YOURSELF

Learn, review and memorize key terms from this section.

ahiṁsā ______

anādi ______

Aṣhṭa Vaidya ______

Aṣhṭāṅga Hṛdaya ______

Aṣhṭāṅga Saṅgraha ______

Atharva Veda ______

Bhaiṣhajya Ratnāvali ______

Bhāva Prakāśha ______

Bhela Saṁhitā ______

Bṛhat Trayī ______

Cakrapāṇi ______

Charaka ______

Charaka Saṁhitā ______

Charaka sampradāya ______

Dṛḍhabala ______

Hārīta Saṁhitā

hiṁsa

Kāśhyapa Saṁhitā

Laghu Trayī

Laghu Vāgbhaṭa

Mādhava Nidāna

nāḍī parīkṣha

Nāgārjuna

Nighaṇṭu

Punarvasu Ātreya

rasa

Rasa Śhāstra

Ṛg Veda

ṛṣhi

Sāma Veda

saṁhitā

sampradāya

Śhāraṅgadhāra Saṁhitā

siddhānta

smṛti

śhruti

Suśhruta

Suśhruta Saṁhitā

Suśhruta sampradāya

Vāgbhaṭa

Veda

Vṛddha Vāgbhaṭa

Yajur Veda

Yogaratnākara

Chapter 18: Review

ADDITIONAL READING

Utilize these references to expand your understanding of the concepts in this chapter.

CLASSICS	1st read	2nd read

REQUIRED READING	Chapters
The Ashtavaidya physicians of Kerala: A tradition in transition, https://www.ncbi.nlm.nih.gov/pmc/articles/PMC3117315/	
Two French Pioneer Historians of Indian Medicine, https://www.ncbi.nlm.nih.gov/pmc/articles/PMC3336532/	
Evolution of medical education in India: The impact of colonialism, https://www.ncbi.nlm.nih.gov/pmc/articles/PMC5105212/	
History of Ayurveda, N.V. Krisnankutty: Origin of Ayurveda, pages 3-23	

OPTIONAL READING	Format
The Interaction of Indian Medicine and Modern Medicine (Colonial Period) - Tom Patterson	
Religious Beliefs and Medical Practices A Sociological Study of Ashtavaidyas of Kerala, chapter 5, by Leela PU	

References

Beckwith, Christopher I. (2009), Empires of the Silk Road, Oxford University Press, p. 30.

Rosu, A. (1993). TWO FRENCH PIONEER HISTORIANS OF INDIAN MEDICINE. Ancient Science of Life, 13(1-2), 2–10.

QUESTIONS & ANSWERS

Record your questions for this chapter here for further research and discussion.

Question:

Answer:

Question:

Answer:

Question:

Answer:

SELF-ASSESSMENT

1. The goal of Āyurveda has always been to
   a. alleviate suffering to pursue life goals
   b. attain *samādhi*
   c. create scholarly work
   d. All of the above
   e. None of the above

2. *Sampradāya* refers to a
   a. collection of classical treatises
   b. practice of *Kāya cikitsā*
   c. school of thought
   d. theoretical model
   e. None of the above

3. Who is the original author of the Charaka Saṁhitā?
   a. Agniveśha
   b. Bhela
   c. Bharadvāja
   d. Cakrapāṇi
   e. Charaka

4. According to the *Suśhruta sampradāya*, the initial teacher was
   a. Agniveśha
   b. Ātreya
   c. Dakṣha
   d. Dhanvantari
   e. Indra

5. The *Charaka sampradāya* focuses on
   a. Internal medicine
   b. Surgery
   c. Toxicology
   d. Both B and C
   e. All of the above

6. The roots of Āyurveda are found in
   a. Atharva Veda
   b. Ṛg Veda
   c. Sāma Veda
   d. Yajur Veda
   e. All of the above

7. Kāśhyapa Saṁhitā is the only surviving Āyurvedic classical work that
   a. is compiled based on Charaka and Suśhruta
   b. specializes in Obstetrics and Pediatrics
   c. specializes in Rasa Śhāstra
   d. All of the above
   e. None of the above

8. Major research and development of Āyurveda during the Rasa Śhāstra period was largely influenced by
   a. British colonialism
   b. Buddhism
   c. original Vedic literature
   d. Śhaṅkarācārya
   e. None of the above

9. During the Rasa Śhāstra period, Āyurvedic scientists developed
   a. annual recitations of Aṣhṭāṅga Hṛdaya
   b. purified mercurial-based medicines
   c. the majority of Āyurvedic literature
   d. All of the above
   e. None of the above

10. The *Nighaṇṭu* section is a specialty of
    a. Bhaiṣhajya Ratnāvali
    b. Bhāva Prakāśha
    c. Mādhava Nidāna
    d. Śhāraṅgadhāra Saṁhitā
    e. Yogaratnākara

Chapter 19 : Āyurvedic literature

KEY TERMS

Aṣhṭāṅga Hṛdaya	Cikitsāsthāna	saṁhitā	Suśhruta Saṁhitā
Aṣhṭāṅga Saṅgraha	Indriyasthāna	Śhārīrasthāna	Sūtrasthāna
Bhāva Prakāśha	Kalpasthāna	Siddhisthāna	Uttaratantra
Charaka Saṁhitā	Nidānasthāna	sthāna	Vimānasthāna
catuṣhka			

The final outcome of Āyurveda's controversial history boils down to what exists today. The significant, persisting records include:

1. The continuity of practice in lineage-based groups in India
2. Written records including complete and incomplete manuscripts

Both of these sources of knowledge are significant for the current development of Āyurveda in their own ways. Lineage-based knowledge can help demonstrate the effectiveness of the science in very specific geographical locations. These methods apply the core principles in specific, ethnic subpopulations within controlled environmental regions and cultural habits. Surviving manuscripts which continue to be used today as the foundations of Āyurvedic medical study and practice across India are equally, if not more important in the context of Global Āyurveda. This is because the variety of classical texts provides a more complete picture of the science, its principles, practices and applications. Classical literature is more readily accessible and available than lineage-based teachers.

For successful professional studies in Āyurveda, it is imperative that students being with a solid foundation in classical literature. Over the course of study, students are required to learn directly from the classics if they expect to gain valid knowledge of the science.

This chapter covers a preliminary introduction to classical literature with instructions on navigating the classical texts. It is an invaluable primer for professional studies.

BACKGROUND

The primary literature for professional Āyurvedic education includes the *Bṛhat Trayī* and *Laghu Trayī*. These works include:

Bṛhat Trayī	Laghu Trayī
Charaka Saṁhitā Suśhruta Saṁhitā Aṣhṭāṅga Saṅgraha Aṣhṭāṅga Hṛdaya	Mādhava Nidāna Śhāraṅgadhāra Saṁhitā Bhāva Prakāśha

At more advanced levels, additional references are regularly used. Students also explore and interpret commentaries in all advanced studies.

Even though these texts are considered the primary foundations for professional Āyurveda today, their history is still unclear. There is controversy over identification of authors and variations that exist between different manuscripts. Changes, additions and deletions have been identified in all texts.

From the *History of Ayurveda*, by N.V. Krisnankutty comes an interesting analysis of the Charaka Saṁhitā on pages 89-90. This briefly introduces the author's extensive research into the complex history of Āyurvedic literature:

"Charaka: Charaka is the redactor of saṁhitās compiled by Agniveśha from the teachings of Ātreya. It is difficult to determine his identity and age. The term caraka is used in many works and on many occasions. Everywhere the meaning is different. It is not possible to assert that there was a particular ācārya or an exclusive Āyurvedic preceptor in that name.

The term caraka: Bhāva Prakāśha contains the following description - Ānanta, a master of all the six vedāṅgas and Āyurveda wandered all over the world in the guise of a sage to learn worldly life. The term caraka is derived from this habit of wandering. It was this Charaka who edited the work of Agniveśha, the disciple of Ātreya.

Some scholars think that the word caraka denotes an expert in medicine and that many physicians are known by that name. The counter argument in that case is that Suśhruta also could very well be designated as Charaka. The name Charaka is associated with the redactor of the works of Agniveśha. This is an individual. Perhaps, in course of time it came to signify a physician in general as we qualify a strong man as the Bhima."

HOW TO USE THE CLASSICAL TEXTS

The classical texts are used today across India throughout all levels of professional Āyurvedic medical education. They provide the foundations of knowledge in core principles for theory and practice, and critical details on best practices in clinical management.

The classics are held in high regard and considered by most to be basic requirements for a professional Āyurvedic career. Although often referred to as "ancient texts," they are so only by sheer age. They are very actively read, studied and practiced today in Āyurvedic hospitals throughout India and other countries.

Navigating the texts can seem daunting at first. The combination of Sanskrit, ambiguous and confusing translations, and seemingly obscure arrangement of information is not user-friendly at first glance for anyone attempting to learn the basics of the science.

The introduction that follows is meant to provide some insight on how the texts are structured, why, and how to approach them for study.

Note the following reminders and recommendations for learning how to effectively utilize the classical texts.

1. All classical Āyurvedic texts were originally composed in Sanskrit.
2. Various texts have been translated to many languages over many centuries, most notably Arabic, Chinese, Tibetan and German. English, however, is a relatively recent language, and only the most significant texts currently have English translations.
3. The quality of English translations varies widely and even with the "best" translations it is still often challenging for newcomers to understand the full depth and breadth of the medical science.
4. The information in the texts is presented in a manner which is very

different from introductory, step-by-step educational materials commonly seen in professional training today. Āyurveda is not presented in a linear fashion to introduce and build knowledge on previous concepts. Instead, it often provides a summary first, with the expectation that the reader is already competent in the full science. Consider instead that information is "contained" in the texts in a way where the reader will fully understand the subject after having completed a thorough study of the entire *saṁhitā*, at a minimum.

5. The texts have been written for the students of the lowest caliber and because of that they have intentionally written the contents in a clear, simple and concise manner in the original Sanskrit. The purpose of this, according to direct statements in the text (Cha. Sū. 4/20, 25/35), is to allow students of the highest caliber to exercise their logic and intellect to realize more than what has been explicitly stated. Infer deeper meanings from the text is generally not possible until the student has completed at least one complete reading of the entire *saṁhitā*.

6. The texts are written with the expectation that the reader already be familiar with the entire science of Āyurveda. The older texts tend to elaborate the concepts in more detail, while later works attempt to better organize the same information and present it in a concise fashion.

7. None of the texts are written for beginner-level introductions.

First, become familiar with the names of the most significant texts and their basic details. These are listed below with their original authors, redactors, contributing authors, significant commentaries and English translations.

Name of the text	Original author	Redactor	Contributing author(s)	Most significant Commentaries	English translations
Charaka Saṁhitā	Agniveśha	Charaka	Dṛḍhabala	Āyurveda Dīpika by Cakrapāṇi Datta	RK Sharma & Bhagwan Dash, or PV Sharma
Suśhruta Saṁhitā	Suśhruta	Nāgarjuna		Ḍalhaṇa, Bhānumatī by Cakrapāṇi Datta, Jejjata	Kaviraj Kunjalal Bhishagratna, or KR Srikantha Murthy, or GD Singhal
Aṣhṭāṅga Saṅgraha	"Vṛddha" Vāgbhaṭa or Vāgbhaṭa I				KR Srikantha Murthy
Aṣhṭāṅga Hṛdaya	"Laghu" Vāgbhaṭa or Vāgbhaṭa II			Arunadatta, Hemādri, Indu	KR Srikantha Murthy
Kāśhyapa Saṁhitā	Kāśhyapa	Jīvaka, Vatsya, Anāyasa			KR Srikantha Murthy
Mādhava Nidāna	Mādhava, Mādhavakāra, or Mādhava-ācarya			Vijayarakṣhita, Sri Kantha Datta	KR Srikantha Murthy, or G J Meulendbeld
Śhāraṅga-dhāra Saṁhitā	Śhāraṅgadhāra				KR Srikantha Murthy, or Dr. G Prabharkar Rao
Bhāva Prakāśha	Bhāvamiśhra			Dr. Bulusu Sitaram	KR Srikantha Murthy
Yogarat-nākara	Anonymous				Asha Kumari, PV Tewari, S. Suresh Babu
Bhaiṣhajya Ratnāvali	Govinda- dāsa	Śhri Brahma Śhankar Miśhra		Shri Ambikadatta Shastri, Shri Brahma Shankar Mishra	Kanjiv Lochan

Each of these texts contributes significantly to the study and practice of Āyurvedic medicine today. And each has its own structure, format and layout which must be understood well in order to fully utilize the information it contains.

Next, review each of the most significant texts to understand its unique purpose, structure and organizational method. While reading the following section, physically open each text whenever possible and follow along with the explanations. Remember, each text typically has a detailed introduction at the beginning which provides more insight into its history, layout and details.

Navigating the Charaka Saṁhitā

The Charaka Saṁhitā has two major English translations that were printed and popularized in the second half of the 20th century. The structure, layout and organization of each translation varies.

The RK Sharma and Bhagwan Dash translation contains 7 volumes with the *Cakrapāṇi* commentary printed in line with the original text. The set typically appears like the first image.

The PV Sharma translation contains 6 volumes with the original text printed in volumes 1-3. The *Cakrapāṇi ṭikā*, or commentary, is printed separately in volumes 4-6. The set typically appears like the second image.

RK Sharma & Bhagwan Dash translation

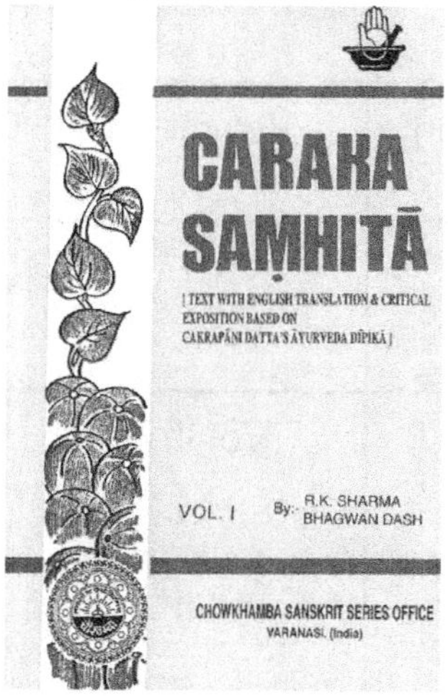

PV Sharma translation

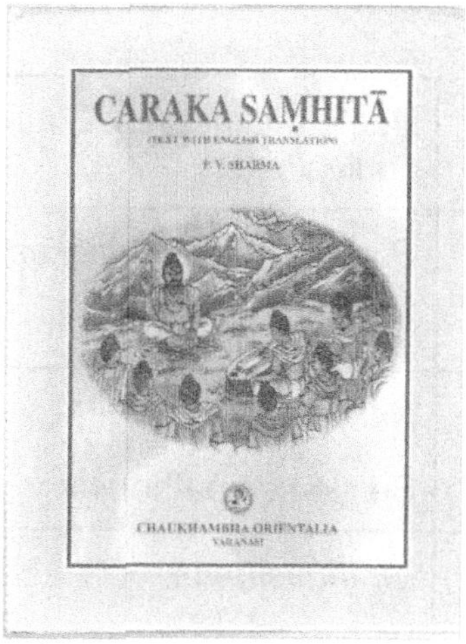

The original Sanskrit contents of both texts are taken from surviving manuscripts. Scholars have made great efforts to review the manuscripts contents and create a consolidated single format. Most surviving manuscripts contain variations and commentators have addressed the issues of modifications, misprints and multiple interpretations.

English translations from each publication vary. At times, one may be easier to understand or interpret than the other. But for the most part, they both attempt to convey a similar meaning.

In Charaka *sūtrasthāna* 30/69-71, several terms are defined which are key to understanding the internal layout of the text.

Praśhna

Praśhna is a question about the contents of the text based on the information presented. Typically, this question is asked by the student to the teacher and appears in dialogue form.

Praśhnārtha

Praśhnārtha is the answer to the question provided. Often this demonstrates the application of *yukti* (logical thought) considering all factors that affect the answer's outcome.

Tantra

Tantra is the subject which provides information on the measures to be followed for health maintenance. This term derives from *tantraṇa*, meaning to sustain the body or observe the rules of health).

Sthāna

Sthāna is a section of the text which focuses on a specific topic, aspect or theme.

Adhyāya

An *adhyāya* is a chapter of a *sthāna* that discusses the details of a specific topic.

The Charaka Saṁhitā is divided into 8 *sthānas*, as explained by the author in *sūtrasthāna* 30/33-68. These sections do not correspond with the printed volumes in a one-for-one manner.

In the RK Sharma and Bhagwan Dash translation, the first *sthāna* is Vol I. *Sthānas* 2 - 5 are printed together in Vol II. The sixth *sthāna* is split across Vol III, IV, and V, and the last two *sthānas* appear in Vol VI. Use the following chart to navigate the text.

Sthāna	Name and nearest English equivalent	Abbreviation	Volume	Chapters
1	*Sūtrasthāna*, or *Śhlokasthāna* Overview, general principles	Cha. Sū.	Vol I	30
2	*Nidānasthāna* Section on pathology	Cha. Ni.	Vol II	8
3	*Vimānasthāna* Proper measurement and proportion	Cha. Vi.	Vol II	8
4	*Śhārīrasthāna* Section on the body	Cha. Sha. / Śhā.	Vol II	8
5	*Indriyasthāna* Fatal diagnoses	Cha. In.	Vol II	12
6	*Cikitsāsthāna* Therapeutics	Cha. Ci.	Vol III, IV, V	30
7	*Kalpasthāna* Formulations for Pañcakarma	Cha. Ka.	Vol VI	12
8	*Siddhisthāna* Section on practical application	Cha. Si.	Vol VI	12

Each *sthāna* focuses on a specific set of related topics within the entire body of the science, with the goal of the full text to cover Ayurvedic medicine from the perspective of *Kāya cikitsā*, or Internal medicine. *Sūtrasthāna* is the most complex of all as it covers a very wide range of topics in a condensed format. However, the order of presentation of topics in *Sūtrasthāna* does not match the order of information presented throughout the rest of the text.

Charaka's *Sūtrasthāna* has a layout which is unique among the classical texts. The 30 chapters that it contains are split into seven *catuṣhkas* or sets of 4 chapters each. These mini-sets, or quadrates, focus on specific subsets of information. Familiarity with the names of each *catuṣhka* provides insight into its purpose and is extremely useful for remembering where information is stored in the text.

Catuṣhka	Nearest English equivalent	Chapters
Bheṣhaja catuṣhka	Therapeutics and medicinal formulations	Ch. 1 - 4
Svasthavṛtta catuṣhka	Maintenance of health	Ch. 5 - 8
Nirdeśha catuṣhka	Specific guidelines for practice	Ch. 9 - 12
Kalpanā catuṣhka	Preparations for management and administration	Ch. 13 - 16
Roga catuṣhka	Overview of disorders	Ch. 17 - 20
Yojanā catuṣhka	Various therapies	Ch. 21 - 24
Annapāna catuṣhka	Food and drink	Ch. 25 - 28

Cikitsāsthāna also contains two chapters which follow a slightly different format from the rest of the chapters in the text. Chapters one and two contain 4 subsections, called *pādas*, and their abbreviation format is typically written as Cha. Ci. 1:2/5, where 1 stands for the first chapter, 2 stands for the second *pāda*, or subsection. These are separated by the forward slash from 5, which represents the line number.

Navigating the Suśhruta Saṁhitā

The Suśhruta Saṁhitā has two major English translations that were printed and popularized in the second half of the 20th century. The structure, layout, and quality of translations vary significantly.

The GD Singhal et al translation contains three large volumes with a more comprehensive inclusion of *Ḍalhaṇa's* commentary with additional notes. The quality of the English translation is excellent. It is noticeably superior to all other English translations of any classical text available at the time of this writing.

The Srikantha Murthy translation contains three volumes with the original text and only select notes based on the *Ḍalhaṇa* commentary. The quality of translation is poor compared to the GD Singhal version.

GD Singhal et al translation

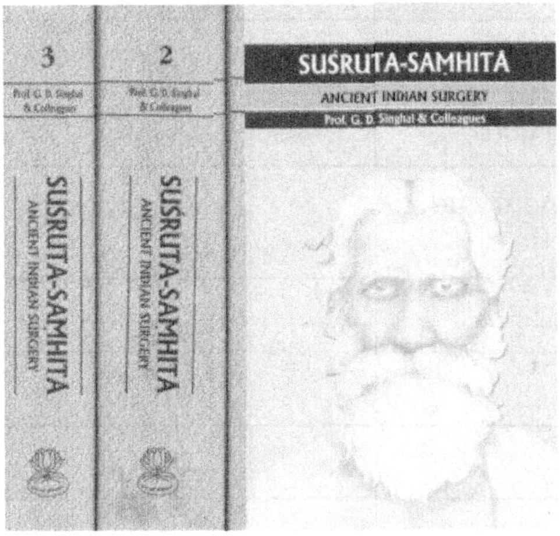

Srikantha Murthy translation

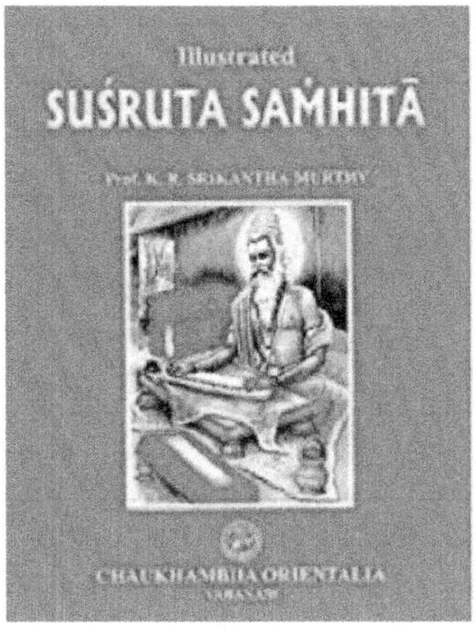

The original contents of both texts are taken from surviving manuscripts and should be identical. However, in some manuscripts slight variations occur and this influences the final translation.

The quality of English is markedly different in the two translations with the GD Singhal version being much easier for native English speakers to understand and digest.

The Suśhruta Saṁhitā is divided into 6 *sthānas*, as described by the author in *sūtrasthāna* 1/40. These sections do not correspond with the printed volumes in a one-for-one manner. In the GD Singhal et al translation, the *sthānas* are arranged as follows:

Sthāna	Name and nearest English equivalent	Abbreviation	Volume	Chapters
1	*Sūtrasthāna* Overview, general principles	Su. Sū.	Vol I	46
2	*Nidānasthāna* Study of diseases	Su. Ni.	Vol I	16
3	*Śhārīrasthāna* Study of the body	Su. Sha. / Śhā.	Vol II	10
4	*Cikitsāsthāna* Therapeutics	Su. Ci.	Vol II	40
5	*Kalpasthāna* Toxicological considerations	Su. Ka.	Vol II	8
6	*Uttaratantra* Final (best) section on additional therapeutics	Su. Utt.	Vol III	66

Each *sthāna* focuses on a specific set of related topics within the entire body of the science, with the goal of the full text to cover Āyurvedic medicine from the perspective of *Śhalya-tantra*, or surgery.

Sūtrasthāna is the most complex of all as it covers a very wide range of topics in a condensed format. However, the order of presentation of topics in *sūtrasthāna* does not match how the topics are presented throughout the rest of the text.

Uttaratantra is the final section dedicated to completing the presentation of knowledge and includes *cikitsā* specific to additional branches of Āyurveda (with a focus on *Śhalya-tantra*).

Uttaratantra (*Aṅga*)	Nearest English equivalent	Chapters
Śhālākya-tantra	Study of diseases above the clavicles	Ch. 1 - 26
Kumāra-bhrtya	Obstetrics and pediatrics	Ch. 27 - 38
Kāya-cikitsā	Internal medicine	Ch. 39 - 59
Bhūtavidya-tantra	Management of mental afflictions	Ch. 60-62
Tantrabhūṣhaṇa	Final supplements	Ch. 63-66

Navigating the Aṣhṭāṅga Saṅgraha

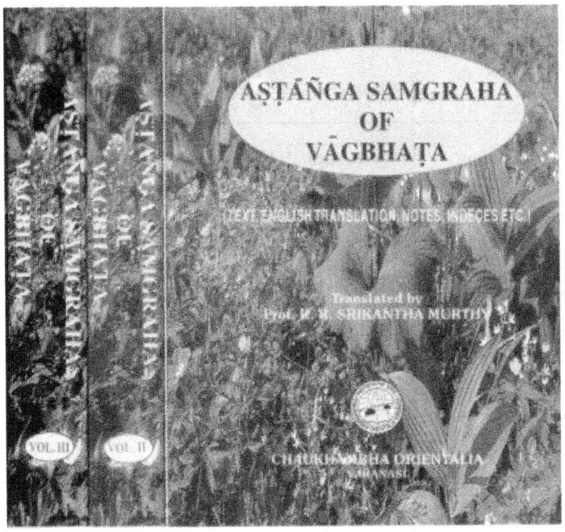

The Aṣhṭāṅga Saṅgraha, the first of two key texts attributed to the author Vāgbhaṭa, has one major English translation which is readily available. Even though it is considered within the *Bṛhat Trayī*, it is not as popular as Charaka, Suśhruta, or Aṣhṭāṅga Hṛdaya.

The Srikantha Murthy translation contains three volumes with the original text and select notes from the translator in *sūtrasthāna*.

The Aṣhṭāṅga Saṅgraha is divided into six *sthānas*, likely influenced by the format of the Suśhruta Saṁhitā. The author describes the layout of the text in *sūtrasthāna* 1/48-63. These sections do not correspond with the printed volumes in a one-for-one manner and are arranged as follows.

Sthāna	Name and nearest English equivalent	Abbreviation	Volume	Chapters
1	*Sūtrasthāna* Overview, general principles	AS Sū.	Vol I	40
2	*Śhārīrasthāna* Study of the body	AS Sha. / Śhā.	Vol II	12
3	*Nidānasthāna* Study of diseases	AS Ni.	Vol II	16
4	*Cikitsāsthāna* Therapeutics	AS Ci.	Vol II	24
5	*Kalpasthāna* Toxicological considerations	AS Ka.	Vol II	8
6	*Uttaratantra* Final (best) section on additional therapeutics	AS Utt.	Vol III	50

Each *sthāna* focuses on a specific set of related topics within the entire body of the science, with the goal of the full text to cover Āyurvedic medicine from all perspectives and specialties by combining knowledge from the authoritative works available at that time. *Sūtrasthāna* is the most complex of all as it covers a very wide range of topics in a condensed format. However, the order of presentation of topics in *sūtrasthāna* does not match how the topics are presented throughout the rest of the text.

Uttarasthāna is the final section dedicated to addressing all branches of *cikitsā*. It includes groups of chapters dedicated to each branch.

Uttarasthāna (*Aṅga*)	Nearest English equivalent	Chapters
Bāla cikitsā	Pediatrics	Ch. 1 - 6
Graha cikitsā	Management of mental afflictions	Ch. 7 - 10
Ūrdhvāṅga	Study of the diseases above the clavicles	Ch. 11 - 28
Śhalya cikitsā	Surgery	Ch. 29 - 39
Damṣhtra cikitsā	Toxicology	Ch. 40 - 48
Jarā or *Rasāyana cikitsā*	Regenerative treatment principles	Ch. 49
Vṛṣhya or *Vājīkaraṇa cikitsā*	Virility and fertility	Ch. 50

Navigating the Aṣhṭāṅga Hṛdaya

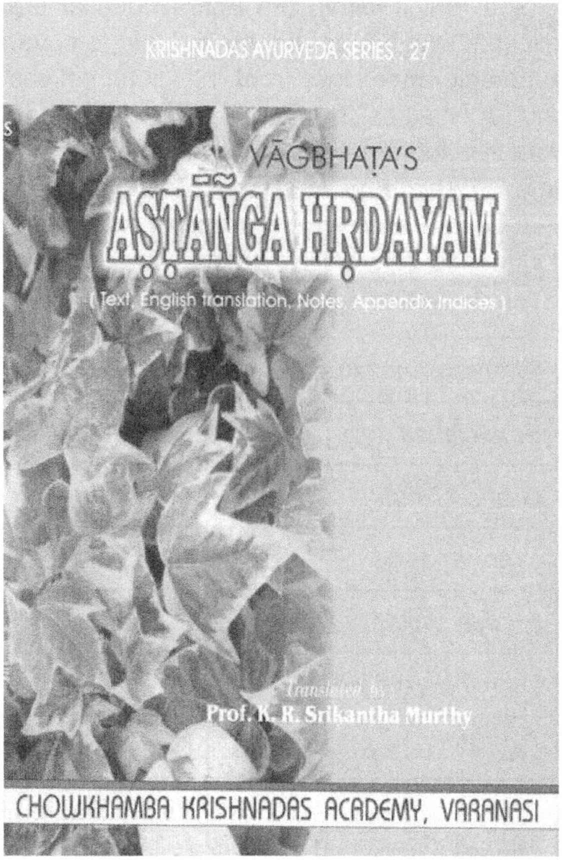

The Aṣhṭāṅga Hṛdaya, the second of two key texts attributed to the author Vāgbhaṭa, may be the most popular classical Āyurvedic text today. It has the most number of recent English translations, although all but one are either incomplete or difficult to acquire outside India. The major English translation by Srikantha Murthy is the most commonly available option and it contains the full text translation.

Its can be attributed to several factors. It is considered to be a concise and accurate condensation of its predecessor, the Aṣhṭāṅga Saṅgraha. Because of this, it contains the essence of the complete science of Āyurveda in the most compact form of any text available. To accomplish this condensation, the detailed explanations of topics are omitted and instead expressed in as short a form as possible. This concise format makes the contents easier to memorize in full.

The Srikantha Murthy translation contains 3 volumes with the original text and select notes from the translator in *sūtrasthāna*.

The Aṣhṭāṅga Hṛdaya is divided into six *sthānas*, as described by the author in *sūtrasthāna* 1/36-48. These sections do not correspond with the printed volumes in a one-for-one manner. In the Srikantha Murthy translation, the *sthānas* are arranged as follows.

Sthāna	Name and nearest English equivalent	Abbreviation	Volume	Chapters
1	*Sūtrasthāna* Overview, general principles	AH Sū.	Vol I	30
2	*Śhārīrasthāna* Study of the body	AH Sha. / Śhā.	Vol I	6

3	*Nidānasthāna* Study of diseases	AH Ni.	Vol II	16
4	*Cikitsāsthāna* Therapeutics	AH Ci.	Vol II	2
5	*Kalpa-Siddhisthāna* Toxicological considerations	AH Ka.	Vol II	5
6	*Uttarasthāna* Final (best) section on additional therapeutics	AH Utt.	Vol III	40

Each *sthāna* focuses on a specific set of related topics within the entire body of the science, with the goal of the full text to cover Āyurvedic medicine from all perspectives and specialties. *Sūtrasthāna* is the most complex of all as it covers a very wide range of topics in a condensed format. However, the order of presentation of topics in *sūtrasthāna* does not match how the topics are presented throughout the rest of the text.

With the text being so concise and compact, it requires that the reader already be familiar with the body of Āyurvedic medical knowledge in order to fully understand it.

Uttarasthāna is the final section dedicated to addressing all branches of *cikitsā*. It includes groups of chapters dedicated to each branch.

Uttarasthāna (*Aṅga*)	Nearest English equivalent	Chapters
Bāla cikitsā	Pediatrics	Ch. 1 - 3
Graha cikitsā	Management of mental afflictions	Ch. 4 - 7
Ūrdhvāṅga	Study of the diseases above the clavicles	Ch. 8 - 24
Śhalya cikitsā	Surgery	Ch. 25 - 34
Damṣhtra cikitsā	Toxicology	Ch. 35 - 38
Jarā or *Rasāyana cikitsā*	Regenerative treatment principles	Ch. 39
Vṛṣhya or *Vājīkaraṇa cikitsā*	Virility and fertility	Ch. 40

Navigating the Mādhava Nidāna

The first of the *Laghu Trayī*, Mādhava Nidāna ushers in a new format for classical Āyurvedic literature. This style moves away from the efforts of the *Bṛhat Trayī's* attempts to consolidate all the knowledge of Āyurveda into one work and instead focuses on an area of specialization. Presenting the knowledge in a concise format was done for ease of reference in clinical applications.

The author of Mādhava Nidāna, named Mādhavakara, thoroughly reviews the concept of *Pañca Nidāna*, or the methodology for assessing pathological processes. The text does not have any sections or parts, and instead is organized into 70 chapters. The first chapter reviews the theoretical aspects of the *Pañca Nidāna* framework. The remaining chapters each cover specific pathological process in detail. In some cases, more than one disease is included within the chapter because they share a common root pathology.

The text was originally named Rugviniśhcaya, or Roga Viniśhcaya, and is still referenced by these names today.

Two English translations are currently available by GD Singhal and by Srikantha Murthy. They include Western medical terms in the translation which can easily create confusion for new readers as they do not convey the full understanding of the classical concepts and pathology.

When citing Mādhava Nidāna as a reference, the abbreviation MN is typically used, along with the chapter number and line number, for example: MN 1/10. No additional *sthāna* or section reference is required.

GD Singhal et al translation

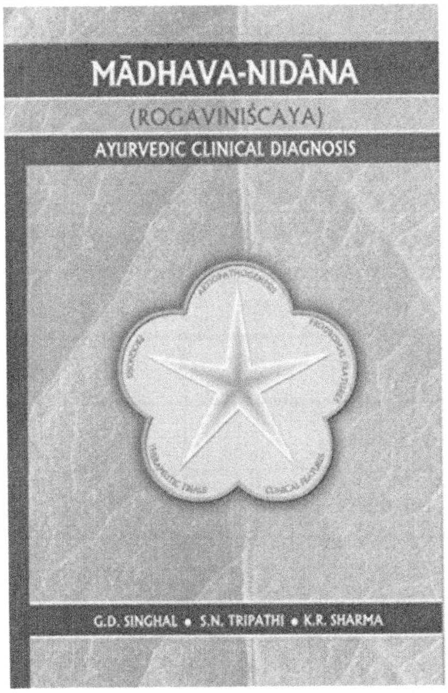

Srikantha Murthy translation

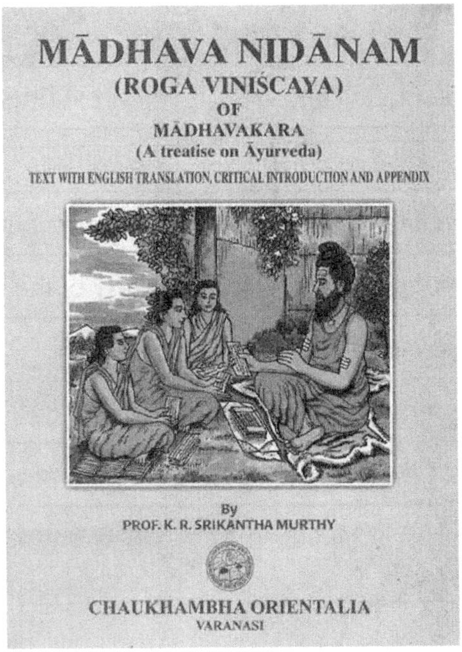

Navigating Śhāraṅgadhāra Saṁhitā

The second of the Laghu Trayī, the Śhāraṅgadhāra Saṁhitā, is ascribed to Śhāraṅgadhāra. The work is famously known for its focus on pharmacology and medicinal formulations.

It includes systems of weights and measures, specific rules for processing medicinal components, *Rasa auṣhadhis* (mercurial and metallic processing and formulations), and many other key concepts of the time period. It is also considered to be the primary resource available today on the practice of *Nāḍī Parīkṣha* in Āyurveda.

The text is organized into three parts with 32 chapters.

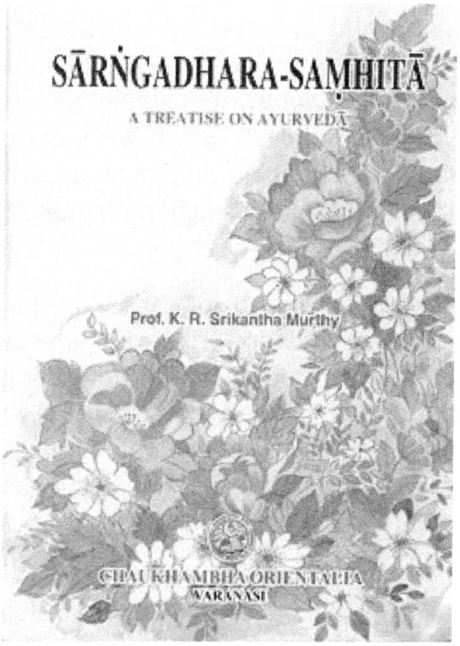

Part	Name and nearest English equivalent	Abbreviation	Chapters
1	*Prathama Khanda* First part Includes general definitions and core methodologies	Śhā. Pr.	7
2	*Madhyama Khanda* Second part Includes specific details for pharmaceutical processes	Śhā. Ma.	12
3	*Uttara Khanda* Third part Includes practical application of medicinal formulations in practice	Śhā. Utt.	13

Navigating Bhāva Prakāśha

The final, and most recent addition to the *Laghu Trayī* is the text *Bhāva Prakāśha* by the author *Bhāvamiśhra*. It is best known for its *Nighaṇṭu* section which serves as a thorough encyclopedia on Āyurvedic *dravya* (Āyurvedic "drugs," or single herbs, and their combinations).

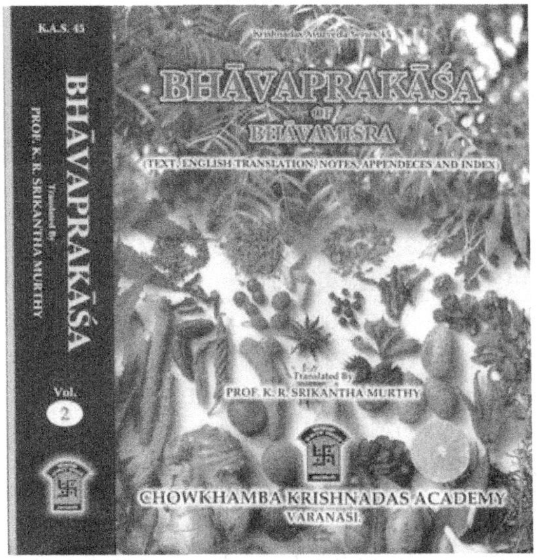

The text is organized into three parts and then divided into six subsections with 80 chapters. Its method of organization is unique among the classical texts. It tends to be more confusing to navigate than other texts because of the additional subsection names and how they are translated.

Part	Name and nearest English equivalent	Abbreviation	Chapters
1	*Pūrva Khanda* (*Prathama Bhāga* & *Dvitīya Bhāga*) First part (first subsection & second subsection) Includes core principles of Āyurveda in an orderly and concise format, followed by the *Nighaṇṭu* section	BP Pū.	7
2	*Madhyama Khanda* (*Prathama Bhāga*, *Dvitīya Bhāga*, *Tritīya Bhaga* & *Caturtha Bhaga*) Second part (first subsection, second subsection, third subsection & fourth subsection) Covers pathological conditions and their management	BP Ma.	71
3	*Uttara Khanda* Third part Includes *Vājīkaraṇa* and *Rasāyana*	BP Utt.	2

Navigating the Bhaiṣhajya Ratnāvalī

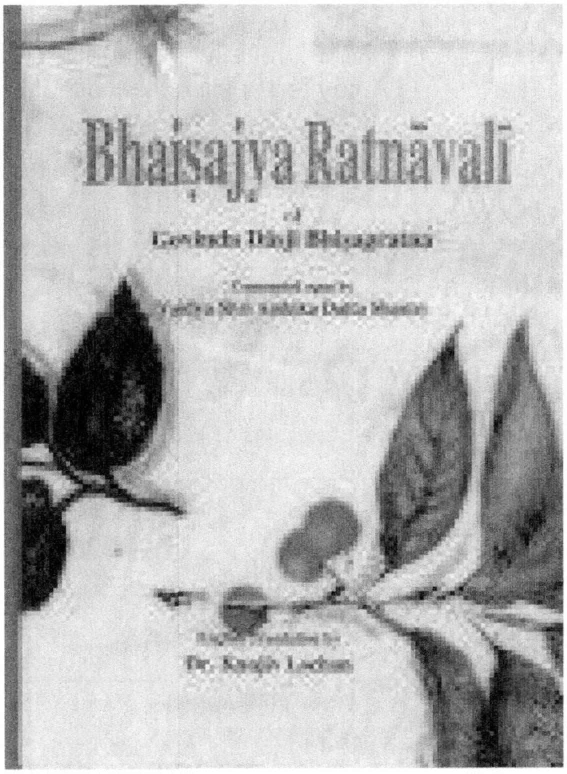

Bhaiṣhajya Ratnāvalī is the most recently written of all of the classical Ayurvedic texts. Authored in the 18th century by Govinda Dāsjī Bhiṣhagratna and commented on by Vaidya Shri Ambika Datta Shastri, it is considered the last great classical text written on Āyurveda. It is a complete encyclopedia divided into three volumes in its English translation by Dr. Kanjiv Lochan.

The text briefly focuses on the origin of Āyurveda and the contents and preparation methods for various types of medicines and traditional formulations. The text does not have any sections or parts, and instead is organized into 106 chapters. Each chapter delves into a detailed review of a disease or common pathology, the subtypes, and comprehensive management. Each volume contains a thorough and easy to navigate table of contents listing the specific diseases covered along with an index. Volume 3 contains a 111 page glossary of technical terms.

TEST YOURSELF

Learn, review and memorize key terms from this section.

Aṣhṭāṅga Hṛdaya

Aṣhṭāṅga Saṅgraha

Bhāva Prakāśha

Charaka Saṁhitā

catuṣhka

Cikitsāsthāna

Indriyasthāna

Kalpasthāna

Nidānasthāna

saṁhitā

Śhārīrasthāna

Siddhisthāna

sthāna

Suśhruta Saṁhitā

Sūtrasthāna

Uttaratantra

Vimānasthāna

INTERPRETING THE CLASSICS

Reading, studying and understanding each of the classical texts is like getting to know a very good friend. Each text has its own train of thought, priorities, goals and methodology. In order to know and understand any one thoroughly, the entire work should be read and analyzed multiple times. This can take years and most Āyurvedic professionals would agree that their interpretation and ability to apply the texts clinically grows with them and their practice over a lifetime.

In the process of analyzing and interpreting the knowledge available, always look at each concept presented and ask the following questions:

1. WHAT is the concept?
   What is the specific name that the author used to describe this concept? Keep in mind that various authors tend to use different names to convey distinct meanings of the concept. Typically, these synonyms should all be analyzed and interpreted to provide a broader and deeper understanding of the complete concept. Their use allows subtle distinctions to be made on many levels especially when applying the concept in practical scenarios.

2. WHO explained it? All authors? Are there any variations?
   Knowing the author who is the primary source of the concept provides insight into the purpose of the concept. For example, concepts described by Charaka are known to operate deeper in the realm of *Kāya*

cikitsā. Those mentioned by Suśhruta are meant to be applied more for *Śhalya tantra*. Each author gives us some insight this way and helps us understand the concept in their train of thought. Variations in the concept across authors are crucial to understanding the applied perspective.

3. WHERE is the concept found in the context of the author's work? What does this placement indicate?

   Placement of concepts through each text follows a specific flow. Each author, especially the later ones, has meticulously and methodically placed each word of their text in a specific order. While reading, analyze and interpret the text, and always consider placement in terms of the *sthāna* (section), *adhyāya* (chapter), line and position of the term or concept. For example, placement of a single concept at the beginning of its group is considered significant so that the first one is like the "leader." The significance of word placement is more profound in prose rather than poetry.

4. WHEN was the topic first mentioned? Does the approximate time period provide any insights?

   Āyurvedic science has been developing and evolving over thousands of years. During its lifetime, it has been influenced by all of the social, political and religious events around it. The information that remains today is a mixture of these influences, and part of the task now is to differentiate the science from other motives. Many of the developments in the science owe their invention to the requirements, needs and external pressures of the time. Considering the influence of these events helps better elucidate the nature of evolution of the knowledge. A good example is the influence of Buddhism on the development of *Rasa Śhāstra*.

5. WHY is the topic significant in the practice of Āyurveda?

   This is a critical question to ask for each topic. It helps to further differentiate the actual scientific knowledge from other information found in the classics which is strongly influenced by a popular political, religious or social agenda. The complete science of Āyurveda is a very sensible body of knowledge when understood in its entirety. Once the full picture can be seen, the odd pieces of information or outliers are much easier to identify.

6. HOW is it presented? Is it a direct list (like facts in a numbered list), discussion, QA, exchange between teacher and student, or group opinion?

   The methodology for presentation can provide insight into how professionals, students and teachers interacted in the past. This is significant because comparing these methods to approaches used today hints at the structure that could be beneficial. In many cases, knowledge is directly stated, as facts. In the older texts of the *Bṛhat Trayī*, interactions such as question and answer sessions, group opinions and discussions are also very relevant. These methods continue to support healthy professional education today and should be utilized whenever possible.

Chapter 19: Review

ADDITIONAL READING

Utilize these references to expand your understanding of the concepts in this chapter.

CLASSICS		1st read	2nd read
Charaka	Cha. Sū. 1/ – 4/ (commentary optional)		
Suśhruta	Su. Sū. 1/ – 4/ (complete)		
	AH Sū. 1/		

REQUIRED READING	Chapters

OPTIONAL READING	Format

References

Śarmā, R. K., & Dāsa, B. Agniveśa's Charaka Saṃhitā. Varanasi: Chowkhamba Sanskrit Series Office; Reprint Edition. 2016.

QUESTIONS & ANSWERS

Record your questions for this chapter here for further research and discussion.

Question:

Answer:

Question:

Answer:

Question:

Answer:

SELF-ASSESSMENT

1. The Bṛhat Trayī includes
   a. 2 treatises
   b. 3 treatises
   c. 4 treatises
   d. 5 treatises
   e. 6 treatises

2. Which text specializes on diagnosis and the framework of disease?
   a. Aṣhtāṅga Hṛdaya
   b. Bhaiṣhajya Ratnāvali
   c. Mādhava Nidāna
   d. Śhāraṅgadhāra Saṁhitā
   e. Yogaratnākara

3. The author of Bhava Prakāśha is
   a. Bhaisajya
   b. Bhāvamiśhra
   c. Charaka
   d. Mādhavakara
   e. Vāgbhaṭa

4. How many *sthānas* does Āṣhṭāṅga Hṛdaya contain?
   a. 3
   b. 6
   c. 7
   d. 8
   e. 10

5. What is unique about the layout of the Charaka Saṁhitā?
   a. It contains Uttara Tantra at the end.
   b. It has 4 quadrates.
   c. It has 7 catuṣhkas.
   d. It has 8 *sthānas*.
   e. None of the above

6. The primary commentary of Suśhruta Saṁhitā is authored by
   a. Ḍalhaṇa
   b. Dṛḍhbala
   c. KR Srikantha Murthy
   d. Nāgarjuna
   e. Suśhruta

7. In classical literature, *sūtrasthāna* typically covers
   a. a general overview of the complete subject
   b. a well-organized outline that the entire text follows
   c. pathology
   d. sections on the body
   e. therapeutics

8. In the Charaka Saṁhitā, which sthānas contain 30 chapters?
   a. indriyasthāna and sūtrasthāna
   b. kalpasthāna and nidānasthāna
   c. nidānasthāna and vimānasthāna
   d. sūtrasthāna and cikitsāsthāna
   e. siddhisthāna and cikitsāsthāna

9. The *Nighantu* section of Bhava Prakāśha is unique because
   a. it contains the only instructions for mercurial medicine preparations
   b. it covers the detailed history and development of Āyurveda
   c. it has 1,000 medicinal formulations
   d. it is the only surviving encyclopedia format of therapeutic dravya
   e. All of the above

10. The most concise, condensed classical text of Āyurveda is
   a. Aṣhṭāṅga Hṛdaya
   b. Aṣhṭāṅga Saṅgraha
   c. Bhāva Prakāśha
   d. Charaka Saṁhitā
   e. Mādhava Nidāna

Unit Review

ORAL EXAM QUESTIONS

Use these questions to prepare answers for the oral examination. You may create written statements or cue cards to memorize the key points that should be included in your response. Scoring is based on your accuracy, brevity, clarity (ABC), use of Sanskrit terms and concepts, and confidence.

1. When was Āyurveda discovered, and how old is it?
2. Discuss the controversial Aryan invasion theory and compare to today's generally accepted Hindu historical account.
3. How have political, social, and other events affected the growth and development of Āyurveda through its recorded history? Do certain types of events have a greater impact? If so, why?
4. Historically, how have cultural beliefs influenced the presentation and perception of Āyurveda in India? Do those beliefs continue to have an impact today?
5. Choose a time period from Āyurvedic history that you find significant and find at least three more pieces of information (factual or controversial) about the period which are not mentioned in this chapter. Explain why these are notable and cite your sources.
6. Compare and contrast the table of contents of one classical Āyurvedic text from each of the time periods in this chapter. What can be understood about the progression of the science over these different time periods based on the remaining literature?
7. Based on what you understand about the classical texts at this point, name one or two texts which would be most appropriate for your current level of professional education and explain why.
8. Compare and contrast the first section of the Charaka Saṁhitā and Bhāva Prakāśha.
9. Create a timeline of classical Āyurvedic literature showing the chronological order of the texts and historical periods. Mention the highlights of each period, and significant contributions of major works.
10. Name at least two positive and negative reasons to study Āyurveda primarily from Aṣhṭāṅga Hṛdaya and explain why.
11. Compare and contrast the first four chapters of Charaka and Suśhruta. Identify the general audience who the authors may be writing to, and the purpose of these chapters.
12. In Aṣhṭāṅga Hṛdaya Sūtrasthāna chapter 1, what does the author state as his purpose for writing the text? Cite the complete reference in abbreviated form including chapter and line numbers.
13. As a new student to Āyurveda, which author or text seems most accessible and easy to relate to? Why?

UNIT IV

Legal Landscape of Traditional Āyurvedic Medicine (TAM)

Chapter 20 : The developing profession and infrastructure

KEY TERMS

professional ethics scopes of practice standards of practice

At the time of this writing, Āyurveda is a developing profession in many countries around the world, including India. It holds the potential to dramatically impact the practice and delivery of health care worldwide. In order to realize this, Āyurveda must mature into a capable, robust and modern system that can demonstrate its efficacy and application today.

Around the world, efforts are increasing towards this goal on many levels. Due to a variety of factors including public perception, legal restrictions and financial regulation, Āyurveda has made more progress in certain countries instead of others. In order for the science to be fully practiced, many systems must be established and recognized. For example, appropriate standards for the profession must be enacted and accepted to self-regulate and maintain accountability. At a minimum, these include:

- standards in education representative of the capacity of Āyurveda as a primary health care system
- scopes of practice
- ethics
- professional values

Even in well-developed professions, these types of standards are regularly reviewed, refined and updated to keep pace with current demands. As an emerging profession and practice, Āyurveda has a unique opportunity to create a vast infrastructure and incorporate improvements learned from modalities that have gone through similar processes in recent decades. Efforts should be put towards expansion of practice before limitations are imposed.

DEVELOPMENT OF ĀYURVEDA

To fully understand the enormity of this issue requires a closer look at the history of the Indian government's policy toward Āyurvedic education and practice during the last century. It's important to know how Āyurvedic Medicine developed in India, before other countries can or should adopt their educational standards.

An examination of the Indian government reports and acts shows how the development of Āyurvedic Medicine was secondary to the development of Allopathic Medicine. Modern India's health care system maintains strong growth toward Allopathic Medicine while Āyurvedic Medicine has been perceived as substandard. Very recently this has begun to change with the rise of global interest and demand along with support from Hindu nationalism.

To understand how this perception developed, review the key reports released through the Indian Government over the last hundred years.

The Usman Report

In 1923, the Usman Report was the first major health report to be published in India. It appeared prior to Independence and was a regional report from Madras. The Usman Report consists of three main sections:

1. A Memorandum on The Science and the Art of Indian Medicine by G. Srinivasa Murti
2. A List of Indian Medical Works Extant (Both Printed and Manuscript) is a valuable survey of well-known medical literature in Sanskrit, Urdu and Tamil in the 1920s.
3. Testimony from many *Vaidyas* and *Hakims* provided in their various original languages. They describe in their own words the Āyurvedic and Unani edical traditions, their importance, the value for their patients, and basic tenets.

The Usman Report shows the clear tension between indigenous and allopathic health care professionals. The report was created by medical doctors who were qualified in both systems of medicine and was printed in several regional languages. The report drew attention from all over India and a three-member sub-committee toured key centers and met with leaders promoting indigenous medicine. The report represented an All-India survey but was published only in Madras.

The Bhore Report

Twenty years later in 1946 just before Independence, the second significant report was commissioned. The Health Survey and Development Committee produced the Bhore Report, which had two main objectives.

1. Survey of the present health conditions and health organizations in British India
2. Recommendations for future developments

The Bhore committee was commissioned to report on all aspects of India's healthcare and medical establishments. There were twenty-four British trained medical participants who prepared the report. The Bhore Report claimed it was the successor to the earlier legislative acts.

Many of the important acts that regulate indigenous medicine were omitted and there was no mention of non-allopathic health care systems. This report followed a common trend of the 19th century that promoted the misconception that Indian culture was ancient and unchanging.

The style in which the Bhore Report was written reflects a committee who lacked serious consideration of the merits of indigenous medicine. The Bhore Report was very influential and paved the foundation for Allopathic Medicine.

The Chopra Report

There was objection to the Bhore Report and two years later in 1948, the Chopra Report was developed. The main objective of the Chopra Report was to recommend a single system for the maintenance of health and prevention and to cure disease. It was prematurely ended due to the partitioning of India. The Chopra Report proposed complete equality in training and practice between indigenous and allopathic practitioners, but was rejected by the government.

Post Partition Reports

In the years following partition a few committees were developed which made attempts to promote Āyurvedic Medicine as a *śhuddha* or pure system in accordance with the traditional science. During the 1950's and 60's a number of committees began to cherry pick from the Chopra Report.

In 1951 the Pandit Report developed research for the validity of indigenous medicines. The Central Institute of Research in Indigenous Medicine and a postgraduate training center for Āyurveda were established in Jamnagar, India.

In 1956 the Dave Report largely discredited the Bhore Report and continued the work of the Chopra Report. This report made 16 recommendations toward the education and practice of *Vaidyas*, *Hakims* and Homeopaths, but the report was never completed.

In 1959 the Udupa Report made another full evaluation of Āyurveda and recommended establishing the Council of Indian Medicine (to regulate educational standards) as well as the Council for Āyurvedic Research. Only the later Council for Āyurvedic Research was established and the committee decided integrated medicine was appropriate.

In 1962 the Mudaliar Report took the opposite view and rejected integrated medicine. This report recommended indigenous medicine should be taught and practiced in its classical form. Unfortunately, Dr Mudaliar was also a member of the Bhore Committee. The committee made a further recommendation that once classical training was complete, they would also be trained in modern establishment medicine (MEM). The Mudaliar Report was fully adopted by the Indian government and laid the foundation for the regulatory systems in place today.

In 1963 the Vyas Report headed by Pt. Sharma, a well-respected Āyurvedic Physician recommended a pure curriculum written in Sanskrit to extend over a four-year period of training.

In 1970 the Central Council of Indian Medicine (CCIM) was enacted to regulate the curricula and syllabi for the Indian Systems of Medicine, this includes Ayurveda, Siddha and Unani Tib and Sowa Rigpa at the under-graduate and postgraduate level. To this day the CCIM remains as the educational regulatory board for Ayurvedic Medicine.

In 1981 the Ramalingaswami Report made five very important recommendations based on the needs of the traditional Indian culture.

- The Hindu concept of varṇāśhrama (stages of life) or "the right attitudes to pain, to growing old and to death"
- Non-consumerist approach to life
- Non-devolved attitude towards health services
- Yoga as an instrument of physical and mental health
- Use of simple homegrown medicines and food

During the last century many attempts were made to endorse Āyurvedic Medicine as *śhuddha* or pure in accordance with the traditional science. The Indian government didn't completely discard Āyurveda but did force the integration of Āyurveda with modern establishment medicine. The Bhore and Mudaliar Reports were the most influential in shaping Āyurvedic education and practice to where it is today. The neglected Usman report deserves a further look being the last indigenous account of Āyurvedic Medicine from a *śhuddha* or pure Vaidya perspective.

INTERNATIONAL DEVELOPMENT OF AYURVEDA

In India today, the integration of Āyurvedic education with modern establishment medicine remains unchanged. The two medical sciences are blended together as if to equate them as proof that Āyurveda is legitimate. As Āyurvedic education migrates to countries outside of India, the integration of the two medical sciences goes with it.

In 2001, the Fundación de Salud Āyurveda Prema in Buenos Ares, Argentina signed a Memorandum of Understanding (MoU) with Gujarat Āyurveda University, Jamnagar,

India. Since then many students have traveled from Central and South American countries to attend short training courses in Jamnagar.

Another program was launched in 2001, called the Āyurvedic Point in Milan, Italy. Developed by Dr. A. N. Narayanan Nambi, a member of ancient Ashtavaidyan family of Thrissur, Kerala. The Āyurvedic Point Program was developed as a template to aid the development of other European programs. Since then three programs were developed, the Rosenberg European Academy of Āyurveda in Germany and the College of Āyurveda and the University of Middlesex in the United Kingdom, these programs offer Āyurvedic education for medical doctors.

Another program developed in Moscow, Russia between 1996 - 2005, called the NAAMI was the first Āyurvedic medical center. It was developed by Dr. S. A. Mayskaya along with several Āyurvedic Doctors from India. During this period, the center provided medical assistance to over 2000 people, but it has since closed.

In spite of a variety of government and societal factors that include public perception, legal restrictions and regulation, Āyurveda is making steady progress across the globe. Countries that recognize medical pluralism with a traditional healing system rooted into their culture are more likely to be open to other traditional systems.

Āyurveda is culturally rooted in India as one of the main traditional healing systems. Due to its long-term establishment and adaptability of the people, Āyurveda is capable of coexisting with Western Medicine.

However, in countries like the United States, the United Kingdom, and Australia the traditional healing system evolved into what is known today as conventional, Western Medicine. These types of countries are much less likely to accept and recognize medical pluralism as seen historically and presently.

Despite many challenges and setbacks over the last few centuries, Āyurveda continues to be capable of serving as a primary health care system. As chronic Illness and higher costs continue to increase worldwide, Āyurveda in its full scope can provide the preventive, mitigative, curative and restorative health care so evidently needed.

Patients and health care providers worldwide are actively seeking effective, preventative and affordable health care services. In 2013 the World Health Organization reported over 100 million Europeans were seeking out traditional and complementary medicine. Āyurveda as a complete health care system has the potential to provide the answer for effective and affordable health care services.

THE FUTURE OF ĀYURVEDA

In order for Āyurvedic Medicine to be practiced in its full scope, many systems must be established and recognized by countries and governments. Appropriate standards for the profession must be enacted and accepted. The profession itself must be capable of self-regulation and maintainence of accountability.

At a minimum, required developments include the following.

1. Standards in education that represent Āyurveda as a primary healthcare system
    - Correct educational standards for Āyurvedic Medicine to prioritize the traditional science
    - Include Western Medical education within Āyurveda as supplementary training
    - Countries outside of India should carefully review and consider their

requirements for professional education instead of haphazardly adopting Indian standards

2. Scope of practice
    - Preservation or protection of health and wellness
    - Prevention of illness
    - Management of illness
    - Restoration of optimal health
3. Levels of practice
    - Vaidya or Āyurveda Āchārya (an Āyurvedic Doctor)
    - Svastha Āchārya (an Āyurvedic Practitioner)
    - Parichāraka (a Pañchakarma Technician)
    - Āyurvedic Pharmacist
4. Infrastructure
    - Outpatient clinic for assessment and treatments
    - In-patient facilities for Pañchakarma, surgery, advanced treatments
    - Pharmacy, dispensary
5. Building Safety
    - Properly constructed building protected from the external environment
    - Sufficient facility space and staff to manage patient requirements
    - Well-ventilated and temperature-controlled facilities
    - Well-equipped with essential supplies, diagnostic tools and medicines
    - Sanitary conditions with routine maintenance and waste removal
6. Ethics and Professionalism
    - Implement appropriate classical and current guidelines for the health care team
    - Implement appropriate practice and ethical guidelines according to each country
    - Implement HIPAA-compliant practices for privacy and protection

All professional standards must be regularly reviewed, refined and updated. As an re-emerging profession and practice, Āyurveda has a unique opportunity to create a vast infrastructure. Careful, proper planning will allow it to incorporate improvements learned from modalities that have gone through similar processes in recent decades. Efforts should be put towards expansion of practice before limitations are imposed.

TEST YOURSELF

Learn, review and memorize key terms from this section.

professional ethics

---

scopes of practice

---

standards of practice

Chapter 20: Review

ADDITIONAL READING

Utilize these references to expand your understanding of the concepts in this chapter.

CLASSICS	1st read	2nd read

REQUIRED READING	Chapters
Modern and Global Ayurveda	3

OPTIONAL READING	Format
Ayurvedic Point, translating tradition into modernity, https://www.ncbi.nlm.nih.gov/pmc/articles/PMC3807956/	Journal article
Ayurveda in Argentina and other Latin American countries, https://www.ncbi.nlm.nih.gov/pmc/articles/PMC3087371/	Journal article
History of the development of Ayurvedic medicine in Russia, https://www.ncbi.nlm.nih.gov/pmc/articles/PMC4850774/	Journal article

References

Ayurveda in Argentina and other Latin American countries, https://www.ncbi.nlm.nih.gov/pmc/articles/PMC3087371/

Ayurvedic Point, translating tradition into modernity, https://www.ncbi.nlm.nih.gov/pmc/articles/PMC3807956/

Central Council of Indian Medicine (CCIM), https://www.ccimindia.org/actandammendment.php

History of the development of Ayurvedic medicine in Russia, https://www.ncbi.nlm.nih.gov/pmc/articles/PMC4850774/

WHO - Traditional Medicine Strategy 2014-2023

Wujastyk, Dominik Jan. 2008. “The Evolution of Indian Government Policy on Ayurveda in the Twentieth Century.” In Modern and Global Ayurveda: Pluralism and Paradigms, edited by Dagmar Wujastyk and Frederick M. Smith, 157–176. New York: Suny Press.

QUESTIONS & ANSWERS

Record your questions for this chapter here for further research and discussion.

Question:

Answer:

Question:

Answer:

Question:

Answer:

SELF-ASSESSMENT

1. Modern India's healthcare system maintains strong growth towards ______ while ______ remains secondary.
   a. Allopathy, Āyurveda
   b. Allopathy, Yoga and Naturopathy
   c. Āyurveda, Allopathy
   d. Āyurvedy, Unani
   e. None of the above

2. What did the Usman Report accomplish?
   a. Completed a survey of known medical literature in Sanskrit, Urdu and Tamil
   b. Demonstrated tension between Āyurveda and Allopathy
   c. Recorded testimony from Vaidyas and Hakims
   d. Both A and B
   e. All of the above

3. What was significant about the Bhore Report?
   a. It influenced the foundation for Allopathic medicine.
   b. It surveyed present health conditions and health organizations.
   c. It was prepared by Allopathic and Indigenous doctors.
   d. Both A and B
   e. Both B and C

4. What did the Chopra Report accomplish?
   a. Create a single system for prevention and management of disease
   b. Equal training and practice for Indigenous and Allopathic doctors
   c. Overcome rejections of the Bhore Report
   d. Both A and B
   e. All of the above

5. Why was the Chopra Report rejected?
   a. Disagreements in government
   b. Disinterest in indigenous medicine
   c. India's partition
   d. Both A and B
   e. All of the above

6. After partition which report greatly influenced modern Āyurveda?
   a. 1951 Pandit Report
   b. 1959 Udupa Report
   c. 1962 Mudaliar Report
   d. 1963 Vyas Report
   e. 1981 Ramalingaswami Report

7. What are the main outcomes of the Mudaliar Report?
   a. Include modern medical training with indigenous medicine
   b. Integrate indigenous medicine with Unani
   c. Teach and practice indigenous medicine in classical form
   d. Both A and B
   e. Both A and C

8. Why was the Central Council of Indian Medicine (CCIM) enacted in 1970?
   a. To regulate curricula of Indian Systems of Medicine
   b. To form a new committee to commission the CCIM Report
   c. To oversee the integration of Allopathic and Indigenous medicine
   d. Both A and B
   e. Both B and C

9. What was the last indigenous account of Āyurvedic Medicine from a *śhuddha* or pure perspective?
   a. the Chopra Report
   b. the Dave Report
   c. the Pandit Report
   d. the Ramalingaswami Report
   e. the Usman Report

10. Āyurveda can advance outside of India with
    a. Applying classical guidelines for professionals
    b. Creating classical educational standards
    c. Encouraging professional ethics
    d. Reducing Allopathic-centric education
    e. All of the above

Chapter 21 : Ethics and values

KEY TERMS

artha	ethics	Nurse Practice Act	professionalism
dharma	kāma	Nursing Care Plan	State Board of Nursing
Duty to the Patient	mokṣha		

Professional ethics and values form the cornerstone of every health care practice. While some of these behaviors come naturally, many must be actively developed in professional character through regular study, training and practice. These skills allow a health care professional to practice effectively and encourage proper respect for themselves and the profession.

The recent quick spread of the term "Āyurveda" in the United States has largely focused on commercial development. Lack of attention to professionalism is due to many reasons, including ignorance of the classical science. For the general public, this can be problematic and dangerous. It is of the utmost importance to emphasize classical Āyurvedic Medicine and prevent false and misleading information.

With this rise of interest in Āyurveda, several people and organizations are pushing to accomplish legalization in the United States quickly. As a result, it is highly questionable if the standardization of Āyurvedic Medicine will be "watered down" and unable to represent its true capacity. Some of these organized groups have created their own standards, rules and guidelines for practice, including education which may not fully preserve the science. Unilateral approach in education and practice creates confusion, competition and separateness. It is crucial to guard Āyurvedic Medicine through the creation and expectation of a strong foundation and stable structure.

Professional Nursing in Western Medicine is an excellent establishment for Āyurvedic health care to emulate. Their strong foundation ensures the standards of practice are followed and the legal nurse title is protected. Studying the profession's history and how it evolved over time into a regulated health care industry, is beneficial in planning, preparing and creating the essential components of a successful health care system.

Review the history and development of the nursing profession in the United States to understand the key required components.

PROFESSIONAL NURSING

History of nursing

During the 19th century, modern nursing began to take shape in Europe and America in various forms. One individual, Florence Nightingale, had a tremendous impact in the foundation of the present day nursing profession.

Florence Nightingale was born in Florence, Italy, on May 12, 1820 to a wealthy family of an affluent British clan. She was well educated in history, mathematics and several languages. At a young age, Florence found her calling in nursing, although her family did not support her.

She attended nursing school in 1850 at the Institute of St. Vincent de Paul in Alexandria Egypt, a hospital run by the Roman Catholic Church. Afterwards, she completed three months of training from Kaiserwerth in

Germany.

A few years later, Florence was asked by the British Secretary of War to supervise a team of nurses to care for soldiers in Turkey during the Crimean War (1853-1856). During this time, she improved the unsanitary conditions and greatly reduced the death rate. Additional changes she instituted included clean, appealing food and a library for intellectual stimulation.

Florence Nightingale was known as the "Lady with the Lamp" as she went bed to bed late into the night, holding her lamp and providing care to the sick.

After the Crimean War, Queen Victoria presented a specially designed brooch to Florence Nightingale as a reward for her work. Since Florence would not accept gifts, the Nightingale Fund for Nursing was founded to commemorate her work in the Crimean War. This provided the means to established St. Thomas Hospital and the first scientifically based nursing school, Nightingale Training School for Nurses in 1860.

Florence used her experiences during the war and published *Notes on Nursing* which sparked worldwide health care reform. In her book, she wrote notes based on standard nurse practice which included observation of the sick, providing pure air and water, nourishing food, efficient drainage, warmth, sunlight, variety in surroundings, cleanliness of patient and bedding, preventing unnecessary noise, and providing hope to the patient.

Another report she wrote, titled *Notes on Matters Affecting the Health, Efficiency and Hospital Administration of the British Army*, was completed in 1858. It was almost a 1,000 pages full of statistics, numerical tables, graphs revealing trends in health care and problems she identified.

In 1907, Florence Nightingale was the first woman to receive the distinguished "Order of Merit" award recognizing her exemplary achievements.

At the age of 90, Florence died. She lead a courageous life, was a revered hero of her time, was known as the founder of modern nursing and forever changed the profession. Her accomplishments cleared the path for middle and upper class women to seek a nursing career, known as an honorable profession.

In 1965, the nursing profession began celebrating "Nurses Day." In her honor in 1974, "International Nurses Day" was chosen to be celebrated on May 12, commemorating Florence Nightingale on her birthday and the important role of nurses in health care.

Ref: Books

Florence Nightingale by Catherine Reef

Notes on Nursing: What it is, and What is Not by Florence Nightingale

[Notes on Matters Affecting the Health, Efficiency and Hospital Administration of the British Army]

Development of professional nursing education

The first nursing school in the United States to follow Florence Nightingale's nursing principles was Bellevue Hospital School of Nursing in New York. It opened in 1873 for six students to be trained in basic cleanliness, neatness, and patient comfort. By the end of the decade, physicians from the hospital were delivering speeches in anatomy, physiology and cleanliness. The school attendance grew quickly and by 1879, there were sixtythree enrolled students.

Ref: Foundation of New York State Nursing

https://www.cfnny.org

Bellevue Hospital School of Nursing Alumnae Association Records,

In 1893, Isabel Hampton lead a group at the Johns Hopkins Training School in laying the foundation for the American Society of Superintendents of Training Schools of Nursing. This was the first nurses association in the United States. By 1912, the association became the National League of Nursing Education. In 1917, they published Standard Curriculum for Schools of Nursing which established acceptable training for the nursing profession.

Later, in 1952 the name changed to what it is known as today, the National League for Nursing. This organization is dedicated to excellence in nursing education by offering professional development, networking opportunities, testing services, nursing research grants, and public policy initiatives.

Their members represent nursing education programs of higher education, health care organizations, and agencies. In 1959, they published the Patient's Bill of Rights: Nursing personnel respect the individuality, dignity, and the rights of every person regardless of race, color, creed, national origin, social or economic status."

Ref. National League for Nursing

http://www.nln.org

The "Associated Alumnae of Trained Nurses of the United States" was founded in 1896. The name was changed in 1911 to what it is known today, The American Nurses Association. This organization represents the interests of all registered nurses, in all 50 states and U.S. territories.

Their purpose is to advance the nursing profession by fostering high standards of nursing practice, expanding the role of nurses, promoting a safe and ethical work environment, bolstering the health and wellness of nurses, obtaining federal funding for nursing education and advocating on health care issues that affect nurses and the public.

Ref: The American Nurses Association

https://www.nursingworld.org

The first nurse registration law was enacted in 1903 in North Carolina to protect the title of nurse and improve the practice of nursing. Following, The Armstrong Act of 1903 was passed in New York, also requiring registration of nurses. The state board of nursing developed nursing exams and issued licenses, although this law did not define the practice of nursing. Eventually, all states were required to have licensure for registered nurses.

Ref: Nurse Practice Acts Guide and Govern Nursing Practice

by Kathleen A. Russell, JD, MN, RN

From the journal of Nursing Regulation

https://www.ncsbn.org/2012_JNR_NPA_Guide.pdf

In 1905, the University of California Board of Regents was granted power by the Legislature to set nursing standards, administer the exams, approve educational programs, issue graduation certificates and reserve the power to revoke them. It became a misdemeanor to use the title, "Registered Nurse" without a certification.

Ref: California Board of Registered Nurses

https://www.rn.ca.gov

The State of Texas formally recognized professional nursing in 1909 with the passage of the first Nursing Practice Act which regulated nursing education, practice and licensure. It also provided enforcement of the Nurse Practice Act rules and regulations.

Ref: Texas Board of Nursing

http://www.bon.texas.gov

Collaboration amongst nursing organizations began in the 1920's in Pennsylvania to build a networking opportunity. This included the National League for Nursing Education, the National Organization for Public Health Nursing, the American Nurses Association, the American Journal of Nursing and the American Social Hygiene Association. By 1937, the National League for Nursing Education published the final version, A Curriculum Guide for Schools of Nursing. It sets objective measures to determine the achievement of educational outcomes.

Ref. National League for Nursing

Link: www.nln.org

Nursing examinations

Unlicensed individuals mislead the public and can cause serious endangerment to patient care. The title nurse is only for those meeting the legal and educational standards, including licensure by examination.

Ref: Nurse Practice Acts Guide and Govern Nursing Practice

by Kathleen A. Russell, JD, MN, RN

From the journal of Nursing Regulation

https://www.ncsbn.org/2012_JNR_NPA_Guide.pdf

There is a process to be followed before taking the exam for licensure with explicit eligibility requirements in the U.S. Applicants must have a social security number, educational requirements per the specific state Board of Nursing (BON), state identification or driver's license card and be fingerprinted for a criminal background check. Applicants with any eligibility issues and criminal offenses will be reviewed.

Ref: Texas Board of Nursing

http://www.bon.texas.gov

Nurse Practice Act

It has been over a hundred years since state governments established boards of nursing to protect the public's health by ensuring safe nursing practice. Each state's Nurse Practice Act is passed by the state's legislature and establishes the state board of nursing with the authority to develop rules and regulations with the full force and effect of the law.

The specificity of the Nurse Practice Act varies in each state but all of them include a definition, the authority, power and composition of their BON, educational program standards, scope of nursing practice standards, types of titles and licenses with requirements, protection of titles, grounds for disciplinary action and violations.

Ref: Nurse Practice Acts Guide and Govern Nursing Practice

by Kathleen A. Russell, JD, MN, RN

https://www.ncsbn.org/2012_JNR_NPA_Guide.pdf

Today, the California Board of Registered Nursing (BRN) describes itself as a state governmental agency established by law to protect the public by regulating the practice of registered nurses. They are responsible for implementation and enforcement of the Nursing Practice Act, including the laws related to nursing education, licensure, practice, and discipline. The Nursing Practice Act, gives them the authority to investigate complaints and take disciplinary action against registered nurses. The Board of Registered Nursing protects and advocates for the health and safety of the public by ensuring the highest quality registered nurses in the state of California.

Ref: California Board of Registered Nurses

https://www.rn.ca.gov

Registered nurse scope of practice

The Nursing Practice Act defines the legal scope of practice for professional registered nurses. "Professional nursing" means the performance of an act that requires substantial specialized judgment and skill, the proper performance of which is based on knowledge and application of the principles of biological, physical, and social science as acquired by a completed course in an approved school of professional nursing. The term does not include acts of medical diagnosis or the prescription of therapeutic or corrective measures.

Ref: Texas Board of Nursing

http://www.bon.texas.gov

Professional nursing involves observation, assessment, planning, intervention, evaluation, rehabilitation, care and counsel, health education for the ill, injured or experiencing changes in normal health processes. This includes the maintenance of health or prevention of illness.

A nurse creates a Nursing Care Plan for each patient, adjusting it as needed. A nurse's focus is Duty to the Patient to provide and coordinate the delivery of safe, effective nursing care through the Nurse Practice Act and Board rules. This duty supersedes any facility policy or physician order.

A nurse is expected to follow the physician's order and proceed with the standard of care in evaluating the order before carrying it out. If the nurse questions the potential harm to the patient, she is expected to keep the patient safe and implement the "chain of command," notifying her direct supervisor first.

The licensed professional nurse takes responsibility and accepts accountability for practicing within the legal scope of practice in accordance with the federal, state and local laws, rules and regulations. This includes policies, procedures and guidelines of the employing health care institution or practice setting. Holding the title of registered nurse, the individual is responsible for providing safe, compassionate, and comprehensive nursing care to patients and their families.

Ref: Texas Board of Nursing

http://www.bon.texas.gov

Nursing standards

General standards of professional practice include education, evidence-based practice and research, quality practice, communication, ethics, leadership, collaboration, practice evaluation and use of available resources.

The Texas Board of Nursing provides a concise list of their nursing standards. These standards are set for the professional nurse to reduce errors, increase quality and continuity of care. They include:

Safe Medication Administration

Administer the right dose of the right medication via the right route to the right patient at the right time for the right reason. These are known as the six right rules.

Documentation

All documentation must be complete, accurate and timely.

Attentiveness, Surveillance

Nurses monitor the patient and staff. They observe the patient's clinical condition. If this is not observed correctly, the nurse cannot identify changes and make knowledgeable discernments and decisions about the patient.

Clinical Reasoning

Nurses interpret patient signs, symptoms and responses to therapies. They must evaluate the changes and adjust appropriately.

Prevention

Nurses follow usual and customary measures to prevent risks, errors, hazards, threats to patient safety and complications due to illness.

Intervention

Nurses properly execute health care procedures aimed at specific therapeutic goals in a timely manner on the right patient.

Interpretation of Authorized Provider's Orders

Nurses interpret authorized provider orders and act accordingly.

Professional Responsibility, Patient Advocacy

Nurses act responsibly in protecting the patient and the family's vulnerabilities. They advocate to see that patient needs and concerns are addressed.

Ref: Texas Board of Nursing

http://www.bon.texas.gov

Rules and regulations

It is the responsibility of a licensed professional nurse to know and understand the rules, regulations and laws to follow. The practice of nursing is a privilege. Although, the right to practice is granted by a state to protect the public receiving care, this right is always accompanied by accountability.

When a nurse provides questionable or unacceptable performance, the Board of Nursing through the authority documented in the Nurse Practice Act, will follow a process to review, investigate and take action. The BON can only take action if it finds sufficient evidence that the nurse violated state laws and regulations.

Disciplinary cases are usually grouped into practice related, drug related, boundary violations, sexual misconduct, abuse, fraud and positive criminal background checks. Every discipline case is considered on an individual basis.

Cases may be handled with a variety of disciplinary actions, including:

- imposing a fine and/or civil penalty
- monitoring practice
- requiring education
- public reprimand or censure for minor violation, usually with no restrictions on license
- limitation on license to practice in role
- setting work hours
- separation from practice for set period of time
- revocation of license

BON actions are public information and federal law requires that adverse actions taken against a health care professional's license be reported to federal databanks.

Ref: Nurse Practice Acts Guide and Govern Nursing Practice

by Kathleen A. Russell, JD, MN, RN

https://www.ncsbn.org/2012_JNR_NPA_Guide.pdf

TEST YOURSELF

Learn, review and memorize key terms from this section.

Duty to the Patient

Nursing Care Plan

Nurse Practice Act

State Board of Nursing

PROFESSIONAL ĀYURVEDA

As a profession today, Āyurveda has much in common with the early years of nursing. Inside and outside India, Āyurveda is at a critical juncture in its establishment and development for various reasons.

Classical records demonstrate that Āyurveda has long held high standards for professional ethics and practice. Today, these same ideals must be considered within the scope of modern, professional Āyurvedic development.

Classical regulations

The purpose of Āyurveda has always been twofold – to maintain health and alleviate suffering. Classically the responsibilities of Āyurvedic professionals to fulfill these goals were considered lifelong duties or careers. Candidates for Āyurveda were carefully selected so that their natural personality corresponded to the demands and expectations of the profession.

Today, assuming the responsibility of a health care provider in almost any capacity often comes along with long hours and demanding work environments. These stressful factors can almost always result in lower levels of health in professionals themselves. It is ironic that committing oneself to professional practice of a health care discipline can become a direct cause for ill health.

Classically, this was never the intention of Āyurveda. In attempting to conform to modern, Westernized standards, the profession today experiences the same pressures of society, overpopulation, unrealistic cultural expectations and many other stress-inducing factors.

Classically, Charaka instructs in *sūtrasthāna* 1/15 that the practice of Āyurveda be directed to supporting the goals of life from a personal and professional level. These *puruṣhārthas* include fulfilling one's *dharma*, *artha*, *kāma* and *mokṣha*.

Dharma	one's life's purpose, work or goal, determined either by society, family or the individual
Artha	accomplishment of material satisfaction
Kāma	enjoyment of material gain
Mokṣha	willful disconnection from the present manifestation of life by satisfactorily completing goals

Although the practice of Āyurveda may present innumerable challenges over the course of a career, it can also provide even more satisfying opportunities for both large and small achievements. The ability to impact another individual's life for the better is a skill that will always be held in the highest regard and one that will provide incomparable satisfaction for a lifetime.

Detailed descriptions of professional ethics,

behaviors and standards are specifically mentioned in Charaka Saṃhitā, *sūtrasthāna* 9/ and Suśhruta Saṃhitā, *sūtrasthāna* 10/. Recommendations address the professional's attitude towards patients, expectations for compensation, behavior toward the opposite sex and obligation to the patient during all stages of treatment.

Developing professionalism and ethics

The Merriam-Webster Dictionary defines professionalism as (Professionalism, 2019):

1. the conduct, aims, or qualities that characterize or mark a profession or a professional person
2. the following of a profession (such as athletics) for gain or livelihood

Ethics are (Ethics, 2019):

1. the discipline dealing with what is good and bad and with moral duty and obligation
2. a set of moral principles : a theory or system of moral values
3. the principles of conduct governing an individual or a group
4. a guiding philosophy
5. a set of moral issues or aspects (such as rightness)

Today, as the Āyurvedic profession grows, it will inevitably need to establish itself clearly through recognized definitions, titles, educational standards, scopes of practice and ethics. Several groups outside of India are making efforts towards this, however the current establishment of Āyurveda is not well organized or united.

With such a heavy emphasis on commercialization of the practice in recent decades, most professionals today have only had access to superficial, incomplete training which prepares them for "cookie-cutter" practice. This style of popularization of Āyurveda as a health care system leads to short-term gains and restriction of scope of practice.

Development of professionalism and ethics needs to come from each individual who calls themselves a professional of Āyurveda. Larger groups who represent the profession and professional body must lead with high standards that are genuine and true to the science.

TEST YOURSELF

Learn, review and memorize key terms from this section.

artha

---

dharma

---

ethics

---

kāma

---

mokṣha

---

professionalism

Chapter 21: Review

ADDITIONAL READING

Utilize these references to expand your understanding of the concepts in this chapter.

CLASSICS	1st read	2nd read
Cha. Sū. 1/15, 9/		
Su. Sū. 10/		

REQUIRED READING	Chapters
Ayurvedic Professionals Association, Ethics and Professional Conduct, https://apa.uk.com/code-of-ethics-and-professional-conduct	Online resource

OPTIONAL READING	Format
Well-Mannered Medicine: Medical Ethics and Etiquette in Classical Ayurveda, Dagmar Wujastyk	Academic book
American Herbalist Guild, Code of Ethics, https://www.americanherbalistsguild.com/ethics	Online resource

References

"Ethics." Merriam-Webster, 2019, https://www.merriam-webster.com/dictionary/ethics

"Ethics and Professional Conduct." 2012. Ayurvedic Professionals Association. https://apa.uk.com/code-of-ethics-and-professional-conduct

"Professionalism." Merriam-Webster, 2019, https://www.merriam-webster.com/dictionary/professionalism

Śarmā, R. K., & Dāsa, B. Agniveśa's Charaka Saṃhitā. Varanasi: Chowkhamba Sanskrit Series Office; Reprint Edition. 2016. Cha. Sū. 1/, 9/.

Singhal, G.D., et al. Suśhruta Saṃhitā of Suśhruta. Chaukhamba Sanskrit Pratiśhthan, Reprint Edition. 2015. Sū. Sū. 10/.

QUESTIONS & ANSWERS

Record your questions for this chapter here for further research and discussion.

Question:

Answer:

Question:

Answer:

Question:

Answer:

SELF-ASSESSMENT

1. What did Florence Nightingale do for the nursing profession?
   a. compiled 1,000 page report on all matters affecting health
   b. defined nursing as an honorable profession
   c. established standards for the nursing profession
   d. set nursing standards that sparked worldwide healthcare reform
   e. All of the above

2. In 1903, the first nurse registration law in North Carolina
   a. implemented exams and licensure
   b. improved the practice of nursing
   c. protected the title of nursing
   d. Both A and B
   e. Both B and C

3. The Armstrong Act of 1903 in New York
   a. defined the practice of nursing
   b. registered nurses
   c. set exams and licensure
   d. Both A and C
   e. Both B and C

4. In 1905, the University of California Board of Regents was granted the right to
   a. administer exams
   b. approve educational programs
   c. issue and revoke nursing certificates
   d. set nursing standards
   e. All of the above

5. What is the purpose of the Nurse Practice Act?
   a. allow each state to pass its own legislature
   b. grant each state definition, authority, power and composition by their BON
   c. set educational standards and define the scope of practice
   d. set types of titles and licenses with requirements
   e. All of the above

6. Which of the following is a requirement in the application for licensure?
   a. education approved by the BON
   b. fingerprint and criminal background check
   c. social security number
   d. state identification or driver's license
   e. All of the above

7. What is a nurse's Duty to the Patient?
   a. evaluate doctor's orders for patient safety
   b. follow the physician's order
   c. provide safe and effective nursing care
   d. Both A and B
   e. Both B and C

8. The legal scope of practice for nursing includes
   a. applying principles of biological, physical, and social science
   b. prescribing therapeutic or corrective measures
   c. using specialized judgment, skill and proper performance
   d. Both A and B
   e. Both A and C

9. Adherence to professional ethics is ultimately the responsibility of the
   a. government administration
   b. patient
   c. professional
   d. regulatory agency
   e. state legislative body

10. Classical Āyurvedic standards for professionalism did not include
    a. attitude towards patients
    b. behavior towards the opposite sex
    c. expectations for compensation
    d. guarantee of alleviation of the disease
    e. obligation to the patient during all stages of treatment

Chapter 22 : Standards in education

KEY TERMS

Āyurveda Ācharya	guru-kula	MD (Ayu)	professionalism
BAMS	guru-śhiṣhya	MS (Ayu)	śhiṣhya
brāhmaṇa	parampara	PhD (Ayu)	vaiśhya
	kṣhatriya		

The term Āyurveda spans far and wide when used in the context of education. Globally, Āyurvedic education ranges from abbreviated portions of natural health information to long-term, professional programs designed to train legally qualified practitioners. Because of the wide usage of the term, it is often unclear and confusing for those new to the subject to determine the quality, depth and scope of education available.

This chapter focuses on a review of professional-level education within and outside India to compare methodologies prevalent at the time of this writing. For a review of Āyurvedic education in other capacities such as self-help, spirituality, etc, refer to Modern and Global Ayurveda.

WITHIN INDIA

Current professional Āyurvedic Medical education in India is legally regulated by CCIM, the Central Council of Indian Medicine. This top-level regulatory body along with the Ministry of AYUSH (Āyurveda, Yoga and Naturopathy, Unani, Siddha and Homeopathy) sets the educational requirements for all licensed medical professions throughout India. These country-wide regulations are then adopted state-by-state and implemented in public and private accredited universities and colleges throughout the country.

When India gained Independence in 1947, "English medicine," Allopathy or Western medicine, was held as the gold standard for current and future medical practice and as an key indicator of the country's development. For traditional systems of medicine, including Āyurveda, it took about ten years after independence for the new Indian government to enact legislation and begin the process of formalizing regulatory bodies for education and practice.

Over the course of British occupation, Āyurveda was reduced to a second-class citizens' health care system in virtually every respect. In education, this sentiment continues to strongly influence the syllabus for standard professional training. With the hope of making Āyurveda more respectable and trustworthy, the syllabus for professional education models Western medicine in duration, structure and content.

Classical Āyurvedic concepts are organized within a framework of Western Medicine. Where discrepancies occur, new "coined terms" are invented in Sanskrit to help Āyurveda fill in gaps as perceived from a Western perspective.

An example of this can be seen in the presentation of diseases in the syllabus where the Western systems approach is followed (i.e., cardiovascular system, skeletal system, immune system, etc.) and Āyurvedic diseases are classified within it. The question naturally arises as to why the authentic classification is ignored.

Between one-third and one-half of the professional Āyurvedic syllabus contents cover Western medicine and include the study of disease, pathology, clinical examination methods, and diagnostic procedures including laboratory tests and imaging.

Students are expected to be competent in Āyurveda and Western medicine, especially if they expect to appear competent to the public. From a practical standpoint, this works very well in India for those who remain within their scope of Āyurvedic practice.

However, many students enter professional Āyurvedic Medical education in India with the intention of primarily practicing Western medicine. This is almost always due to the availability of steady jobs, income and societal acceptance. Reliable, continuous employment in the Āyurvedic sector has historically been extremely weak although that position is beginning to change as international demand increasingly drives the market.

The pathway for Āyurvedic medical education in India consists of three recognized degrees, at the Bachelor's, Master's and PhD level, all of which allow successful graduates to become licensed in their state and nationally through CCIM. Additionally, specialty diploma courses are available to BAMS graduates for short-term, specialized study and practice.

Around 2010, regulations were updated to require that all BAMS-level faculty complete a minimum education level of an MD or MS in Āyurveda to qualify for any teaching position. This created a massive growth of MD/MS (Ayu) programs across India because teaching positions are one of the few reliable employment avenues available to Āyurvedic professionals that provide consistent income.

Level 1	Bachelor's of Āyurvedic Medicine and Surgery (BAMS)	A 5.5-year course of study including a 1-year mandatory internship. This degree grants the title of *Āyurveda Ācharya* and allows one to legally practice as a *Vaidya* or Āyurvedic Doctor.
Level 2	MD or MS in Āyurveda, abbreviated as MD (Ayu) or MS (Ayu)	A 3-year course of study, including dissertation, in one of fifteen specialties in non-surgical (MD) or surgical (MS) fields. This level is often called "Post-Graduate" in India and students will typically refer to this level of study as "PG." This degree grants the title of *Āyurveda Vachaspati*.
Level 3	PhD in Āyurveda, abbreviated as PhD (Ayu)	A minimum 3-year course of study, including research and dissertation (2-7 years), for super-specialization. This degree grants the title of *Āyurveda Varidhi* rather than Doctor of Philosophy.

Only when students complete each level of BAMS, MD (Ayu) and PhD (Ayu) are they legally recognized as a qualified *Vaidya* in India.

While the BAMS level is named as a Bachelor's degree, its study and practice requirements far exceed a normal Bachelor's of Arts or Science in a standard four-year collegiate education. The naming of the BAMS degree is likely a misnomer. It is actually a First Professional degree, corresponding to a Doctor of Medicine (MD), Doctor of Jurisprudence (JD), Doctor of

Chiropractic (DC), etc (Structure of the U.S. Education System: First-Professional Degrees, 2008).

The BAMS degree takes a minimum of 5.5 years to complete. It consists of 3,500 hours of theoretical instruction plus 2,000 hours of supervised, clinical internship. This is the equivalent of 300 semester credit hours within the US higher educational system. It is currently the most advanced professional Āyurvedic training available globally. Its graduates are likely the best prepared to practice Integrative Medicine because of the heavy emphasis on Western Medicine.

TEST YOURSELF

Learn, review and memorize key terms from this section.

Āyurveda Ācharya

BAMS

MD (Ayu)

MS (Ayu)

PhD (Ayu)

professionalism

OUTSIDE INDIA

The export of Āyurveda from India in the form that is popular today began in the 1970's and 1980's. It has produced a variety of offshoots over the past few decades, many of which are strongly lineage-based. Several chapters in *Modern and Global Ayurveda* cover these topics thoroughly.

With education, supply in the West has risen to meet demand and the perceived notion of the science. From approximately 1980 through the early decades of 2000, those who found Āyurveda valuable were often in need of practical and effective personal healing solutions. Often, solutions from Western medicine did not provide relief. This resulted in the disproportionate rise of self-help style education aimed towards a disenfranchised group of people.

Ultimately, it obscured the bigger picture of Āyurveda's full capacity. Although many believe that the positive outcomes of spreading the word outweigh the negative side of misinformation, the opposite is growing more apparent each day.

From a liability perspective, it is much easier and safer to promote Āyurvedic education than Āyurvedic medical practice outside of India for many reasons. Because of the nature of Āyurveda and the large amount of information that is almost always shared to provide health-promoting services, the line between educating and practicing is often grey. These details will be covered in Chapter 12: Legal Landscape.

Many countries around the world are considering Āyurveda more seriously and a few have already enacted legislation to practice their "version" of the science. Typically, this consists of a subset of the full scope of Āyurveda which conforms to a role as a Complementary, Alternative or Integrative system auxiliary to Western medicine.

Several educational providers attempt to bolster this approach by additionally offering "training in India" programs which typically last a few weeks or less. On deeper review, a significant portion of these programs appear to be more like foreign, cultural immersion programs which do not require students to deal with actual challenges of professional education in India.

Many barriers and obstacles exist that prevent those of non-Indian origin from gaining substantial knowledge and practice in India, especially in a short time frame. At a minimum, these include language, food, climate, culture, transportation, and training formats.

Popular educational programs can directly influence professional educational standards by setting incorrect expectations and promoting a false image of Āyurveda. The current, popular perception of Āyurveda includes such a heavy emphasis on self-healing which puts a major limitation on the actual practice of the full science. There is a serious gap in professional understanding and application of the science outside of India which should be thoroughly addressed before this limited perspective of the science becomes solidified into recognized standards.

Many of the professional educational programs in the United States today fall into one of the three categories as recommended by the National Ayurvedic Medical Association (NAMA). These include the Ayurvedic Health Counselor, the Ayurvedic Practitioner and the recently added Ayurvedic Doctor.

The creation of syllabus contents for these courses was done in large part by non-Indians with partial Āyurvedic medical training typically centered around a single teacher or limited circle of teachers. The inclusion of a few Indian Āyurvedic doctors in this process has been cited as sufficient justification that the program contents are genuine and authentic.

However, a cursory review of the syllabus compared to the classical texts and BAMS syllabus would make it evidently clear that many important topics are missing and/or misrepresented.

The development of this provisional approach came largely out of the hope to avoid or minimize some of the challenges in teaching authentic, classical Āyurveda. The primary obstacle is the use of Sanskrit, but without it much of the value and knowledge of the entire science becomes unavailable. The concepts and presentation of Āyurvedic Medicine are also distinctly different from the Western train of thought, thus requiring their own appropriately designed framework and presentation.

In some ways, the development of professional education in the West has echoed India's educational approaches. Both systems have created education which intends to conform to existing infrastructure rather than provide a clear, direct view of the science in its own holistic framework.

Many people are intrigued with Āyurveda today and decide to study it for a variety of reasons. Often times, these reasons relate to a personal health issue that the individual has experienced either for themselves or a loved one, and they turn to Āyurveda with hopeful eyes for the answer. Although this has helped Āyurveda gain attention and spread outside India, it is not the best reason for one to opt to study the science on a professional level.

The Āyurvedic classics contained strict rules on the selection of candidates to maintain high standards of education and practice. Traditionally, professional Āyurvedic education was conducted following the *guru-śhiṣhya parampara*, or *guru-kula* format. *Śhiṣhyas*, or students, were accepted through a formal review and inducted by a *Vaidya* based on their familial lineage (most often a high caste, Brahmin family) or through personal merit, qualities and capabilities. *Vaidyas* were primarily responsible for the selection process and for the student's development throughout the duration of education and practical training. This personal, direct responsibility allowed the experienced *Vaidya* to more closely monitor the student's progress, capabilities and ethics.

Adhering to such standards today is unfortunately not the norm. With the exception of a handful of highly rigorous and competitive institutions in India, almost anyone, anywhere can apply to an Āyurvedic professional program, be accepted, and proceed to practice.

Many practitioners are forced to adapt their services for self-promotion and financial gain. While new developments and advancements of the science should always be fostered, they are currently too heavily dependent on immediate financial return. This presents a number of major issues for the profession. This topic must be recognized and discussed within the professional community to prioritize high standards, ethics and professionalism over shortcut methods for commercialization.

TEST YOURSELF

Learn, review and memorize key terms from this section.

guru-kula

guru-śhiṣhya parampara

śhiṣhya

CLASSICAL CANDIDATE REQUIREMENTS

Suśhruta dedicates the second chapter of his thorough treatise completely to the selection and initiation of the student (Su. Sū. 2/). He recommends that students be:

- from a family (lineage) of *brāhmaṇa*, *kṣhatriya*, or *vaiśhya* caste
- young, in the prime of life
- of good character, courageous, clean, well-mannered, humble, energetic and vigorous
- intelligent, mentally stable (steadfast), strong in memorization, equipped with sensible judgement, and capable of acting appropriately in all types of situations

Additional important physical characteristics are delineated as well. These were likely applicable at the time to help increase the student's chances of success in their practice and life-long career.

Once the student was selected, he became the responsibility of the teacher for the duration of the education. The student was expected to live with the teacher in strict accordance with their rules. All activities of the student were to be approved by the teacher first including eating, studying, sleeping and travel outside the residence.

Students were expected to not only be educated in the science but also were required to be trained in behavior, mannerisms, and character appropriate to the profession. This was the expectation and practice of classical *guru-śhiṣhya paramparā*, the tradition of teacher and disciple.

Charaka elaborates on the expectations of the student during their training in Cha. Vi. 8/5-8.

Many of these qualities and techniques may be relevant today. As the profession grows, these aspects of the classical science should also be appropriately considered in shaping requirements for study and practice which will ultimately reflect the image of the profession. Recognizing and respecting this long-standing tradition and actively working to maintain it must be a priority of the re-emerging profession.

TEST YOURSELF

Learn, review and memorize key terms from this section.

brāhmaṇa

---

kṣhatriya

---

vaiśhya

LEARNING ĀYURVEDA TODAY

Learning Āyurveda today requires a distinct thought process compared to standard Western sciences. Āyurveda utilizes a combination of holism, expansionism and reductionism which strongly reflects in the structure of the codified knowledge and application of its scientific principles.

Many classical expectations for qualities of students continue to stand as absolute requirements today. Strong memorization skills, quickness, agility, rapid, accurate logical processing, and sharp discernment skills must be present for success today. Additionally, students should be capable of reading accurately, quickly and efficiently, coalescing concepts in a holistic fashion, and retaining large amounts of information for long periods of time.

Many of these skills also develop over the course of study. Students often find that their own perspectives change from reductionist to holistic, expansionist thinking. This happens gradually and improves as familiarity with classical concepts increases. The classical teaching methods improve this process by providing similes to demonstrate concepts within the body to relatable, recognizable events in nature.

The study of Āyurveda on a professional level requires competency in the foundational subjects of Sanskrit and several key Western sciences such as anatomy, physiology, biology, chemistry, physics, astronomy, earth science and environmental science.

While it is helpful to have a background in Western medical sciences, it should be remembered that the knowledge of Western medicine in no way precludes or exempts the student from studying all aspects of classical Āyurveda. Professionals with training in multiple medical disciplines often face additional challenges in grasping authentic concepts unless they can overcome common, deeply trained behaviors to compare and contrast sciences instead of understanding each from its own perspective.

The study of Āyurvedic medicine also requires a basic, functional command of Sanskrit. At a minimum level, all Āyurvedic professionals must be fluent with the ĀYUT transliterated form of the *Devanāgarī* script and a minimum vocabulary of approximately 300 Āyurvedic terms. The advanced study of Sanskrit grammar and sentence translation becomes more important in advanced professional studies that extend beyond one year.

The basic command of reading and writing using transliteration, along with basic vocabulary creates a bridge to access classical knowledge in its original form and opens the doors to the study of the true science including its concepts and logical thought patterns. This allows the student opportunities to learn the genuine principles rather than attempting to correlate knowledge through other disciplines and methodologies.

Certain skills provide additional, specific advantages in studying and mastering Āyurveda. These include being:

- multilingual, or having a natural affinity towards languages
- objective, with scientific and logical discrimination
- capable of objective, critical analysis
- capable of applying complex analysis and math
- patient, determine and confident to succeed

The foundational portion of study of Āyurveda primarily involves memorization as any large body of scientific knowledge requires. Traditionally, this period of memorization would continue for as long as required to complete it satisfactorily. Today, a high level of quality in professional practice can be established as a direct outcome of rigorous education.

Classical Āyurvedic literature recognized that students could be categorized in one of three levels, low, medium or high, based on intellectual capacity and learning abilities. In several instances, the texts specifically state that they have been written for students of the low category. Information in the classical texts is presented accordingly. Students of higher categories are expected to extrapolate further meanings and deeper understandings from the basic information that has been explicitly mentioned.

A specific example is found in Charaka *sūtrasthāna* 25/35. The teacher, Punarvasu Ātreya, directly states that the information provided in the context of the chapter will be presented for students of low and medium categories. These direct explanations make the knowledge clear at a basic level. For students of the high category, the information provided allows them to apply logical reasoning and infer more meanings to realize new perspectives.

In Cha. Sū. 30/17-19, instructions are provided for students of all three categories. The material in the text is meant to be read, understood, and recited in the correct order by all students. Once this has been accomplished, each student must then interpret the meanings appropriately. Applied knowledge was intended to be advanced by:

- elaborating and expanding concepts
- contracting and condensing concepts
- proposing theories
- testing theories through applied reasoning
- providing valid demonstrations of theories
- subsuming concepts in a structured hierarchy of organized theoretical knowledge
- correlating and concluding results

These exercises are intended to be performed by all levels of students to enhance the depth, breadth and comprehension of knowledge.

Classically, in a *guru-kula* style educational format, the teacher would directly observe the student and their progression of knowledge over time. As the ability to monitor students individually reduced with larger class sizes in modern, institutionalized educational formats, this organic approach to student growth could not be sustained by a single teacher.

Today, it has been replaced with examination formats that provide a standardized approach to assessing students. Professional Āyurvedic education would more ideally be suited to a combination of styles which draw the benefits of both methods.

Finally, at the completion of Āyurvedic education, the student was expected to be able to explain the nuances of the entire text within the context of individual sections and chapters. By memorizing the full contents of the text, the student could then be considered equipped to engage in various types of discussions and debates which would help advance the science in various ways.

Suśhruta succinctly summarizes the need for depth of understanding in *sūtrasthāna* 4/4 by likening the heavy weight of knowledge to a burdensome load carried by a donkey unaware of the value of the contents. Memorization, comprehension and application were all required to fully apply the learned science.

Chapter 22: Review

ADDITIONAL READING

Utilize these references to expand your understanding of the concepts in this chapter.

CLASSICS		1st read	2nd read
Charaka	Cha. Sū. 30/17-19 Cha. Vi. 8/5-8		
Suśhruta	Su. Sū. 2/, 4/		

REQUIRED READING	Chapters
Modern and Global Ayurveda	6, 7

OPTIONAL READING	Format
The Ayurveda Education in India: How Well Are the Graduates Exposed to Basic Clinical Skills?, https://www.ncbi.nlm.nih.gov/pmc/articles/PMC3095267/	
Global challenges of graduate level Ayurvedic education: A survey, https://www.ncbi.nlm.nih.gov/pmc/articles/PMC2876920/	u
The Rosenberg European Academy of Ayurveda – Quality in Ayurvedic education in German-speaking Europe, https://www.ncbi.nlm.nih.gov/pmc/articles/PMC3117322/	
Benchmarks for Training in Ayurveda, http://apps.who.int/medicinedocs/en/d/Js17552en/	

References

Ayurveda Syllabus/Curriculum, 2014. Central Council of Indian Medicine. Retrieved 2019 from https://www.ccimindia.org/ayurveda-syllabus.php.

Śarmā, R. K., & Dāsa, B. Agniveśa's Charaka Saṃhitā. Varanasi: Chowkhamba Sanskrit Series Office; Reprint Edition. 2016. Cha. Sū. 30/, Cha. Vi. 8/.

Singhal, G.D., et al. Suśhruta Saṃhitā of Suśhruta. Chaukhamba Sanskrit Pratiśhthan, Reprint Edition. 2015. Sū. Sū. 2/, 4/.

Structure of the U.S. Education System: First-Professional Degrees, February 2008. International Affairs Office, U.S. Department of Education. Retrieved 2019 from https://www2.ed.gov/about/offices/list/ous/international/usnei/us/professional.doc

QUESTIONS & ANSWERS

Record your questions for this chapter here for further research and discussion.

Question:

Answer:

Question:

Answer:

Question:

Answer:

SELF-ASSESSMENT

1. The BAMS degree completes theoretical study in
   a. 4 years
   b. 4.5 years
   c. 5 years
   d. 5.5 years
   e. 6 years

2. MS (Ayu) specializes in
   a. *Agada tantra*
   b. *Kaumārabhṛtya*
   c. *Kāya cikitsā*
   d. *Prasūti Tantra*
   e. *Śhalya-tantra*

3. In the *guru-śhiṣhya parampara*, who is responsible for the student's education and training?
   a. parents of the student
   b. *śhiṣhya*
   c. teacher
   d. the student's caste
   e. None of the above

4. Advanced mastery of Sanskrit grammar is most relevant for
   a. advanced, BAMS-level professional Āyurveda
   b. all levels of professional Āyurveda
   c. entry-level professional Āyurveda
   d. self-help Āyurvedic education
   e. All of the above

5. Which characteristic is not mentioned classically for students?
   a. accurate logical processing
   b. agility
   c. memorization
   d. physical strength
   e. sharp discernment

6. Classical Āyurvedic literature is primarily written for students of the
   a. high category
   b. low category
   c. medium category
   d. All of the above
   e. None of the above

7. Āyurvedic education in India is regulated by
   a. AYUSH
   b. BAMS
   c. CCIM
   d. Medical Council of India
   e. World Health Organization

8. To complete the highest level of professional Āyurvedic education in India requires a minimum of
   a. 6 years
   b. 8 years
   c. 10 years
   d. 12 years
   e. 15 years

9. The BAMS degree covers a total of _____ hours.
   a. 3,000
   b. 3,500
   c. 4,500
   d. 5,000
   e. 5,500

10. Outside India, Āyurvedic education
    a. closely resembles Indian Āyurvedic education
    b. is strongly focused on self-help education
    c. often lacks deep, classical Āyurvedic training
    d. Both A and B
    e. Both B and C

Chapter 23 : Standards in practice

Professional Āyurvedic practice also takes on many forms and presentations in different locations. Classically, and traditionally, the most advanced practice of the complete science has been centered in the Indian subcontinent. With growing interest and development globally, Āyurvedic practice is increasing and improving on many levels.

EXPECTATIONS OF A VAIDYA

Classically, the expectation of successfully completed Āyurvedic education is a life-long career as a *Vaidya*. Charaka states that a *Vaidya* should be proficient in theory, experienced in practice, dexterous and clean (or pure) in presentation, behavior, thought and all aspects (Cha. Sū. 9/6).

Upon completion of studies, Charaka also states that the graduate continuously work to improve their knowledge and understanding of the science (Cha. Sū. 9/20-23).

Practice of Āyurveda in the classical model was meant to be performed by the professional according to their caste. Charaka instructs in *sūtrasthāna* 30/29 that *Brāhmaṇa* individuals were expected to utilize the knowledge of Āyurveda to provide benefit (ie, relief from suffering) for all living beings and creatures. *Kṣhatriya* individuals applied it for their own protection of health. And *Vaiśhya* individuals were expected to earn a living from the practice.

In order to fully comprehend the significance of these implications today, one must understand how the caste system was intended to work and society's perceptions and expectations of individuals at various levels.

Notice that the lowest caste, the *Śhūdra* caste, was not mentioned by Charaka. These individuals were almost always restricted from learning and practicing Āyurveda, in addition to many other exclusions from society. Suśhruta, however, recognizes in *sūtrasthāna* 2/5 that according to some teachers, an occasional exception for very worthy *Śhūdra* students was acceptable.

Classical authors also recognized the need to study and understand allied sciences and disciplines in order to enhance knowledge and practical skills in Āyurveda. Suśhruta makes this point clear twice.

First, in *sūtrasthāna* 4/7, he reminds the reader that it would be impossible to cover all aspects of all scientific disciplines in one single treatise, and the student should always seek opportunities to learn from specialists in other fields. Although not directly stated, the intention is to include allied sciences as well as other branches and specialties within Āyurveda.

In *sūtrasthāna* 34/14, he again reminds the student that an expert surgeon is well-respected when he is cross-functionally trained. Here he specifically emphasizes the need for training in other branches of Āyurveda, such as *Kāya Cikitsā*, for overall success.

WITHIN INDIA

Recently, the opportunities for gainful employment have been growing for Āyurvedic graduates in India. Previously, BAMS graduates were limited to opening their own clinic or working under an established doctor for much needed practical training. With the growth of the herbal pharmaceutical industry, these graduates now find more opportunities, such as formulating, developing and testing Āyurvedic products, especially cosmetics.

General practice poses many challenges for BAMS-level graduates in India. Public perception of Āyurveda as a second-class citizens' health care system over the last few centuries is perhaps one of the biggest obstacles.

Western medical doctors with similar education and experience typically and readily charge consultation fees 10-25 times higher than their Āyurvedic counterparts. Worsening this situation is the public impression that Āyurvedic doctors ought to perform *seva* or service to society otherwise they are considered greedy. This leads to a very dangerous state of practice as it financially destabilizes the profession at the direct expense of individual practitioners and their families.

The perception that Āyurveda is "natural" leads to another misconception that it is not as valuable as Western, synthetic medicine. For an Āyurvedic doctor trying to support a family this creates an extremely difficult financial situation which necessitates turning to other means of reliable income.

One of the quickest and most common ways to boost income is for an Āyurvedic doctor to practice Western medicine. This is extremely common especially in certain areas of India.

The Āyurvedic doctor may have already gained sufficient, basic knowledge of Western pathologies and diagnoses during training in BAMS, and by using these terminologies with patients, along with prescribing Western pharmaceuticals, they can project the impression that they are a "real" doctor.

To qualify for teaching positions and other permanent jobs in hospitals and institutions, BAMS graduates must continue studies and complete at least the next level of Āyurvedic training, a Post-Graduate MD or MS.

Placement into one of these programs, especially with an affordable tuition (typically in a government college), is like playing the lottery. Each year, thousands of applicants apply through an extremely competitive multiple choice examination, and only about 100 are accepted for government-funded seats nationwide.

A few remaining management seats with tuition rates often five to ten times higher are left for those whose families can afford them. But the struggle is certainly worth it because the higher level degree almost certainly guarantees permanent employment and financial stability.

Another significant and growing niche in the Indian Āyurvedic business world is medical tourism and the spa industry. With rising foreign demand for Āyurveda, many centers have popped up in tourist zones like Kerala and Himachal Pradesh. BAMS graduates who present well to foreigners can find steady employment in these centers, and in very high end resorts they can expect monthly salaries at least 5-10 times higher than teaching positions. Financial stability and recognition in one's community are often the biggest drivers for choosing a career path.

Because of the high degree of competition within the field, Āyurvedic doctors in lineage-based practices have been known to guard their secrets very tightly. With so many challenges to face in India, it becomes extremely difficult for Āyurveda to project an image as a successful health care system relevant on the international stage today. With the Modi government, a much stronger focus on Hindu traditions has developed and serious financial investment is beginning to flow into Āyurveda. Time will tell how far this helps to develop the infrastructure, perception and advancement of the science.

OUTSIDE INDIA

The practice of Āyurveda outside India takes on many forms. With growing interest and commercial demand, the name Āyurveda is being attached to many types of products and services to increase their market value. This gives the appearance that Āyurveda is spreading outside India, however the truth is that the deeper knowledge and practice of the subject lags considerably behind.

With so many short courses, self-development programs, and miniaturized versions of practitioner training available, many individuals graduate each year and go on to promote themselves as Āyurvedic professionals in various manners. The diversity of approaches to practice are again largely driven to meet consumer demand and often focus on diet and lifestyle advice, beauty regimes, cleanses and detoxes, spa, massage and body treatments, and general approaches designed to promote "balance" and "self-healing." Many of these miss the entire point of Āyurveda completely and can even cause considerable harm when applied injudiciously.

Among many issues with currently popular Western approaches to professional Āyurvedic training are two that stand out prominently. First, none of the current institutions or professional organizations openly provide support for professionals in practice. Many practitioners try to overcome this obstacle by staying in contact with their teachers, or establishing new mentors, but all of these are very informal arrangements.

Second, many institutions portray the image that graduates are capable of practicing the "full scope" of Āyurveda after as little as two years of study. Projecting the idea that diagnosis, management and prescription of custom herbal formulae can be managed competently with minimal education is extremely dangerous and likely to become a major reason for required professional regulation.

Additionally these expectations set the graduate up to immediately feel a lack of confidence from insufficient training leading many to abandon the profession. This trend has been common with self-help style educational programs in various disciplines of natural health and coaching, and is certainly not limited to Āyurveda alone.

OBSTACLES TO THE PRACTICE OF ĀYURVEDA OUTSIDE INDIA

There are quite a few major issues that limit the practice of Āyurveda outside India. This general overview covers the main categories:

- Legal regulations
- Financial investment
- Infrastructure
- Professional presentation
- Public expectations

Most countries do not currently recognize Āyurveda as a legal practice of health care, commonly leaving practitioners at risk of practicing medicine without a license. In the US, this is a felony offence. To circumvent this, many practitioners purposely maintain a status "under the radar" and limit themselves, their offerings, and abilities to avoid attention. This leads to stunted individual careers and limited professional growth on a larger scale. Additionally, the lack of regulation makes it difficult for practitioners to qualify for full-coverage professional liability insurance.

For a genuine Āyurvedic practice and business to be truly successful, financial backing, investment and support are all required. Materializing funds at these levels cannot be expected from individual practitioners and must be done with community support and professional involvement. Serious financial investment is required to improve standards, infrastructure and tools in education and practice. Financial aid for higher studies would help attract younger students who could advance the profession as a long-term career.

Lack of infrastructure leads to a disjointed professional network creating a climate of discontinuity and unhealthy internal competition. The lack of clearly defined roles within the Āyurvedic professional community, coupled by the lack of clarity regarding professional education and qualification has led to the current scenario where individuals prioritize lineage-based teachings over a well-rounded education. Not only does the professional community remain stagnant, it also sends wrong messages about the purpose and capabilities of Āyurveda as a primary health care system to observers. The result is that the professional community appears to consist of groups of followers focused on belief-based healing rather than scientific methods.

This strongly influences public perception of Āyurveda as an almost “magical” healing modality unrooted in a strong scientific foundation. This unfortunate misrepresentation could not be further from the truth and even worse could cost Āyurveda its standing as the formidable, complete health care system that it is. A broad team of highly educated and seasoned practitioners are needed to collaborate and communicate effectively on the international level about the depth and breadth of the science.

Chapter 23: Review

ADDITIONAL READING

Utilize these references to expand your understanding of the concepts in this chapter.

CLASSICS		1st read	2nd read
Charaka	Cha. Sū. 9/, 30/29 Cha. Vi. 8/5-8		
Suśhruta	Su. Sū. 2/, 4/		

REQUIRED READING	Chapters
Modern and Global Ayurveda	Chapter 11

OPTIONAL READING	Format
Development of minimum standards of clinical establishments Ayurveda, http://clinicalestablishments.gov.in/WriteReadData/86.pdf	

References

Śarmā, R. K., & Dāsa, B. Agniveśa's Charaka Saṃhitā. Varanasi: Chowkhamba Sanskrit Series Office; Reprint Edition. 2016. Cha. Sū. 9/, 30, Cha. Vi. 8/.

Singhal, G.D., et al. Suśhruta Saṃhitā of Suśhruta. Chaukhamba Sanskrit Pratiśhthan, Reprint Edition. 2015. Sū. Sū. 2/, 4/, 10/.

QUESTIONS & ANSWERS

Record your questions for this chapter here for further research and discussion.

Question:

Answer:

Question:

Answer:

Question:

Answer:

SELF-ASSESSMENT

1. According to Su. Sū. 2/, students were generally not allowed from which caste?
   a. *brāhmaṇa*
   b. *kṣhatriya*
   c. *śhūdra*
   d. *vaiśhya*
   e. None of the above

2. Traditionally, completion of professional Āyurvedic studies lead to
   a. a career as a *Vaidya*
   b. a career in teaching
   c. additional, mandatory apprenticeship
   d. cross-functional training
   e. specialization within the field

3. Today, BAMS graduates typically
   a. are highly respected
   b. are in high demand
   c. become teachers immediately
   d. face many challenges to practice
   e. work as equals with Western medical counterparts

4. A recent, major driver for demand of Āyurvedic professionals is
   a. Āyurvedic hospitals
   b. community health centers
   c. herbal product development
   d. *Pañcakarma* centers
   e. surgical wards

5. Full-scope practice of Āyurveda outside India is limited by
   a. abundant Āyurvedic medicines
   b. lack of BAMS graduates
   c. lack of health care demand
   d. lack of infrastructure
   e. lack of public interest

6. Public perception of Āyurveda strongly caters to
   a. balance and self-healing
   b. beauty services
   c. massage and treatments
   d. spa services
   e. All of the above

7. Insufficient professional training produces practitioners who are
   a. capable of creating proper custom formulations
   b. confident in all levels of practice
   c. prepared for clinical training in India
   d. All of the above
   e. None of the above

8. Lack of professional infrastructure leads to
   a. a disjointed professional network
   b. professional abandonment
   c. unrealistic expectations for single practitioners
   d. All of the above
   e. None of the above

9. In the US, practicing certain aspects of Āyurveda may leave the practitioner liable of
   a. injury to the patient
   b. practicing medicine without a license
   c. providing classical *Pañcakarma*
   d. All of the above
   e. None of the above

10. Professional Āyurvedic practice outside India generally
    a. lacks classical foundations
    b. lacks professional support
    c. requires mentors
    d. All of the above
    e. None of the above

Chapter 24 : Legal considerations

KEY TERMS

Alternate License Education Health Freedom	medical pluralism practicing medicine without a license prima facie	Regulatory Exemption Safe Harbor	Traditional & Complementary Medicine Whole Medical Systems

As a rapidly growing field in the US, the legal landscape of Āyurveda can change quickly and is often influenced by external, competing groups and established boards. Keep in mind that the information presented below may have changed since the time of publication of this work. The reader is strongly encouraged to use the Additional Reading reference list at the end of this section for updated, current information.

The study of the legal landscape that governs the practice of Medicine and Complementary and Alternative Medicine ("CAM") in the US is complex. At the time of this writing, Āyurveda is neither recognized nor licensed as a professional practice in any of the 50 states. Ultimately, the law which takes precedent in a practitioner-patient relationship is that of the patient's home state, unless modifiable by the practitioner's contractual agreement. This leads to additional complexities with the wide variety of state-by-state legislation for unlicensed practitioners and can significantly alter legalities of practice.

OVERVIEW OF LEGAL CONSIDERATIONS

In general, the main avenues for safe, legal practice include four primary methods with varying limitations. Before discussing each of these methods in detail, it is important to review the legal ground rules that apply to all.

Education

Providing educational services under the auspices of free speech

Alternate License

Practicing under an alternate license (see Appendix 1)

Health Freedom

Under a state's Health Freedom Act, if available

Regulatory Exemption

As a practitioner of a regulatory-exempt organization

Each of these methods has its benefits and drawbacks, and the onus lies with the individual practitioner to choose the method most appropriate to their personal, professional and legal requirements.

The practice of medicine in the US is regulated by federal and state governments which define specific legal boundaries that determine a variety of permissible activities, limitations and restrictions throughout the country.

Recognize first that the absence of a license to practice Āyurveda does not make it directly illegal. That line is crossed only when an individual is determined to be "practicing medicine without a license" by written or recorded evidence which demonstrates usage of specific medical terms or claims. This type of evidence is called prima facie.

Because the practice of medicine within the US is very tightly regulated by the government, it is very restrictive. The legal framework established by federal and state governments has largely closed avenues for other medical systems. Unlike many other countries, the US does not readily recognize medical pluralism. This is the root cause of the issue and is beginning to change with passage of Health Freedom Acts.

MEDICAL PLURALISM

In the US, medical pluralism has been be defined as "the employment of more than one medical system or the use of both Western and Complementary and Alternative medicine (CAM) for health and illness." (Wade, 2008). Recognition of medical pluralism in the US has changed dramatically since the late 1800's with the establishment of the American Medical Association and the efforts to homogenize the practice of health care and medicine throughout the country. Today, medical pluralism is becoming the norm for many nations and has been declared a basic human right of indigenous peoples by the United Nations (Burford, 2010).

The shift in perspective and acceptance bears great significance for all practices which currently fall under the umbrella of Complementary and Alternative Medicine. These systems will continue to realize growth with increasing demand from the general population for a variety of health issues, personal preferences and beliefs. As recognition for these systems continues to grow, professional organizations who represent these systems will be expected to establish appropriate levels of standards for quality education and full scope of practice.

With greater acceptance of medical pluralism, the classification of Complementary and Alternative Medicine should instead be recognized as Whole Medical Systems (WMS). These include Traditional and Complementary Medicine (T&CM) or Traditional and Complementary and Alternative Medicine (TCAM/CAM). Several of these consist of complete systems of theory and practice that have developed through many global cultures over time independently from Western Medicine (Whole Medical Systems, 2019).

As global demand continues to rise for Whole Medical Systems and they are studied scientifically, evidence and outcomes bears out their efficacy. Āyurveda is well-positioned to demonstrate positive outcomes as it is well-established and recognized in India alongside Western Medicine and the two systems have a long history of independent and collaborative training and practice. These approaches will help reshape the practice of medicine if Whole Medical Systems are allowed to function on equal standing with Western Medicine.

TEST YOURSELF

Learn, review and memorize key terms from this section.

medical pluralism

---

practicing medicine without a license

Traditional & Complementary Medicine

Whole Medical Systems

PRIMA FACIE

In the United States, prima facie is the legal phrase for evidence that demonstrates the practice of medicine without a medical license. One of the most common methods for prosecuting an unlicensed practitioner is by demonstrating verbal and/or written evidence that shows intent or practice of medicine without a license. This type of evidence is often found in promotional materials describing the practice. Prima facie can be qualified by using terms and phrases like:

- "consult with patients"
- "treatment of disease or illness"
- "prescribe remedies"
- "diagnose illness"
- "cure illness"
- "provide therapy"
- "administer medicine"
- "relieve symptoms"

Any recorded format or presentation that bears evidence to these or similar phrases and terms can be used as evidence of the practice of medicine. Without having a recognized license to practice medicine in the state where the evidence exists, one may be prosecuted by local, state or federal governmental agencies as well as private organizations or individuals for practicing medicine without a license.

Evidence of prima facie can consist of any evidence that is considered proof of the practice of medicine. Each state has the power to define the practice of medicine according to their own laws and boards.

The clear, safe strategy is to avoid the possibility of having any evidence which could be considered or even misconstrued as prima facie. Always avoid describing any Āyurvedic practice using words, images, symbols or marks that would traditionally be reserved for the medical profession. Focus on ways to communicate that the goal is to educate clients to improve health rather than address disease.

The following chart can be used as a guide to help frame thought processes and communication in a way which is less likely to be considered prima facie.

Avoid phrases like:	Prefer phrases like:
Consult, meet, work with or treat patients	Educate clients, members, students (or a phrase specific to the business service provided)
Prescribe, advise or administer medicines, remedies, herbs or therapies	Recommend natural products, formulations, supplements
Diagnose illness, pathology	Provide education on Āyurvedic knowledge and perspectives on health and traditional perspectives on dysfunction
Treat, manage, provide therapy (therapeutic intervention) or cure for specific illness, pathology	Provide education and recommendations on health improvement and general traditional techniques according to Āyurveda
Relieve symptoms	Improve, support and promote health and its functions
Avoid causative factors for disease	Educate on how to make better choices for positive health and quality of life

In a strict Āyurvedic context, many of the terms and phrases on the "Avoid" list can even be replaced with the classical Āyurvedic terms that are appropriate to the specific situation. However, care must be taken to avoid translations that use restricted medical terms. Not only can this can convey an inappropriate understanding to the client, but it can also quickly create legal risk for the practitioner.

TEST YOURSELF

Learn, review and memorize key terms from this section.

prima facie

GENERAL LEGAL PROTECTIONS

There are certain best practices that should be employed by any practitioner when planning to operate a business related to health and wellness. These include forming a separate legal entity to manage all finances and business operations, obtaining appropriate insurance, and ensuring that all health-related services are properly informed with signed and recorded consent.

The simplest way to form a separate legal entity is to submit Articles of Incorporation to create a Limited Liability Company (LLC) in the state of residence or state of primary business operations. Generally, this is accomplished by filing with the Secretary of State and then creating an internal Operating Agreement.

In more complex cases, the entity may be formed as a different type such as C-Corp, S-Corp, Limited Liability Partnership (LLP), Non Profit or other, appropriate entity type.

This determination must be made based on the requirements and future plans for the business and the individuals involved.

The state of incorporation may also be different from the location of business operations if no business presence can be established. In some cases, a foreign entity certificate must also be obtained to operate a business in another state. This may be useful to provide extra legal protection for the entity in various situations, particularly concerning "piercing the corporate veil" which can place personal assets at risk in the event of litigation. In special circumstances like these and for any specific advice, proper legal counsel should always be obtained.

Once the business entity is established, a federal EIN (Employer Identification Number) can be registered free of charge online. Local permits and sales tax registration may also be required depending on the products and services offered.

Insurance coverage should always be maintained for general liability, professional liability and any additional needs. Although it has been challenging in recent years to find steady insurance providers for Āyurvedic practice, more options are becoming available. At the time of this writing, Alternative Balance offers a package for Āyurvedic students and professionals including general and limited professional coverage. Refer to their website for current options.

Finally, detailed records of business transactions must be maintained. The specifics of what these records must include depends largely on how a professional chooses to practice. At a minimum level, these records typically contain direct contact information about the parties involved in any financial transaction along with details of the products and/or services provided. Beyond this, additional information can include signed informed consent statements, disclosures of intention, the professional's education, and more. There are many opinions on what should be recorded, and the final decision is often based on the approach to practice and requirements of the state.

The importance of legal structure, documenation and record keeping is highlighted in one of the few cases against a Western Herbal practitioner that went through litigation. Review the detailed account from the Rocky Mountain Herbal Institute to see these legal issues in action:

https://www.rmhiherbal.org/aa/f-ahr3-rights.html

LEGAL PATHWAYS TO PRACTICE ĀYURVEDA

Because of the wide range of legal complexities in the United States, it is imperative that Āyurvedic professional clearly and properly understand the legal pathway to practice that is most appropriate for them.

Review each of the four most common pathways below. Consider factors specific to your personal situation and how these can impact your ideal method of practice.

Option #1: Education

This is the most widely recognized method for practice that is valid throughout the United States. The practitioner represents themselves as an educational provider, and can include their own educational credentials for validation. This is the most common method for individuals possessing a doctorate-level degree, or an unrecognized doctor title (but not licensed as a doctor in the US). In appropriate academic settings, the use of the "Dr." title before a name is justified based on a qualified degree.

To further emphasize the educational nature

of services, instruction is commonly provided in a group format through books, workshops, online trainings. These formats provide a broader, generalized approach with is less personalized.

The main contingencies here are that the practitioner may not provide direct, individualized advice, guidance or recommendations as this could potentially be construed as a doctor-patient relationship. Even in one-on-one coaching sessions, all verbal and written information should always be presented as an educational experience. The professional must avoid any statements that appear to be direct, personal instructions. The individual receiving the services must recognize that they are being informed and educated through the process to make final decisions on their own.

This method requires informing the client in advance that they are agreeing to educational services. Typically this is done with a waiver, release of liability or other type of agreement form which the client is required to read, understand and sign before services begin.

In many cases, this is the safest legal scenario for practice, however it limits the practitioner's ability to detail the depth or quality of their services. The FDA exemption statement from the DSHEA Act is typically included on all documents or publicly available materials as a precaution. The language included is based on:

"This statement has not been evaluated by the Food and Drug Administration. This product is not intended to diagnose, treat, cure, or prevent any disease." (Public Law 103-417, 103d Congress).

Various groups of health educators have been able to utilize this method successfully. Perhaps the most notable group in this category includes those who practice Health Coaching. The International Association for Health Coaches™ has compiled a considerable amount of legal research including a full report titled "*Health Coaching: Your Right to Practice Guide*." These are excellent resources for better understanding the legal rights and limitations of practicing in an educational scope (Advocacy - IAHC).

The American Herbalist's Guild is another professional group which strives to disseminate quality information through herbalism education for more effective use of naturally available herbs and other substances. The AHG Code of Ethics includes a statement that registered practitioners act as educators. They recognize that "AHG members shall assume the role of educators, doing their best to empower clients in mobilizing their own innate healing abilities and promoting the responsibility of clients to heal themselves." (Code of Ethics, American Herbalists Guild)

With the growth of online resources for health education, many groups are recognizing the opportunity to provide services through platforms where multiple professionals can connect with clients and work together in a collaborative fashion. These service providers make their roles and limitations very clear through a wide range of legal consent statements that the onus of responsibility of health lies with the individual (client) accessing or receiving the services. It is worthwhile to review an example of a Terms and Conditions page to better understand how language can be crafted to protect the practitioner (Terms and Conditions of Use, Noom Inc.).

Liability insurance is always an intelligent business option even when working as an educator. In addition to general insurance (slip and fall, accidents, etc) specific professional insurance as a health or wellness educator should be sought and obtained wherever available. Care must be taken to review the policy in detail to understand coverage incidents, limits and exclusions. In many cases, herbs and supplements are not included in the educator's coverage but rather handled by the herbal retailer or distributor.

Practicing as an educator offers many benefits but is restricted by standard limitations on the ability to make claims for management of health conditions. This method may be a viable option for practitioners especially in situations where services are offered in multiple states through an online format.

Option #2: Alternate License

Many practitioners who do not want to be limited in their ability to make claims about what they can do, treat, or manage, prefer to provide services under an alternate license that is recognized by the state where they practice. This requires additional time and financial investment to complete training and receive licensure, but may be worth the extra effort especially to those who plan to practice in a specific geographical area (typically in a single state or confined geographical location). Professional liability insurance with more comprehensive coverage is generally easy to obtain for established professions. Refer to Appendix 1 for a list of practices and modalities that can be considered in this approach.

With this method, practitioners should always follow good documentation practices and require patients to read, understand and sign an informed consent, agreement, release of liability, or other legal form before services begin. The practitioner's scope of practice can vary widely according to state law and in certain cases, more than one license is needed to fully "cover" the complete range of services that can be provided by an Āyurvedic professional.

The major uncertainty with this method is whether a practitioner will in fact be protected under the alternate license in the event of litigation. Often times, the licensing board and professional insurance will only effectively cover therapeutic services included in the scope of practice of the recognized license. This would leave the professional vulnerable personally and professionally, running the risk of losing insurance coverage, their license and potentially more.

Practicing under an alternate license may still be worthwhile if the practitioner intends to limit their application of Āyurveda to basic education and simple protocols. Care can always be taken to work with patients who are already leaning towards an Āyurvedic approach so that provided recommendations are more educational in nature.

Option #3: Health Freedom

The concept of health freedom is based on the fact that the practice of medicine in the United States is overly and broadly defined while being limited to conventional Western, synthetic, or bio-medical care. Because of these overly restrictive medical laws, Traditional and Complementary Systems, such as Whole Medical Systems, including Āyurveda, have had undue and unnecessary limitations imposed on their practices which have limited their inherent rights to operate.

Establishment of "Health Freedom Acts" also known as "safe harbor practitioner exemption" laws intends to overcome the undue restrictions on health practice laws and to some degree, restrictions on medical pluralism. This is possible when the modalities practiced under Safe Harbor Exemption Laws do not pose imminent risk of harm to the public and do not involve the performance of any prohibited acts according to defined medical practice (Protecting Your Access To Health Care Freedom In Massachusetts, 2019).

The Health Freedom Movement is based on

the natural rights of individuals to access a form of health care that they prefer, even if it is not recognized or accepted within the definitions or scope of Western medicine. Acceptance and availability of multiple modalities is precisely the objective of medical pluralism as already practiced legally in many other countries.

The mission of the Health Freedom Movement is to promote access to all health care information, services, treatments and products that individuals deem beneficial for their own health and survival. This can be accomplished by promoting legislative reform of the laws impacting the right to health care access and choice. Ultimately, the goal is to promote the health of the people while allowing each person the support and freedom to choose how to manage their health.

A second main objective of the Health Freedom Movement is to prevent alternative products including vitamins, minerals, herbals, botanicals, amino acids and other food supplements from falling under government and pharmaceutical regulation and restriction. If regulated, companies could then be required to spend millions on research for products that are commonly used today. Instead, the dietary supplement industry wants these products to remain classified as food and be readily available to the public.

At the time of this writing, ten US states offer the right to practice under a Health Freedom Act or Law, and an additional six are actively pursuing legislation. Each state writes their own law with most being favorable to the consumer rather than the practitioner. While a Health Freedom Act can allow unlicensed practitioners protection against the charge of practicing medicine without a license, it also restricts certain professional activities which are typically controlled by existing state boards. These most commonly include prohibited acts based on the state's defined practice of medicine.

Successful health freedom legislation can accomplish key steps towards greater acceptance of medical pluralism by:

- providing parameters of practice for professionals and allowing unlicensed professionals an opportunity to share their services with the health care consumer more openly and freely
- increasing consumer awareness about alternative health professionals through more open advertisement and public service campaigns
- allowing a broader range of professional and public health care dialogue
- establishing potential for collaborations among professions to provide improved options and opportunities for public health

The National Health Freedom organizations collaborate with all states to encourage legislation by providing templates, language and support through experience.

Health freedom law timeline

Since 1976, states have recognized the need to allow consumers their choice in health care. The timeline of legislation over the past few decades demonstrates the increase in recognition of Health Freedom and its implementation.

2015 – Nevada A.B. 295: The Healing Arts Bill for Wellness Services

2013 – Colorado Senate Bill 13-215 – Colorado Natural Health Consumer Protection Act

2009 – New Mexico Enacted the Unlicensed Health Care Practice Act

2008 – Arizona Revised Statutes Sections 32-2911 Amended

2005 – Louisiana Revised Statutes 20-37 VI-B

2003 – Rhode Island Statute 23-75 – Unlicensed Health Care Practices

2001 – California SB 577 – California Complementary and Alternative Health care Practitioners

1999 – Minnesota Statute 146A – Minnesota Freedom of Access to Complementary and Alternative Health care Practitioners

1994 – Oklahoma Statute 59-480 (Oklahoma Parameters for Jurisdiction of Physician Licensing Act) – Oklahoma Allopathic and Surgical Licensure and Supervision Act.

1976 – Idaho 54-1804 (Idaho Exemptions to the Medical Practice Act) – Unlicensed Practice. Penalties and Remedies Relating to Unlicensed Practice

Health Freedom legislation varies from state to state but generally includes the following parameters:

- The freedom of the public to choose and have access to a variety of practitioners and modalities of health care
- Legal protections for unlicensed practitioners from violations of state-level Medical Practice Acts while requiring that they provide written disclosure and consent statements to their clients making it clear that they are not licensed medical doctors

It is important to recognize that Health Freedom legislation does not protect an unlicensed practitioner from the following (Health Freedom Laws, National Health Freedom Coalition):

- Engaging in practices specific to state-licensed doctors such as surgery, prescribing or stopping pharmaceutical prescriptions, utilization of modern medical diagnostic techniques including x-rays, and overt, specific, and willful conventional medical diagnosis
- Liability in the case of having caused real and demonstrable harm to one's patients or clients

For professionals who do not hold an active license with a state medical board, practicing under Health Freedom can be a very attractive option. The professional should be well-versed in the Health Freedom law that applies and be sure to meet all requirements with documentation and avoid all restricted activities. Access to professional liability insurance is available in a similar manner as it is with practicing under the option of education.

However, as with the option of practicing under Education, practitioners licensed in alternate health care professions must fully understand the allowances and restrictions of the practice laws in their state.

Option #4: Regulatory Expemption

Organizations which obtain federally-exempt status from public regulation and FDA governance are allowed to operate independently provided that they meet guidelines which include mechanisms for internal arbitration and resolution of practitioner-patient litigation. Very few of these organizations currently exist in the US, but their presence is significant.

These groups fall under two general categories: religious and tribal (Native American). Examples of religious groups include the Amish, Christian churches, Mennonites and others. The tribal category includes all bands of Native American Tribes, either recognized (at the federal or state level) or unrecognized.

Both groups of organizations, religious and tribal, are allowed exemption from standard government regulation (including the FDA and other state-recognized boards) because of their ability to self-govern and handle arbitration internally. In both cases, the practitioner and patient must agree to conduct their transaction under the regulations of the religious or tribal organization and essentially exit federal and state jurisdiction. This waives the regulations, oversight and control of the US government within the terms of the transactions that occur under the signed agreement.

Included in religious and tribal self-government is the responsibility to manage all health care practitioners within the organization. This is often accomplished by granting titles of certification for practitioners after scrutinizing their education and practice, running a thorough background check and meeting other criteria. Practitioners are bound to ethical practice within the scope defined by the organization with the fundamental principle of "do no harm."

Although there are few organizations operating with regulatory exemption, their presence is significant as it may provide the most protection for health care professionals practicing an unlicensed profession. The procedures required to become a practitioner within such an organization tend to be difficult and lengthy, and practitioners often need to spend additional time to educate their patients on the benefits of this type of relationship. But once the relationship is established, both the practitioner and patient can work together more openly and honestly than under any of the other options for practice.

The following review covers two of the main organizations that represent each approach (religious and tribal). Other organizations may operate differently.

Pastoral medical association

The Pastoral Medical Association is a unique professional organization that offers licensure for those practicing natural medicine or natural health and wellness within the context of religious affiliation. The Pastoral Medical Association offers licensure to practitioners who are state-licensed or unlicensed.

For practitioners with a currently active state-licensed medical practice, the PMA license provides the opportunity to work in a broader scope and includes natural health services which may not be allowed within the scope of the state license (Benefits of PMA Licensing).

The PMA recognizes the challenges of an individual practitioner in providing health and wellness services and claims that by joining their association, practitioners can overcome common obstacles such as:

- Reduced income in direct-pay models for Western medical professionals
- Too few clients
- Confusion about scope of practice for alternative protocols and ability to practice outside of the standard medical license scope
- Marketing and business management for independent practice

Pastoral Science and Medicine is the term devised by the PMA to describe the system of natural approaches founded upon spiritual principles used by PMA-licensed practitioners for promoting and improving physical, mental and spiritual health. Clients of PMA practitioners achieve health improvements by making positive lifestyle changes and following other natural procedures that are biblically sound, scientifically based and professionally administered pursuant to acceptable standards of care.

Pastoral Science and Medicine is not Western Medicine nor does it involve the practice of Western Medicine. Specifically, PMA-licensed practitioners do not examine, diagnose, treat, or cure any mental or physical disease, disorder or illness, or physical deformity or injury. No medications or pharmaceutical drugs are prescribed. Pastoral Science & Medicine services are completely separate from and not related to, approved by or dependent upon any secular federal or state governmental licensing authority or any other health care license the practitioner may have.

License protections

The Pastoral Medical Association strives to protect those practitioners who are unlicensed in a state by:

- Offering a legal path to ministerial practice in all US States and many foreign jurisdictions
- Offering access to the PMA professionally drafted patient-client agreement that provides extra protection for providing services
- Offering access to professional practice liability insurance that is designed exclusively for PMA licensees from a top-rated insurance company
- Offering access to affordable legal assistance through a top national firm experienced in protecting personal and religious freedoms which can advise on legal structure and issues raised by a state agency
- Providing a listing in the PMA professional directory to promote services to prospective clients nationwide
- Providing a professionally designed wall certificate and license suitable for framing
- Providing a professional ID card as a PMA licensed provider
- Providing options to lease a customizable website to promote a practitioner's PMA services, separating this business from secular medical and alternative health care services. This includes appropriate descriptions, disclaimers and disclosures to existing and prospective clients and governmental licensing authorities.
- Continuing to protect and advance the rights to practice Pastoral Science and Medicine; identifying and giving access to resources that will help practitioners deliver more effective clinical services and proven health-related products.
- Including access to information, educational programs, resources and tools to help practitioners improve professional knowledge and skills to promote and expand practice more effectively, serve clients better, and run business more efficiently and profitably.

License requirements and scope of practice

PMA licensing requires the practitioner to pass the PMA licensing process and adhere to PMA's scope of license, standards of care, and rules for providing services. The organization is established as an ecclesiastical association and uses its own arbitration process to address professionalism issues and resolve disputes.

It provides protection for the public in a manner similar to the secular government's regulation professional practices through licensure.

PMA's license requirements include being over 21 years of age, clearing a comprehensive background review, having a defined spiritual orientation, meeting specific education and experience criteria, and attaining a high passing grade on PMA's license exam (new as of January 1, 2017). Applicants must also be willing to confirm the statement of PMA Practitioner Shared Beliefs, Accepted Responsibilities & Pledge, as a license requirement.

There are two levels of PMA licenses. The first is the Diplomat of Pastoral Science & Medicine (D. PSc.) and the second is the Doctor of Pastoral Science & Medicine (PSc.D).

The cost of a PMA license varies and involves a comprehensive process where multiple factors are evaluated. The staff time required, as well as the actual cost to complete the practitioner profile and background investigation vary with each practitioner. Therefore, the cost of processing license applications varies as well. The application fee and annual license fee are evaluated and determined based on these variables in the licensing process. The PMA does maintain a flexible "no practitioner left behind" program to assure that every qualifying practitioner can afford a PMA license.

All forms of Natural Medicine qualify for PMA licensing, Health care service that abide by the "Practitioner Pledge" and demonstrate safe practice using natural substances and/or therapies are more likely to be approved within the scope of the PMA license.

No unnatural substances or harmful mechanical devices are allowed within the practice. Touch therapies are completely natural and generally fall within the scope of practice.

If practicing in a state with the Health Freedom law, the PMA license may still be valuable because of limitations and restrictions imposed by specific state law. A small number of states have now passed health freedom legislation, but those laws are not uniform in their terms and the interpretation of the various provisions of those laws by governmental agencies can result in a variety of outcomes in determining scope of health care services, advertising, and compliance. In this context, the PMA license offers an additional avenue for legal safety.

An example of the patient-client agreement form can be reviewed here: https://pmai.us/wp-content/uploads/2017/03/AgreementforWellnessServices-2017.pdf

Turtle Healing Band

The Turtle Healing Band is a member of the Indigenous HealthCare Practitioners Organization with the ability to grant licenses under the power of Native American Tribal sovereignty, or the inherent right to self-government. Unlike religiously-affiliated organizations, practicing members in the Turtle Healing Band and patients are not required to adhere to a specific religion or spiritual practice. Additionally, they are not required to be of Native American ethnic descent.

The Turtle Healing Band maintains the traditional perspectives of the Native American people and views the geographical region of North America as "Turtle Island." State boundary lines are not recognized in this traditional perspective, as Tribes span varying geographical areas. However, sovereignty varies among tribes based on their federal or state recognition. This can create a complex issue of authority in certain states.

Recognition and licensure through the Turtle Healing Band allows the practitioner to operate under sovereignty of the Native American Tribes. The process for licensure and method of practice is similar to the Pastoral Medical Association. Here, practitioners and patients sign an agreement to conduct business under the authority of the Tribes which is outside the purview of federal, state and other US regulatory agencies. This provides a way for practitioners and patients to speak more freely and openly about the services being provided, and honestly share information and professional recommendations.

TEST YOURSELF

Learn, review and memorize key terms from this section.

Alternate License

Education

Health Freedom

Regulatory Exemption

Safe Harbor

Chapter 24: Review

ADDITIONAL READING

Utilize these references to expand your understanding of the concepts in this chapter.

REQUIRED READING	Chapters
Appendix 1: Health care systems and modalitites	
Case study - Practicing medicine without a license?, http://www.rmhiherbal.org/aa/f-ahr3-rights.html#preface	
International Association for Health CoachesTM Advocacy page and Health Coaching: Your Right to Practice Guide, https://iahcnow.org/advocacy/	
National Health Freedom Coalition, http://www.nationalhealthfreedom.org/Index.html	

OPTIONAL READING	Format
Terms and Conditions example for online platform, https://www.noom.com/terms-conditions-use/	
PMA Practitioner-Patient Agreement, https://pmai.us/wp-content/uploads/2017/03/AgreementforWellnessServices-2017.pdf	

References

Wade, C., Chao, M., Kronenberg, F., Cushman, L., & Kalmuss, D. (2008). Medical Pluralism among American Women: Results of a National Survey. Journal of Women's Health, 17(5), 829–840. http://doi.org/10.1089/jwh.2007.0579

Burford, G. (2010). Citizen's choice of preferred system of healthcare as a fundamental human right. Journal of Ayurveda and Integrative Medicine, 1(1), 22–25. http://doi.org/10.4103/0975-9476.59823

"Public Law 103-417, 103d Congress." gpo.gov. Accessed July 31, 2017. https://www.gpo.gov/fdsys/pkg/STATUTE-108/pdf/STATUTE-108-Pg4325.pdf

"Advocacy - IAHC." iahcnow.org. Accessed July 31, 2017. https://iahcnow.org/advocacy/

"Code of Ethics, American Herbalists Guild." americanherbalistsguild.com. Accessed July 31, 2017. https://www.americanherbalistsguild.com/ethics

"Terms and Conditions of Use, Noom Inc." noom.com. Accessed July 31, 2017. https://www.noom.com/terms-conditions-use/

"Health Freedom Laws, National Health Freedom Coalition." nationalhealthfreedom.org. Accessed July 31, 2017. http://nationalhealthfreedom.org/infocenter/health-freedom-laws-passed/health-freedom-laws/

"Benefits of PMA Licensing." pmai.us. Accessed July 31, 2017. https://pmai.us/pma-licensing-benefits/

"Benchmarks for Training in Ayurveda." http://apps.who.int. Accessed July 31, 2017. http://apps.who.int/medicinedocs/en/m/abstract/Js17552en/

"WHO traditional medicine strategy: 2014-2023." http://apps.who.int. Accessed July 31, 2017. http://apps.who.int/medicinedocs/en/m/abstract/Js21201en/

"Mission Statement – National Ayurvedic Medical Association." http://www.ayurvedanama.org. Accessed July 31, 2017. http://www.ayurvedanama.org/page/Mission_Statement

Whole Medical Systems versus the System of Conventional Biomedicine. https://www.ncbi.nlm.nih.gov/pmc/articles/PMC5530407/

Protecting Your Access To Health Care Freedom In Massachusetts. https://www.spiritofchange.org/Spring-2019/Protecting-Your-Access-To-Health-Care-Freedom-In-Massachusetts/.

QUESTIONS & ANSWERS

Record your questions for this chapter here for further research and discussion.

Question:

Answer:

Question:

Answer:

Question:

Answer:

SELF-ASSESSMENT

1. Which of the following states offers a Safe Harbor Exemption law?
   a. Alaska
   b. Michigan
   c. New Mexico
   d. Texas
   e. Vermont

2. Practicing Āyurveda under an alternate medical license
   a. allows Āyurvedic surgeries to be performed
   b. constitutes legal practice under Safe Harbor laws
   c. could result in losing the alternate medical license
   d. is fully insured under the alternate medical license
   e. prevents the practitioner from being sued

3. Professional insurance should cover
   a. general liability
   b. individual requirements
   c. professional liability
   d. All of the above
   e. None of the above

4. Āyurvedic professionals in the US are allowed to
   a. consult with patients
   b. diagnose Āyurvedic diseases
   c. educate clients on traditional Āyurvedic health care
   d. treat clients with Āyurvedic therapies
   e. None of the above

5. Protecting personal liability in the US for Āyurvedic practice is accomplished by
   a. operating as a business entity
   b. registering as a foreign corporation
   c. registering as an Āyurvedic professional in a national organization
   d. All of the above
   e. None of the above

6. Providing Āyurvedic services through education allows professionals to
   a. exercise their first Amendment rights
   b. form a doctor-patient relationship
   c. provide direct, personalized health recommendations
   d. use the "Dr." title in all marketing materials
   e. All of the above

7. Health Freedom Acts (Safe Harbor Exemption laws) essentially pave the way for
   a. expansion of prohibited medical acts
   b. freedom of medical practice
   c. licensure for Āyurveda
   d. medical pluralism
   e. universal health insurance coverage

8. Practicing under Safe Harbor Exemption laws does not allow one to
   a. discontinue a prescription
   b. perform or prescribe X-ray diagnostics
   c. prescribe pharmaceutical medicines
   d. provide specific medical diagnoses
   e. All of the above

9. Practicing within the PMA requires one to
   a. adhere to PMA's scope of license
   b. affiliate with a defined religion
   c. agree to arbitration under PMA
   d. complete a comprehensive background check
   e. All of the above

10. Health Freedom Acts generally require that practitioners
    a. be a previously licensed medical professional
    b. clearly state their level of education
    c. meet each patient in person initially
    d. obtain special federal or state clearance
    e. None of the above

Chapter 25 : Communication and documentation

Health care communication for Āyurveda presents an array of unique challenges in all areas of practice. The language, concepts and presentation of Āyurveda require specific, specialized vocabulary and perspective. These terms, concepts and attitudes towards holistic health care affect everyone involved in the process including clients and Āyurvedic health care professionals.

While Āyurvedic health care professionals ideally learn the science in a classical, traditional manner that is distinct from Western approaches, clients may not be as familiar with the true, holistic system. A large portion of clients' involvement in Āyurveda requires and comprises education to learn concepts and understand the reasoning behind the science.

From a professional perspective, communication and documentation are areas that currently require five to ten years of dedicated attention and development for Āyurveda. The first step towards this effort is creating a language set that is commonly known and understood among Āyurvedic professionals.

In 2016, there were more than 400,000 documented Āyurvedic professionals practicing worldwide (4). With no formal digitized system to record patient and client records, it is believed that most record their patients' health information via an independent format developed by each practice.

Utilizing current technology, Western Medicine has developed digitized data systems for patient information and communication, called the Electronic Health Record (EHR).

The integration of the EHR across health care providers has fast changed the future of Western Medicine by providing the capability to maintain a patient's EHR from birth to death. Responsible sharing of this information between providers theoretically allows patients easier interaction with the health care system.

If the Āyurvedic profession were to adopt an integrated EHR system it could quickly transform the practice of Āyurvedic medicine. Unfortunately, this is not occurring in an organized fashion. One of the major obstacles to creating such infrastructure is the enormous cost of designing, developing and producing an appropriate system (4).

PATIENTS RIGHT TO PRIVACY

Protecting personal and medical information gathered in association with the care of a patient is a core value in health care. There are several ways a patient's privacy should be protected. A patient's right to privacy includes their personal space, personal data, personal choices and/or decisions, and personal relationships with family and friends (2).

The care of a patient also includes accurate communication of relevant information among all attending health care professionals. The recent advancement of communicating through electronic records, recordings and retrieval technology has created many challenges around protecting a patient's right to privacy. Breaches of a patient's health information can have serious personal and reputational consequences for both patients and health care professionals (2).

HIPAA, PHI AND NPP RULES

The Health Insurance Portability and Accountability Act (HIPAA) rules provide national protection for Patient Health Information (PHI) within the United States.

HIPAA applies to all health care, administrative, billing and insurance professionals. HIPAA grants all patients the right to access their own PHI and the right to be notified if a breach of their PHI has occurred. Patients must also be given a Notification of Privacy Practices (NPP), which states how the health care professional protects their PHI. The NPP must describe all the ways the PHI is used, disclosed, and protected (3).

In addition, a health care professional must obtain the patient's written permission to share their PHI with other health care professionals, insurance companies, friends and family, or for the collection of data for a directory or any other purpose.

It is important to understand that HIPAA is a federal law and in states where a more protective law exists the HIPAA rules do not override such state laws. For example, some states allow minors between the ages of 16 – 18, the right to their own privacy if it concerns their reproductive health (3). It is important to abide by both the HIPAA rules and state rules where the health care professional practices.

References

2. American Nurses Association - https://www.nursingworld.org/~4ad4a8/globalassets/docs/ana/position-statement-privacy-and-confidentiality.pdf

3. The Office for the National Coordinator for Health Information Technology. Guide to Privacy and Security of Electronic Health Information.

https://www.healthit.gov/sites/default/files/pdf/privacy/privacy-and-security-guide.pdf

4. A visual grid to digitally record an Ayurvedic Prakriti assessment; a first step toward integrated electronic health records - https://www.sciencedirect.com/science/article/pii/S2225411016300451

Chapter 25: Review

ADDITIONAL READING

Utilize these references to expand your understanding of the concepts in this chapter.

REQUIRED READING	Chapters
A visual grid to digitally record an Ayurvedic Prakriti assessment; a first step toward integrated electronic health records, https://www.sciencedirect.com/science/article/pii/S2225411016300451	
American Nurses Association Position Statement on Privacy and Confidentiality, https://www.nursingworld.org/~4ad4a8/globalassets/docs/ana/position-statement-privacy-and-confidentiality.pdf	

OPTIONAL READING	Format
AyurEHR, http://www.erxsolutions.in/	
Guide to Privacy and Security of Electronic Health Information, https://www.healthit.gov/sites/default/files/pdf/privacy/privacy-and-security-guide.pdf	

References

QUESTIONS & ANSWERS

Record your questions for this chapter here for further research and discussion.

Question:

Answer:

Question:

Answer:

Question:

Answer:

SELF-ASSESSMENT

1. Communication among Āyurvedic health care professionals can
   a. appear quite different from Western medical terminology
   b. be unfamiliar to non-professionals
   c. include specialized Āyurvedic terminology
   d. All of the above
   e. None of the above

2. Formal records of Āyurvedic practice are generally
   a. available to Āyurvedic doctors only
   b. electronic health records
   c. only written in Sanskrit
   d. recorded independently in various practices
   e. shared through a worldwide network

3. A major challenge in standardizing Āyurvedic health records is
   a. lack of international regulation
   b. lack of standard record format
   c. overuse of technology
   d. All of the above
   e. None of the above

4. EHR for Āyurveda would be best to establish where
   a. advanced Āyurveda is practiced
   b. Āyurvedic doctors are not legally recognized
   c. health care companies are highly advanced
   d. in Asia
   e. All of the above

5. Protection of personal and medical information is
   a. a core value in health care
   b. a strong reflection of ethical and professional practice
   c. considered a patient's right to privacy
   d. All of the above
   e. None of the above

6. Making patient's EHR available to other health care providers carries inherent risks such as
   a. advanced care in critical emergencies
   b. data breaches
   c. doctor's access to patient history
   d. loss of data during power outages
   e. patient's access to their own data

7. Implementation of HIPAA in Āyurvedic practice is
   a. a minimum requirement for practice
   b. a standard type of PHI
   c. challenging due to financial requirements
   d. the patient's choice in services
   e. None of the above

8. Under HIPAA, PHI is protected by
   a. administrative health care professionals
   b. billing departments of health care
   c. doctors, nurses and staff
   d. health care insurance providers
   e. All of the above

9. In Āyurvedic practice that is not HIPAA compliant, PHI should be
   a. discussed openly in professional forums
   b. made available only to the client
   c. shared with anyone who requests it
   d. shredded immediately
   e. stored in an unlocked cabinet

10. A patient's right to privacy covers
    a. personal choices
    b. personal data
    c. personal relationships
    d. personal space
    e. All of the above

Chapter 26 : Advancing the Āyurvedic profession

SVASTHA ĀCĀRYA COMPETENCY GUIDELINES	
2.5.0	Health care standards for Āyurveda
2.5.2	Explain methods for advancing Āyurveda and provide examples of valid methods for demonstrating outcomes
2.5.3	Define anecdotal evidence and explain its common usage and limitations

KEY TERMS

anecdotal evidence

"The research paradigm in Āyurveda needs to lean more towards studies of efficiency instead of 'evidence'. We need to let go of the thought of trying to prove something to people who don't believe (more because of the paradigm than because of the evidence)."

- Freedom Cole, May 12, 2018

For over one hundred years, the professional Āyurvedic community in India has been expressing the need for improved standards in education and practice. To advance the profession, the foundation of students, practitioners, researchers, scientists and others involved needs to cooperate and collaborate in a productive way. Because of many obstacles, these advancements have been delayed and debated for decades with little improvement.

Today, with the relatively quick global spread of Āyurveda, the same needs are now being amplified. With current tools and technology, Āyurveda has an even greater potential to develop into a global, professional practice. The first half of the 21st century will hopefully see major changes and developments for Āyurveda.

ADVANCING ĀYURVEDA

Many possibilities exist for advancing Āyurveda today. The range of these methods span from tried and tested approaches to truly radical reform.

Considering these options, it is important that the recent history of Āyurveda be critically reviewed. Over the last few centuries the influence of colonialism has lead to severe marginalization of Āyurveda. This attitude has consciously and subconsciously become deeply engrained in virtually every aspect of the science. Āyurvedic professionals in India have and continue to struggle to break free from this position. The long-lasting effects of colonialism continue to dampen the authentic spirit of the science and limit its potential for true innovation.

If well-established in a creative, bold environment that supports advancement and innovation, Āyurveda is poised to develop rapidly. Advancement of the science intends to maintain its solid foundations in classical principles and practice while integrating modern perspectives and approaches.

A few examples of methods for advancing Āyurveda include:

- utilitizing technology
- forward thinking approaches
- refraining from using language like ancient
- focusing on adaptability and applicability in modern cultures

Research and development are prime areas for advancement of Āyurveda. However, the approach to designing study models must reflect the inherent intelligence of the holistic framework. It cannot simply base itself in Western frameworks and attempt to modify or adjust in certain ways to accommodate Āyurveda. This is the exact behavior which has denigrated the science for centuries and professionals must be ready to separate themselves from these approaches.

Rather than continue to "prove" Āyurveda to an establishment that typically views it with an inherent bias, Āyurvedic professionals should completely ignore any need for justification from the Western scientific community. Instead, they should establish themselves as Āyurvedic scientists and direct their tefforts toward establishing a proper foundation rooted in the authentic, holistic framework of Āyurveda.

Through these efforts of trial, error, research and refinement, true advancement of the science is possible. Valid scientific methodologies can be applied logically, accurately and most importantly, creatively, to demonstrate outcomes that are true to Āyurvedic science.

Many methods that are considered commonly accepted today are not relevant for an Āyurvedic framework. These include methods and approaches utilized in Randomized Controlled Trials and Evidence-based Medicine. The inherent nature of holistic systems is structured in a circular, non-linear fashion compared to reductionist approaches. These inherent differences demand that testing architecutres be designed specifically to reflect the nature of the system accurately.

Lastly, to bolster the reputation and respect of Āyurveda, professionals must caution the common, widespread use of anecdotal evidence. The Merriam-Webster Dictionary defines anecdotal evidence as (anecdotal evidence, 2019):

1. evidence in the form of stories that people tell about what has happened to them

While these types of "success stories" often help convince individuals to try Āyurveda for themselves, they do little to support the image among the scientific community. Instead, Āyurvedic professionals must recognize and accept responsibility to advance the science and its practice using means that are true and authentic to the original system.

TEST YOURSELF

Learn, review and memorize key terms from this section.

anecdotal evidence

Chapter 26: Review

ADDITIONAL READING

Utilize these references to expand your understanding of the concepts in this chapter.

REQUIRED READING	Chapters
Vaidya-scientists: catalysing Ayurveda renaissance, https://www.researchgate.net/publication/235330134_Vaidya-Scientists_Catalysing_Ayurveda_Renaissance	

OPTIONAL READING	Format

References

"Anecdotal evidence." Merriam-Webster Dictionary, 2019, https://www.merriam-webster.com/dictionary/anecdotal%20evidence.

Patwardhan, Bhushan & Joglekar, Vishnu & Pathak, Namyata & Vaidya, Ashok. (2011). Vaidya-Scientists: Catalysing Ayurveda Renaissance. Current science. 100. 476-486.

QUESTIONS & ANSWERS

Record your questions for this chapter here for further research and discussion.

Question:

Answer:

Question:

Answer:

Question:

Answer:

SELF-ASSESSMENT

1. Research frameworks for Āyurveda that are based on Western science are inherently
   a. factual
   b. holistic
   c. precise
   d. reductionist
   e. standardized

2. Colonial influence has negatively impacted Āyurveda's
   a. advancement
   b. innovation
   c. practical scope
   d. research
   e. All of the above

3. Western science typically perceives Āyurveda
   a. ancient
   b. as unscientific
   c. with inherent bias
   d. All of the above
   e. None of the above

4. Western research methodologies limit Āyurveda's
   a. classical literature
   b. inherent holism
   c. linear-based approach
   d. All of the above
   e. None of the above

5. Anecdotal evidence is beneficial for Āyurveda's
   a. advancement in Western Medicine
   b. demonstration of scientific outcomes
   c. large-scale research
   d. mass marketing appeal
   e. All of the above

6. Referring to Āyurveda as "ancient" promotes an image within scientific communities of
   a. lack of research and development
   b. natural wisdom
   c. static nature
   d. Both A and B
   e. Both A and C

7. Scientific innovation in Āyurveda
   a. has been prevalent since colonialism in India
   b. is largely absent globally
   c. occurs commonly today
   d. requires Western scientific methodologies
   e. All of the above

8. Research models that accurately represent Āyurveda include
   a. evidence-based medicine
   b. holistic models
   c. randomized controlled trials
   d. All of the above
   e. None of the above

9. Advancement of Āyurveda could occur with
   a. cutting-edge technology
   b. innovative perspectives
   c. scientific, classical methodologies
   d. All of the above
   e. None of the above

10. Anecdotal evidence should be utilized in Āyurveda to
    a. demonstrate efficacy
    b. highlight the need for valid research
    c. prove outcomes scientifically
    d. All of the above
    e. None of the above

Chapter 27 : Professional Āyurvedic community

The professional Āyurvedic community includes many levels and varieties of organizations and individuals on local, national and global levels. These vary largely by country to meet the demands and expectations of professional education and practice.

INTERNATIONAL ORGANIZATIONS

The most prominent international organization that represents Traditional Medicine including Āyurveda is the World Health Organization. The WHO has been publishing information and recommendations on the education and practice of Āyurveda as Traditional medicine since the early 2000's.

As part of the 2003 WHO resolution on Traditional medicine, member states were urged to organize and utilize their Traditional medical practices on a national level and provide regulation for licensing and practice. To better support these efforts, the WHO published Benchmarks for training in Ayurveda in 2010 to provide guidance and recommendations on a number of issues. In 2013, the publication WHO traditional medicine strategy: 2014-2023 was published as an update to the 2002 strategy.

One of the significant differences with the WHO approach is in the wording used for classification. Systems like Āyurveda are considered "Traditional Medicine" rather than "Complementary and Alternative." This is an important distinction which allows complete systems of medicine to be recognized as Whole Medical Systems capable of providing primary health care.

http://apps.who.int/medicinedocs/documents/s17552en/s17552en.pdf

http://apps.who.int/gb/archive/pdf_files/WHA56/ea56r31.pdf

http://www.searo.who.int/entity/health_situation_trends/who_trm_strategy_2014-2023.pdf?ua=1

UNITED STATES OF AMERICA

Within the US, several organizations exist on national and state levels. Primary aims and objectives of most of these groups include professional representation, establishment of standards, definitions of scopes of practice and other regulatory efforts.

National organizations

Three notable organizations currently exist on the national level in the US. Each represents Āyurveda in varying degrees and approaches.

ĀYU Council

ĀYU Council represents the diverse profession of Āyurveda in the United States of America. It recognizes the full scope of Āyurveda for primary, holistic and sustainable health care.

ĀYU Council adheres to classical foundations of Āyurveda and promotes the growth and establishment of the science as a complete medical system. It acknowledges the need for adapting the practice of Āyurveda to the American culture rather than strictly following Indian standards of implementation.

ĀYU Council is establishing the most competent levels of education and practice for Āyurveda outside of India. It certifies professionals at the following levels:

1. Svastha Āchārya (SA)

2. Parichāraka (PC)
3. Āyurveda Āchārya (AA)

Each of these levels is rooted in the classical Āyurvedic health care infrastructure. All three can work independently and collaboratively to provide primary and integrative Āyurvedic health care.

ĀYU Council actively works to maintain classical authenticity and bring innovation to the field. ĀYU Council promotes the practice of Āyurveda under the scope of Health Freedom to avoid unnecessary efforts towards licensure and the inherent limitations that it imposes.

https://www.ayucouncil.org/

NAMA

The National Ayurvedic Medical Association (NAMA) is a national organization representing the Āyurvedic profession in The United States of America. Its mission includes goals to establish and maintain standards of education, ethics, professional competency and licensing.

The organization has been operating since 2000 to support Āyurvedic education and practice, and is developing scopes of practice, national exams and other means to promote coherence within the Āyurvedic profession around its structure of three levels of professionals:

1. Ayurvedic Health Counselor (AHC)
2. Ayurvedic Practitioner (AP)
3. Ayurvedic Doctor (AD)

NAMA is actively and prematurely pursuing accreditation and licensing of Āyurveda based on insufficient standards for education and practice.

Historically, however, the organization has largely supported and defended the proliferation of New Age Āyurveda within the United States. It has resisted many of the challenges inherent in proper classical Āyurvedic training by ignoring key, required components such as Sanskrit.

It has grossly underestimated the potential of Āyurveda as a primary health care system and demonstrates repeatedly that it acts primarily to protect its commercial educational base.

https://www.ayurvedanama.org/

AAPNA

The Association of Ayurvedic Professionals of North America (AAPNA) is an organization representing the Āyurvedic profession in North America. The organization has established many titles for various levels of practice and awards them to individuals who can demonstrate that they have completed a certain amount of training.

https://www.aapna.org/

State organizations

Several state organization currently exist in the US. Their representative are closely tied to NAMA and are presently working towards unrealistic goals for the profession.

The California Association of Ayurvedic Medicine (CAAM) represents the Āyurvedic profession in the state of California. It takes a strongly superficial approach to the education and practice of the profession and largely promotes New Age Āyurveda.

The Colorado Ayurvedic Medical Association (COLORAMA) represents the Āyurvedic profession in the state of Colorado. It has developed mainly from lineage-based proponents of Āyurveda.

A few additional state organizations exist throughout the country. It should be clearly noted here that the major drivers behind the long-standing national and state organizations in the US are built upon incomplete and inconsistent training in the practice of classical Āyurveda.

If the efforts of these organizations succeed in establishing Āyurveda's legal scope within the US, there will likely be significant, long-term repercussions due to their lack of understanding of the complete science and their ability to properly represent its full scope of practice.

ADVOCACY GROUPS

In addition to the groups mentioned earlier, there are several advocacy groups who promote concepts including medical pluralism, sustainable healthcare, and natural, non-invasive approaches to health care. Professionals in natural and holistic health care should be aware of these groups and others and utilize them as a resource as needed.

Alliance for Natural Health

The Alliance for Natural Health USA (ANH-USA), is part of an international organization dedicated to promoting sustainable health and freedom of choice in health care through good science and good law.

They protect the right of natural health practitioners to practice and the right of consumers to choose the health care options they prefer. Since 1992, they have worked to shift the medical paradigm from an exclusive focus on surgery, drugs and other conventional techniques to an "integrative" approach incorporating food, dietary supplements and lifestyle changes. ANH-USA is paving a path toward sustainable health care through preventive health measures and bringing the cost of health care back to a reasonable level.

ANH-USA is committed to sustainable health and recognizes the environment and physical health are inextricably related. The ANH-USA understands human health will suffer if air and water are polluted, and human consumption and exposure to synthetic chemicals in food, products and medicine continues. ANH-USA is working to ensure individuals have the right to choose a sustainable and preventive approach to health along with nutritional integrative health care. The organization lobbies Congress and state legislatures, acts as a government watchdog, files comments on proposed rulings, and educates the public, press and other decision-makers.

Sustainable health also applies to the environmental ethic of conservation of the physical body designed to live in tune with nature. A high-quality diet, appropriate supplements, exercise and the avoidance of toxins are especially important tools in building and maintaining health. Sustainable health is also about financial sustainability. Higher health care costs lead directly to higher unemployment and lower standards of living, both of which can lead to obstacles in health management. Western medicine is too often defined as taking more drugs and vaccines at an earlier and earlier age. The concept of sustainable health lies with disease prevention while improving the vitality of humanity and dramatically reducing the cost of sick care.

http://www.anh-usa.org/

https://www.anhinternational.org/

Chapter 27: Review

ADDITIONAL READING

Utilize these references to expand your understanding of the concepts in this chapter.

REQUIRED READING	Chapters

OPTIONAL READING	Format

References

QUESTIONS & ANSWERS

Record your questions for this chapter here for further research and discussion.

Question:

Answer:

Question:

Answer:

Question:

Answer:

SELF-ASSESSMENT

1. The WHO Benchmarks for Training in Ayurveda state that training for Āyurvedic practitioners begins with
   a. Hindi
   b. Sanskrit
   c. Vedic spirituality
   d. All of the above
   e. None of the above

2. According to the WHO Benchmarks for Training in Ayurveda, Āyurvedic education started becoming institutionalized in the
   a. 7th century
   b. 14th century
   c. 16th century
   d. 19th century
   e. 20th century

3. The WHO classifies Āyurveda as
   a. Alternative medicine
   b. Complementary health care
   c. Integrative medicine
   d. Siddha medicine
   e. Traditional medicine

4. In 2003, the WHO urged member states to
   a. approve licenses for international practitioners
   b. expand natural treatment modalities
   c. formulate and implement national policies and regulations on traditional medicine
   d. increase production of medicines for global distribution
   e. train practitioners according to WHO guidelines

5. The WHO Benchmarks for Training in Ayurveda recognizes professionals at the levels of
   a. Āyurveda dispensers
   b. Āyurveda distributors
   c. Āyurveda practitioner
   d. Āyurveda therapist
   e. All of the above

6. The Āyurvedic profession is represented in the US by
   a. AAPNA
   b. ĀYU Council
   c. NAMA
   d. All of the above
   e. None of the above

7. The US organization that represents Āyurveda based on classical practice methodologies is
   a. AAPNA
   b. ANH-USA
   c. ĀYU Council
   d. NAMA
   e. WHO

8. The longest running national organization that represents Āyurveda in the US is
   a. AAPNA
   b. ANH-USA
   c. CAAM
   d. ĀYU Council
   e. NAMA

9. The concept of sustainable health care was first recognized by
   a. AAPNA
   b. ANH-USA
   c. CAAM
   d. ĀYU Council
   e. NAMA

10. Premature licensing of Āyurveda in the US will most likely
    a. create long-term repercussions for legal Āyurvedic practice
    b. ignore the full potential of Āyurveda as a Whole Medical System
    c. limit its scope of practice
    d. All of the above
    e. None of the above

Unit Review

ORAL EXAM QUESTIONS

Use these questions to prepare answers for the oral examination. You may create written statements or cue cards to memorize the key points that should be included in your response. Scoring is based on your accuracy, brevity, clarity (ABC), use of Sanskrit terms and concepts, and confidence.

1. How can commitment to Āyurveda as an ethical profession help fulfill one's puruṣhārthas?
2. Consider the progress of Āyurvedic education where you live and cite three reasons that have influenced its development.
3. Identify three ideal qualities that you want to develop in yourself over the course of your professional education. Create a plan with specific, attainable goals that will help you succeed in professional and personal development.
4. Do you view market demand for Āyurveda outside India as a beneficial or detrimental driver for the growth of authentic Āyurveda? Explain your reasoning using examples from the context of general society or within your community.
5. Choose one of the obstacles to the practice of Āyurveda outside India and elaborate on it. Explain how it can directly affect individual professionals. Provide solutions or work-arounds.
6. Have you considered what types of Āyurvedic professional activities might be appropriate for you after completing professional education and training? Identify benefits and drawbacks for these possibilities.
7. What are five accusations of prima facie and explain the defense statements that a practitioner could use against such accusations. What is the most important action to take when accused?
8. Consider the current practice of Āyurveda in India and compare it to the types of modalities listed in Appendix 1. What is an appropriate classification for Āyurveda - as a complete system or disparate practice? Cite the reasons within the context of medical pluralism.
9. Is communication between Āyurvedic professionals in India and the US important? Why or why not?
10. What do you see as the top three areas of focus for development of professional Āyurveda? Identify them and briefly explain how they could be implemented.
11. Research the educational requirements listed by the WHO, NAMA and AAPNA at any one professional level. Compare and contrast the expected outcomes of students at similar levels of education.

MODERN AND GLOBAL AYURVEDA

1. What stands out from this chapter for you on a personal or professional level?
2. Do you think Svoboda's account of education is still accurate today?
3. What significant insights does Welch provide about the professional Āyurvedic educational system in India?
4. Considering the shortcomings mentioned by Welch in this chapter, are there opportunities for improvement? Where?
5. Do you believe that Āyurveda should strive for "standardization"? Why or why not?

UNIT V

Sanskrit Prerequisites for Āyurveda

Chapter 28 : Indic languages

KEY TERMS

Devanāgarī	Hindi	Malayalam	Tamil
Gujarati	Kannada	Marāṭhi	

A basic understanding of Indic languages is key to accessing many levels of knowledge and practice within Āyurveda. The development of Āyurvedic science has been deeply intertwined with the language and culture of the Indian subcontinent for thousands of years and its practice today reflects these connections.

From the earliest records of Āyurveda, Sanskrit has been the primary language. It holds a high place in Vedic and Hindu societies as the most respected language of scholars and practitioners.

Permanent records of Āyurveda and most streams of classical Vedic knowledge have always been retained and guarded in Sanskrit. Based on these original records, supplementary materials in local languages have been written to spread the science regionally.

SANSKRIT'S ORIGINS AND USE TODAY

Similar to Āyurveda, the true origins of the Sanskrit language may never be fully known. Many historians have presented various theories and views to explain the history and origins. The two major proposed theories argue the Indo-Aryan origin versus the Indian subcontinent origin.

One group states that evidence exists to demonstrate that Sanskrit originated in the areas currently known as Syria, Turkey and Iraq, as a Proto-Indo-European language. As its peoples migrated east, it transformed in the Indo-Iranian form, which became the foundation for the Vedic Sanskrit that was used to record the Vedas. From here, the language found a more permanent home in the Indian subcontinent and has since been known as Sanskrit. This theory is more often adhered to by proponents of a European-centric view of world history.

Another group states that the language was born in the Indian subcontinent and arose from there. They consider the lack of evidence prior to the Vedas, or non-acceptance of evidence, sufficient to support this view. This is the perspective more commonly supported by Indian historians who claim the language, culture and origins to have originated in the Indian subcontinent.

Various forms of historical evidence may help estimate the time periods that surviving texts can be ascribed to. For example, the Vedas are generally accepted to have been recorded around the time of the 5th century BCE or earlier. Based on this, additional texts may be placed in approximate time ranges by also considering their content, references to other texts and major events.

One significant text which continues to hold a primary position is the compilation of the rules of Sanskrit grammar codified by Pāṇini, who is considered to be the father of Sanskrit grammar. His work lays out all of the details of the language in a manner which is more succinct and efficient compared to any other grammarian to date (O'Connor, J. J. and Robertson, E. F., 2000).

Sanskrit itself has not survived as a very

popular language for everyday communication, however. Its main uses today include transmission of Vedic knowledge, continuation of classical texts and manuscripts, and recitation for religious functions.

There are very few villages in India which continue to use it as a primary means of communication today. According to the 2011 Census of India, approximately 25,000 people in the entire country reported Sanskrit to be their first or mother language (Census of India, 2011).

The Modi government is working to change this by promoting a "Sanskrit revival" as part of its overall agenda to promote traditional Hindu culture. It is working to popularize the language for common use and on a national level. The language is also attracting popularity outside India where universities in some countries, including Germany, are offering more courses to meet student demand.

Sanskrit likely appeals to Germans because of commonalities in both languages in their structure and order. Sanskrit has been a focus for German scholars for centuries. Recently, Germany has also established advanced training and practice for Āyurveda.

MODERN INDIC LANGUAGES

As one of the oldest, continuously used languages of the Indian subcontinent, Sanskrit provides the base for many modern Indian languages. Many of these derivative languages continue to use the *Devanāgarī* script with minor modifications to their written forms and speech.

For example, the Vedic *Devanāgarī* Sanskṛit alphabet is slightly larger than the currently used *Devanāgarī* alphabet of Hindi. And with both languages, pronunciation rules differ in subtle but significant ways.

The Indian subcontinent is one of the more culturally and linguistically rich areas in the world today. Over 19,000 languages and dialects are in use today (Census of India, 2011).

Virtually any of the Indic languages, their scripts and alphabets can be used in conjunction with Āyurveda. The official languages of India that are commonly used with Āyurveda include:

Gujarati	state of Gujarat
Hindi	common language of many states in North India
Kannada	state of Karnataka
Malayalam	state of Kerala
Marāṭhi	state of Maharashtra
Tamil	state of Tamil Nadu

Each of these languages, and many others, shares a similar vocabulary with Sanskrit and classical Āyurvedic terminology.

Additionally, they all find similarities in their alphabet, some more than others. For example, Hindi uses a somewhat smaller alphabet written in the same *Devanāgarī* script. Other languages like Gujarati, Kannada, Malalayam and Marāṭhi follow the same or similar alphabet phonetically but are written in a different script.

In addition to slight variations between Sanskrit's Vedic *Devanāgarī* script and modernized scripts for local languages, pronunciation variations also exist. To native speakers of any of these Indian languages, these minor pronunciation variations are clear and obvious enough to easily identify an individual's native location within the country.

Native Hindi speakers follow abbreviated pronunciation rules compared to Sanskrit. This typically results in the shortening of classical Āyurvedic terms when they are mixed with Hindi.

Native Malayalam speakers generally add an "uhm" sound to the endings of many words. This becomes quickly apparent when classical Sanskrit terms are spoken within Malayalam because of the conspicuous extra ending sound.

In written formats, both of these alterations to classical Āyurvedic terminologies also become quickly apparent. These variations can help explain the wide variety of spellings seen in common terms when they are written using the Roman alphabet.

Examples for these variations will be reviewed in detail in the following chapters along with the concepts of translation and transliteration.

Compare the various scripts used to write some of these languages:

Gujarati is written in Gujarati script.

Gujarati = ગુજરાતી

Hindi is written in *Devanāgarī* script.

Devanāgarī = देवनागरी

Kannada is written in Kannada script.

Kannada = ಕನ್ನಡ

Malayalam is written in Malayalam script.

Malayalam = മലയാളം

Marāṭhi is written in *Devanāgarī* script.

Marāṭhi = देवनागरी

Tamil is written in Tamil script.

Tamil = தமிழ்

TEST YOURSELF

Learn, review and memorize key terms from this section.

Devanāgarī

Gujarati

Hindi

Kannada

Malayalam

Marāṭhi

Tamil

Chapter 28: Review

ADDITIONAL READING

Utilize these references to expand your understanding of the concepts in this chapter.

REQUIRED READING	Chapters
Panini, http://www-history.mcs.st-andrews.ac.uk/Biographies/Panini.html	

OPTIONAL READING	Format
The Genomic Formation of South and Central Asia https://www.biorxiv.org/content/biorxiv/early/2018/03/31/292581.full.pdf	

References

Census of India, 2011. http://censusindia.gov.in/2011Census/C-16_25062018_NEW.pdf

O'Connor, J. J. and Robertson, E F. November 2000, "Panini." JOC/EFR. School of Mathematics and Statistics University of St Andrews, Scotland http://www-history.mcs.st-andrews.ac.uk/Biographies/Panini.html

QUESTIONS & ANSWERS

Record your questions for this chapter here for further research and discussion.

Question:

Answer:

Question:

Answer:

Question:

Answer:

SELF-ASSESSMENT

1. The origins of Sanskrit
   a. are dated to 5 BCE
   b. are explained by the Indo-Aryan origin theory
   c. are in modern-day Syria
   d. may never be fully known
   e. All of the above

2. Modern Hindi is written in
   a. *Devanāgarī*
   b. Hindi alphabet
   c. Pāṇinī
   d. Sanskrit
   e. None of the above

3. Vedic *Devanāgarī* is _______ than modern *Devanāgarī*.
   a. different
   b. larger
   c. smaller
   d. the same size as
   e. None of the above

4. Which modern Indian language uses the *Devanāgarī* script?
   a. Gujarati
   b. Hindi
   c. Malayalam
   d. Marāṭhi
   e. Tamil

5. The Census of India (2011) recorded a total of approximately
   a. 121 languages
   b. 10,000 languages
   c. 14,000 languages
   d. 19,000 languages
   e. 25,000 languages

6. Interest in Sanskrit and development of Āyurveda is seen today in
   a. France
   b. Germany
   c. Italy
   d. South America
   e. the United Arab Emirates

7. Today in India, Sanskrit is spoken mostly in
   a. business offices
   b. government buildings
   c. large cities
   d. North India
   e. only a few villages

8. Who is considered the father of Sanskrit?
   a. Charaka
   b. *Devanāgarī*
   c. Kālidāsa
   d. Pāṇini
   e. Suśhruta

9. A modern Indian language that adds an "uhm" sound to classical Āyurvedic terms is
   a. Gujarati
   b. Hindi
   c. Kannada
   d. Malayalam
   e. Marāṭhi

10. Since its earliest records, Āyurveda has been written in
    a. Hindi
    b. Sanskrit
    c. Vedic *Devanāgarī*
    d. Both A and B
    e. Both B and C

Chapter 29 : Goals and expectations

Learning Sanskrit for professional Āyurveda has distinct goals and expectations at various levels of study and practice. Depending on the duration and depth of study, and the intended scope of practice, Sanskrit requirements can differ greatly.

At a minimum level, Āyurvedic professionals who have not previously studied Sanskrit should expect to:

1. Learn the origins, background and significant history of the language.
2. Memorize the complete Vedic *Devanāgarī* (the Sanskrit alphabet) in ĀYUT-transliterated form for use in English.
3. Understand the core, mechanical differences between the *Devanāgarī* and Roman or Latin alphabets.
4. Pronounce each *akṣhara* (syllable) of the *Devanāgarī* alphabet and explain its method of proper pronunciation.
5. Identify all types of *akṣharas*, schwa, *virāma*, half consonants, conjunct consonants and *sandhi*, and explain the usage of each.
6. Demonstrate *akṣhara* notation.
7. Combine *akṣharas* to create words.
8. Dissect words to their component *akṣharas*.
9. Read and write Sanskrit through ĀYUT-transliteration.
10. Continue to learn additional transliteration methods.

One common misconception is that Āyurvedic professionals are required to read and write the original *Devanāgarī* script and be able to translate it. This level of Sanskrit study takes years for basic competency and adds a significant amount of time onto the total study duration.

For professionals levels including the Āyurvedic Health Coach, the Svastha Āchārya and the Parichāraka, an advanced requirement for Sanskrit is not necessary. It is much more important for these levels to have a strong vocabulary providing a broad and deep understanding of Āyurvedic concepts so they can be thoroughly explained to a variety of audiences.

In advanced Āyurvedic studies and practice at the Āyurveda Āchārya and above, reading and writing in the original *Devanāgarī* script is required. Advanced levels also must have a basic understanding of grammar. Translation becomes much more important as it opens the door to accessing the classical texts in a deeper way, allowing one to read and comprehend the intention of original classical texts. It also makes the commentaries accessible. These are critical for fully understanding and applying the science at advanced levels.

Over time, more classical Āyurvedic works will likely be translated into English. However, the quality of translations must also be considered when expecting to learn the original information. Until the original concepts become accessible in a language other than Sanskrit, it is best for true students and practitioners to appreciate and understand the need for learning Sanskrit.

Resources such as the free, online e-Samhitas from the Central Council for Research in Āyurveda and Siddha (CCRAS), New Delhi, are providing much needed access to classical literature.

Chapter 29: Review

ADDITIONAL READING

Utilize these references to expand your understanding of the concepts in this chapter.

CLASSICS	1st read	2nd read

REQUIRED READING	Chapters

OPTIONAL READING	Format
Charaka Saṁhitā, e-Samhita (CCRAS) http://niimh.nic.in/ebooks/ecaraka/	Online
Suśhruta Saṁhitā, e-Samhita (CCRAS) http://niimh.nic.in/ebooks/esushruta/	Online

References

QUESTIONS & ANSWERS

Record your questions for this chapter here for further research and discussion.

Question:

Answer:

Question:

Answer:

Question:

Answer:

SELF-ASSESSMENT

1. The expectation to learn Sanskrit depends on the
   a. depth of study
   b. duration of study
   c. intended scope of practice
   d. All the above
   e. None of the above

2. A basic Sanskrit skill required by entry-level Āyurvedic professionals is to
   a. be proficient in grammar
   b. combine *akṣharas* to create words
   c. create and translate sentences
   d. memorize the original *Devanāgarī* script
   e. All of the above

3. For Svastha Āchāryas, the primary use of Sanskrit is for
   a. enumeration of numbers
   b. grammar
   c. terminology
   d. All the above
   e. None of the above

4. Why is learning the original *Devanāgarī* script useful?
   a. to learn proper Sanskrit pronunciation
   b. to read classical commentaries
   c. to recite *mantras*
   d. All the above
   e. None of the above

5. For entry-level Āyurvedic training, the Vedic *Devanāgarī* script must be memorized
   a. in ĀYUT transliterated form
   b. in its modern, Hindi form
   c. in its original form
   d. All of the above
   e. None of the above

6. Sanskrit is required for professional Āyurveda because
   a. all classical texts are translated in English
   b. classical translations in English are always accurate
   c. only classical commentaries are in Sanskrit
   d. All of the above
   e. None of the above

7. The *Devanāgarī* alphabet is pronounced through
   a. *akṣharas*
   b. consonants
   c. schwa
   d. *virāma*
   e. vowels

8. For most Westerners, learning to fluently read and write classical Sanskrit in the original *Devanāgarī* script often requires
   a. about six months
   b. one month of full-time study
   c. one year of part-time study
   d. several weekend courses
   e. years of dedicated study

9. Learning a comprehensive vocabulary of classical Āyurvedic terms allows a professional to
   a. communicate concepts to larger audiences
   b. speak Sanskrit fluently
   c. spell all words correctly in Sanskrit
   d. All of the above
   e. None of the above

10. For non-Āyurvedic professionals, Sanskrit is
    a. a required subject to master
    b. an exclusive tool only available to serious candidates
    c. helpful to understand holistic Āyurvedic concepts
    d. necessary for complete treatment
    e. All of the above

Chapter 30 : Translation and transliteration

KEY TERMS

akṣhara	lossless matching	syllable	vaṭa
diacrtitical mark	Saṁskṛta	translation	vāta
ĀYUT	Sanskrit	transliteration	

Since the earliest written records of Āyurveda, Sanskrit has been the language of choice. It has encapsulated and encoded the science using poetry and prose, and conveyed many layers of knowledge with a highly specialized vocabulary. Over time this knowledge and its written formats were highly refined. Maintaining continuity of advanced practice has been challenged over the last several hundred years. The full depth of understanding has reduced, leaving fewer specialized individuals to practice today.

Additionally, the hyper-specialization of the science presents a challenge to translate the information thoroughly and effectively into other languages, especially English.

Because of these challenges, some level of Sanskrit must be learned by all who study and practice Traditional Āyurvedic Medicine in a professional capacity. The majority of learning required is memorization of vocabulary terms with their correct transliteration and spelling.

Each term is often accompanied by one or more conceptual meanings which can vary according to context, rather than single word-for-word translations. Sanskrit study at this level provides the jargon of the profession with specialized terminologies.

In Sanskrit, knowledge is layered using terms with multiple meanings. To understand the full implications of the original statements, translation often requires contextual disambiguation with multiple passes. This is one reason why the key to understanding authentic Āyurvedic knowledge lies in the ability to understand the original Sanskrit.

In Charaka Saṁhitā *sūtrasthāna*, chapter 6, the student Agniveśha asks his teacher Punarvāsu Ātreya who the text is written for. The teacher responds that it is intended for the lowest level of students (on a scale of low, medium, and high), so that it is accessible in its most basic level.

Students at the medium and high levels are expected to grasp additional meanings of the text in deeper ways, depending on their ability to understand the language and apply their logical thought processes. Those who can extract multiple accurate meanings and interpretations from the text have a clear advantage to understanding the full depth and breadth of the science.

TRANSLATION AND TRANSLITERATION

Two terms that will be used throughout the career of an Āyurvedic professional are translation and transliteration. Review and memorize the definitions of each of these terms with their distinctions.

The Merriam Webster Dictionary defines translation as (Translation, 2018):

1. An act, process, or instance of translating: such as
    a. a rendering from one language into another; also :

the product of such a rendering

b. a change to a different substance, form, or appearance

Translate means (Translate, 2018)

1. To turn into one's own or another language
2. To transfer or turn from one set of symbols into another : transcribe
3. To express in different terms and especially different words : paraphrase
4. To express in more comprehensible terms : explain, interpret

Applied in the context of Āyurvedic medical education, translation is essentially the process of converting any original content or information from its existing form (often in Sanskrit) into another language, while maintaining its original meaning, quality and intention.

Maintaining originality and authenticity can be easy or difficult depending on the language that it's being translated into. For example, translating classical texts into most modern Indian languages like Hindi or Malayalam is relatively easy, whereas translating the same content accurately into English is often difficult or impossible. This is mainly due to the availability of terms that accurately express the specific meaning and completeness of the concept. English lacks in many of these terms whereas most modern Indian languages find them in common use today.

The Merriam Webster Dictionary defines transliterate as (Transliterate, 2018):

1. To represent or spell in the characters of another alphabet

Transliteration allows the original *akṣharas* of Sanskrit terms to be taken from the *Devanāgarī* alphabet and represented accurately using letters from the Roman alphabet.

Because *Devanāgarī* contains more *akṣharas*, or syllables than the letters in the Roman alphabet, additional representations are required to fully and accurately express all of the sounds as letters in the Roman alphabet.

To do this, several Roman letters are modified by adding diacritical marks. This creates additional letters that allow the two alphabets to be mapped in a unique, one-to-one fashion. This is called lossless matching.

Transliteration methods

There are several international methods of transliteration. They include:

1. ĀYUT

   Āyurvedic Universal Transliteration

2. IAST

   International Alphabet of Sanskrit Transliteration

3. Harvard-Kyoto
4. ITRANS
5. SLP1

ĀYUT is the transliteration method used through this textbook. It is based on IAST and is adapted to provide more user-friendly pronunciation. It is simpler than IAST and faster for students who are not studying advanced Sanskrit.

IAST is the standard transliteration method used in academics since the early 20th century. While this transliteration method is one of the most common for scholarly publications, others are also commonly used in various applications, especially for digital representations of Sanskrit.

Several variant transliteration schemes are used within specialized areas of study, including Āyurveda. With regular use of transliteration, the subtle but significant differences in transliteration schemes will become easier to recognize.

All methods follow clear rules that allow Sanskrit to be represented accurately in the Roman alphabet with lossless matching.

The following table describes the diacritical marks used in ĀYUT transliterated Sansrkrit.

Type of diacritic	*Akṣharas*
Long bar	ā, ī, ū, ṝ, ḹ
Over-dot	ṅa, aṁ
Tilde	ña
Under-dot	ṛ, ṝ, ḷ, ḹ aḥ ṭa, ṭha, ḍa, ḍha, ṇa ṣha
Accent mark	śha

Whenever these diacritical marks are present, they indicate a specific, single *akṣhara*. This also indicates the method of pronunciation. This pronunciation can vary significantly from the way letters are pronounced in English.

The following example demonstrates some of the variations in transliteration using different methods ("Help." Monier-Williams Sanskrit-English Dictionary, 2019).

Read each slowly to notice the differences in representation of letters. How should each be pronounced? Which ones are easier or harder to pronounce?

Transliteration method	Representation of terms
ĀYUT	saṁskṛta devanāgarī aṣhṭāṅga
IAST	saṁskṛta devanāgarī aṣhṭāṅga
Harvard-Kyoto	saMskRta devanAgarI aSThAGga
ITRANS	saMskRita devanaagarii aShThaa~Nga
SLP1	saMskfta devanAgarI aSTANga

Compare each of these transliteration methods to the *Devanāgarī* script in the following section. The transliteration of Sanskrit in Latin letters is not the same as reading the original *Devanāgarī* script.

TEST YOURSELF

Learn, review and memorize key terms from this section.

diacrtitical mark

ĀYUT

---

lossless matching

---

translation

---

transliteration

SANSKRIT VERSUS SAṀSKṚTA

The word Sanskrit (alternately, "Sanskṛit," "Sanskrut," or "Sanskruth") is the translated English form of the original term, *Saṁskṛta*. The word *Saṁskṛta* is the ĀYUT transliterated form of the original term, written using Roman characters with diacritical marks instead of the *Devanāgarī* script.

The terms Sanskrit and *Saṁskṛta* can be used interchangeably in writing and speech. Generally, however, the English form of the word is preferred when used in written and spoken English. This is the standard notation followed throughout this textbook series.

The correct usage of terms in each script can be expressed as:

	ĀYUT Transliteration (Roman alphabet)	Original *Devanāgarī* script
English form of the word	Sanskrit	n/a
Original (Sanskṛit) form	*Saṁskṛta*, or *Saṁskṛtam*	संस्कृत, संस्कृतम्

TEST YOURSELF

Learn, review and memorize key terms from this section.

Saṁskṛta

Sanskrit

LEARNING SANSKRIT FOR ĀYURVEDIC MEDICAL PRACTICE

There are very specific objectives when learning Sanskrit for Āyurvedic medical practice. These goals will vary according to the intended level of practice. For an entry-level professional capacity, the major requirements include:

1. A complete understanding of the language and its components
2. Fluid reading and writing of the transliterated *Devanāgarī* script in ĀYUT form. Reading and writing the original *Devanāgarī* script is not required for entry-level professions.
3. Ability to form and dissect words
4. Understanding the concept of *sandhi*
5. Ability to identify *sandhi* in basic forms and create and split simple examples
6. Understanding how Sanskrit is represented in prose and poetry

In advanced studies of Āyurvedic Medicine, students are expected to memorize the complete *Devanāgarī* script and be able to read and write fluidly from the classical texts in their original form.

The ability to fully master grammar is not as high of a priority as that requires deep, long-term study in Sanskrit alone. Memorization of a large vocabulary and wide knowledge of contextual meanings is much more essential for successful Āyurvedic studies.

Learning Sanskrit, even in its transliterated

form alone, can present specific challenges to Western students, especially those who do not speak or write languages other than English.

One of the main challenges is that mastering reading and writing the transliterated *Devanāgarī* script requires learning the Roman alphabet in a different way. With transliteration, Roman characters which may appear to be the same (but have diacritical marks added to them) are pronounced distinctly. And, the meaning of words can change depending on the diacritical marks used to write the word.

For example, the following words may appear to be the same when the diacritical marks are ignored. However, in the original Sanskrit, each of these words is distinct and conveys a very different meaning.

Correct ĀYUT Transliteration	Loose Transliteration	Meaning	Original *Devanāgarī*
vata	vata	uttered, sounded, spoken	वत
vāta	vata	one of the three *doṣhas*	वात
vaṭa	vata	a variety of Banyan tree	वट

For native Indians who read and speak at least one Indic language, this difference is clear and obvious because the words are pronounced is distinctly. Traditionally, Indic languages are primarily phonetic instead of written. For native speakers, acute sound recognition develops at a very young age.

Native speakers of Indic languages will hear the differences while native English speakers usually will not. This is a normal obstacle and one of the biggest challenges in the learning process for many Western students.

A similar effect can also be seen in English where native speakers will understand the differences in sentences like "polish the Polish furniture" or "farms produce produce" whereas non-native English speakers may struggle.

Additionally, the *Devanāgarī* alphabet does not technically consist of "letters" like the Roman alphabet does. Instead, each syllable in *Devanāgarī*, which appears to be a "letter" is actually called an *akṣhara*. The *akṣharas* may be a single vowel, or consonant plus a vowel, which forms a syllable.

These combine to form sounds and ultimately words. The mechanics of the *Devanāgarī* alphabet are significantly more complex than English and most Roman-based languages.

TEST YOURSELF

Learn, review and memorize key terms from this section.

akṣhara

____

syllable

____

vaṭa

____

vāta

____

Chapter 30: Review

ADDITIONAL READING

Utilize these references to expand your understanding of the concepts in this chapter.

CLASSICS	1st read	2nd read

REQUIRED READING	Chapters

OPTIONAL READING	Format

References

"Help." Monier-Williams Sanskrit-English Dictionary, April 22, 2019, https://www.sanskrit-lexicon.uni-koeln.de/monier/help.html.

"Translation." Merriam-Webster, 2018, https://www.merriam-webster.com/dictionary/translation

"Translate." Merriam-Webster, 2018, https://www.merriam-webster.com/dictionary/translate

"Transliteration." Merriam-Webster, 2018, https://www.merriam-webster.com/dictionary/transliteration

QUESTIONS & ANSWERS

Record your questions for this chapter here for further research and discussion.

Question:

Answer:

Question:

Answer:

Question:

Answer:

SELF-ASSESSMENT

1. Sanskrit encapsulates
   a. highly specialized concepts in Āyurveda
   b. many layers of knowledge
   c. Vedic knowledge
   d. All the above
   e. None of the above

2. The Merriam-Webster dictionary defines translation as
   a. making a written copy
   b. rendering a word from one language to another
   c. representing letters in another alphabet
   d. spelling in the characters of another alphabet
   e. None of the above

3. *Saṁskṛta* is _____ while Sanskrit is _____ .
   a. translated, transliterated
   b. transliterated, transcribed
   c. transliterated, transcripted
   d. transliterated, translated
   e. None of the above

4. Basic Sanskṛit is required for Āyurveda to
   a. accurately convey concepts
   b. learn diacritical marks
   c. read *Devanāgarī* script
   d. understand grammar
   e. None of the above

5. Correct ĀYUT transliteration avoids
   a. contextual disambiguation
   b. diacritical marks
   c. searching in the dictionary
   d. pronunciation
   e. translation

6. Which professional level of Āyurvedic Medicine requires reading and writing the *Devanāgarī* script?
   a. Āyurveda Āchārya
   b. Āyurvedic Health Coach
   c. Paricharaka
   d. Svastha Āchārya
   e. None of the above

7. Which transliteration method is primarily used in academia?
   a. ĀYUT
   b. Harvard-Kyoto
   c. IAST
   d. ITRANS
   e. SLP1

8. Accurate transliteration must be one-to-one with
   a. *akṣhara* identification
   b. *Devanāgarī* script
   c. diacritical marks
   d. lossless matching
   e. None of the above

9. Examples of transliteration schemes can be found in
   a. *Devanāgarī* alphabet maps
   b. Roman alphabet maps
   c. the Monier-Williams Sanskrit-English Dictionary help files
   d. translation
   e. None of the above

10. Which of the following terms indicates one of the three *doṣhas*?
    a. *vata*
    b. *vaṭa*
    c. *vāta*
    d. All of the above
    e. None of the above

Chapter 31 : Resources and tools

Many resources are available online to help students learning Sanskrit. Several useful ones are listed here. Each resource should be practiced regularly so that the student gains proficiency and ease in use, especially with the Monier-Williams dictionary.

DICTIONARIES

Two main dictionaries are freely available online to translate Sanskrit to English, and English to Sanskrit: These are:

1. The Monier-Williams Sanskrit-English Dictionary

   http://www.sanskrit-lexicon.uni-koeln.de/monier/

2. Spoken Sanskrit Dictionary

   http://spokensanskrit.org/

The MW Dictionary is more difficult to use than Spoken Sanskrit, however it provides additional depth in translations and information. It also ensures exact matches for search terms, unlike Spoken Sanskrit. When unsure about the correct transliteration for a term, search for it first in Spoken Sanskrit.

Each dictionary allows various transliteration method inputs and displays. Output in MW can be set to a specific transliteration scheme.

Use the following examples to look up terms and their variations in each dictionary:

1. doSa, dosha
2. dhAtu, dhatu
3. mala
4. srotas

While learning transliteration schemes and becoming accustomed to their input methods, it is normal to not find any results in the MW Dictionary. Always check the input type and enter the search term according to that type's transliteration scheme. Use the help link to match the *akṣharas* of the *Devanāgarī* script to the corresponding letters of the Roman alphabet.

Searching for terms in the Spoken Sanskrit Dictionary can appear relatively easier for new students. The search algorithm in this dictionary is much more forgiving and allows for multiple variations of transliteration methods simultaneously. However, it often returns many more possible matches. Each of these must be reviewed carefully to determine which is the exact search term.

TYPING

Typing with correct, accurate transliteration schemes presents challenges on most types of computers today. Keyboard layouts for computers in English-speaking locales are set by default to the Roman alphabet, rather than the *Devanāgarī*.

Keyboards can be customized to allow for specific entry of each *Devanāgarī akṣhara*. This type of setup and usage is generally less user-friendly and requires some computer skills.

Depending on the operating system of the device, certain methods for entering transliterated Roman alphabet characters are easier than others. Review some of the most common methods below.

Transliterated typing on a PC

Typing in ĀYUT transliterated form with diacritics on PCs can be done in several ways. The easiest method is to simply copy and paste the desired character. Maintaining a list of the entire transliterated *Devanāgarī* alphabet is the most efficient way to do this.

More extensive methods of transliteration can be accomplished by setting custom dictionaries in word processors to automatically replace certain terms with their transliterated forms. Although this is quite time consuming to setup, it can save time in the long run.

Keyboard input types can also be changed to different alphabets. Shortcut keys can allow switching between input methods easily. Additional shortcut keys allow entry of specific letters. Once these combinations are memorized, typing in *Devanāgarī* can be quick and easy.

Finally, special keyboard shortcuts can be programmed directly into the operating system to produce Roman alphabet characters with diacritical marks. These keyboard shortcuts are usually not short combinations and are more cumbersome to use compared to switching the keyboard input method.

Transliterated typing on MAC OS

Typing in ĀYUT transliterated form with diacritics on MAC OS can be somewhat easier because of the built-in character sets which are automatically programmed to the Option key. Many key combinations exist to produce Roman alphabet characters with diacritics. Use the following list for reference.

<u>Vowels (option A)</u>

Ā	option A + A
ā	option A + a
Ī	option A + I
ī	option A + i
Ū	option A + U
ū	option A + u
Ṝ	option A + R
ṝ	option A + r
Ṛ	option A + R + Delete
ṛ	option A + r + delete
Ḹ	option A + L
ḹ	option A + L
Ḷ	option A + L + Delete
ḷ	option A + l + Delete

<u>Enye (option N)</u>

Ñ	option N + N
ñ	option N + n

<u>Dot above a letter (option W)</u>

Ṅ	option W + N
ṅ	option W + n

<u>Dot below a letter (option X)</u>

Ḥ	option X + H
ḥ	option X + h
Ṃ	option X + M
ṁ	option X + m
Ṭ	option X + T
ṭ	option X + t
Ṇ	option X + N
ṇ	option X + n
Ṣh	option X + S
ṣh	option X + s

<u>Accent mark (option E)</u>

Śh option E + S

śh option E + s

Typing in Devanāgarī script

Using transliteration schemes, Roman characters can be entered to produce *Devanāgarī* script. To type in *Devanāgarī*, the program must support the character set and the keyboard input type must be changed.

Additionally, the LexiLogos website allows character entry using one alphabet and it transforms it to another. For Sanskrit, the website provides a page speicifically for *Devanāgarī*.

http://www.lexilogos.com/keyboard/sanskrit_devanagari.htm

The interface also allows for entry using the mouse by clicking on the buttons that represent each *akṣhara*. To type accurately in *Devanāgarī* script using this tool requires advanced knowledge of Sanskrit.

For additional details on transliteration, review the following reference.

https://ipfs.io/ipfs/QmXoypizjW3WknFiJnKLwHCnL72vedxjQkDDP1mXWo6uco/wiki/International_Alphabet_of_Sanskrit_Transliteration.html

Chapter 31: Review

ADDITIONAL READING

Utilize these references to expand your understanding of the concepts in this chapter.

CLASSICS	1st read	2nd read

REQUIRED READING	Chapters
International Alphabet of Sanskrit Transliteration, https://ipfs.io/ipfs/QmXoypizjW3WknFiJnKLwHCnL72vedxjQkDDP1mXWo6uco/wiki/International_Alphabet_of_Sanskrit_Transliteration.html	
Monier-Williams Sanskrit-English Dictionary, https://www.sanskrit-lexicon.uni-koeln.de/scans/MWScan/2014/web/webtc/indexcaller.php	
Spoken Sanskrit Dictionary, http://spokensanskrit.org/	

OPTIONAL READING	Format
SARIT: Search and Retrieval of Indic Texts, http://sarit.indology.info/exist/apps/sarit/works/	

References

Glashoff, K. (n.d.). Sanskrit Dictionary for Spoken Sanskrit. Retrieved from http://spokensanskrit.org/

International Alphabet of Sanskrit Transliteration. (2016, December 3). Retrieved from https://ipfs.io/ipfs/QmXoypizjW3WknFiJnKLwHCnL72vedxjQkDDP1mXWo6uco/wiki/International_Alphabet_of_Sanskrit_Transliteration.html

Monier Williams Sanskrit-English Dictionary (2008 revision). (n.d.). Retrieved from https://www.sanskrit-lexicon.uni-koeln.de/monier/

Sanskrit Multilingual Keyboard. (n.d.). Retrieved from https://www.lexilogos.com/keyboard/sanskrit_devanagari.htm

QUESTIONS & ANSWERS

Record your questions for this chapter here for further research and discussion.

Question:

Answer:

Question:

Answer:

Question:

Answer:

SELF-ASSESSMENT

1. The Monier-Williams Sanskrit-English Dictionary does not use
   a. ĀYUT
   b. Harvard-Kyoto
   c. IAST
   d. ITRANS
   e. SLP1

2. The Monier-Williams Sanskrit-English Dictionary allows for
   a. translation from English to Sanskrit
   b. translation from Sanskrit to English
   c. transliteration from English to Sanskrit
   d. All the above
   e. None of the above

3. The Spoken Sanskrit Dictionary
   a. allows for partial word input
   b. helps match terms in *Devanāgarī* only
   c. is easier for beginners to use than MW
   d. shows many variations of terms
   e. All of the above

4. Terms that are entered into MW but not transliterated properly will return
   a. alternate terms
   b. link to help file
   c. not found message
   d. reminder to check transliteration scheme
   e. the nearest equivalent

5. The Spoken Sanskrit dictionary displays results in
   a. *Devanāgarī*
   b. translation
   c. transliteration
   d. All of the above
   e. None of the above

6. Typing diacritical marks on MAC OS can be done using
   a. lowercase letters only
   b. the caps lock key
   c. the command key
   d. the option key
   e. uppercase letters only

7. LexiLogos *Devanāgarī* Sanskrit keyboard allows
   a. checking spelling
   b. looking up Sanskrit terms
   c. producing output in *Devanāgarī* script
   d. producing output in Roman letters
   e. All of the above

8. Entering the term "dhatu" into the MW dictionary returns
   a. a not found message
   b. links to the pronunciation key
   c. one definition of dhatu
   d. three definitions of dhatu
   e. None of the above

9. The Spoken Sanskrit dictionary often returns
   a. less results than needed
   b. more results than needed
   c. only exact matches
   d. results in multiple transliteration schemes
   e. None of the above

10. Entering the term "dhatu" into the Spoken Sanskrit dictionary returns
   a. 0 results
   b. 1 results
   c. 3 results
   d. 10 results
   e. more than ten results

Chapter 32 : Basic Devanāgarī

KEY TERMS			
akṣhara	Devanāgarī	schwa	Vedic Sanskrit
anusvāra	diphthongs	semivowel	virāma
aspirate	long vowel	short vowel	visarga
combined vowel	monophthong	sibilant	vowel
consonant	phonemic orthography	simple vowel	vowel add-on

The *Devanāgarī* script is the official script and alphabet of Sanskrit. Its complete form in Vedic Sanskrit is more elaborate than its current, slightly smaller, modern form. For thorough study of classical Āyurveda, the older Vedic *Devanāgarī* alphabet is used. This fully covers the classical and modern literature of Āyurveda.

BASIC MECHANICS OF THE ALPHABET

Phonetics

Sanskrit is a language that is spoken as it is written and written as it is spoken. In linguistics, it is considered to be a language with high phonemic orthography.

Each syllable, or *akṣhara*, of the *Devanāgarī* alphabet represents how a specific and unique sound is produced. This makes reading and writing Sanskrit easier than many other languages, including English, once the *Devanāgarī* alphabet is memorized fluently. Vedic Sanskrit has strongly influenced most modern Indian languages today which are also largely phonetic-based.

Akṣharas: the syllables of the alphabet

The *Devanāgarī* alphabet consists of *akṣharas*, which can be best equated to syllables. These include vowels, consonants, semivowels, sibilants and an aspirate. Each of these syllables contains either one or two beats (also called counts) to create a short or long duration sound when pronounced. A single count is made by using a short vowel, while a double count is made by using either a long vowel or diphthong.

All *akṣharas*, except vowels, include an inherent, or implicit "a" sound as a single beat. This is pronounced more like the phrase "uh" rather than a normal English hard "a" or "ah." The presence of this inherent "a" or "uh" sound is called schwa. All transliterated *akṣharas* except the vowels must include this inherent schwa sound and are therefore always expressed followed by the letter "a" to represent this sound explicitly.

In some cases, the inherent schwa must be stopped, or suppressed. To do that, a special mark is added to the syllable, called a *virāma*. It can be used with any of the syllables except vowels. It is typically only written when the original *Devanāgarī* script is used and appears as a small, diagonal line placed under the syllable and directed down towards the right side. In transliteration, however, the *virāma* is not required because Roman letters are represented without the inherent schwa.

ĀYUT transliterated term	Original *Devanāgarī* term	Explanation of *virāma*
Bhiṣhak	भिषक्	The original term ends in a consonant with the schwa stopped. The *virāma* stroke is placed just below the final consonant pointing down towards the right. This is only required in the original *Devanāgarī* script.

With transliteration, also notice that uppercase and lowercase representation has no significance, unlike English. Throughout this series of textbooks, uppercase letters will be used wherever required for proper English. This distinction has no effect on the original *Devanāgarī*.

TEST YOURSELF

Learn, review and memorize key terms from this section.

akṣhara

Devanāgarī

phonemic orthography

schwa

Vedic Sanskrit

virāma

THE DEVANĀGARĪ ALPHABET

The complete *Devanāgarī* alphabet used in Vedic Sanskrit includes 49 *akṣharas*. These are grouped into vowels, vowel add-ons, consonants, semivowels, sibilants and an aspirate.

Akṣhara classification

English name	Sanskrit name	Number	Description
Vowels	*Svara (hrasva, dīrga)*	14	A vowel is a class of speech sounds in which the oral part of the breath channel is not blocked and is not constricted enough to cause audible friction.
Vowel add-ons	*Svara (anusvāra, visarga)*	2	Vowel add-ons can only be added onto an existing vowel. They extend the vowel's sound with a closing sound of "uhm" or "uh."
Consonants	*Vyañjana (sparśha)*	25	A consonant is a class of speech sounds characterized by constriction or closure at one or more points in the breath channel.

Semivowels	*Vyañjana (antaḥsthā)*	4	A semivowel has the articulation of a vowel but is shorter in duration and is treated as a consonant in syllabication.
Sibilants	*Vyañjana (ūṣhman)*	3	A sibilant has, contains or produces the sound of or a sound resembling that of the "s" or the "sh" in sash.
Aspirate	*Vyañjana*	1	The aspirate is a consonant having aspiration as its final component.

Vowels

In Sanskrit, the entire group of 14 vowels plus the two vowel add-ons are collectively called *svara*.

Each vowel has its own specific pronunciation method. The duration of pronunciation may be expressed as either one beat (short) or two beats (long).

Vowels are pronounced somewhat like they are in English. They often are pronounced softer, sounding more similar to romance languages like Spanish and Italian.

Each vowel sound is produced by opening the mouth to allow the sound to be generated. The vowels in the *Devanāgarī* alphabet are written in subgroups that follow specific patterns.

Vowels are roughly grouped into three main sections in classical Vedic *Devanāgarī*.

The first subgroup includes short and long vowels. These are pronounced and held for one or two beats.

a	"uh"	b**u**t
ā	"uuh"	h**a**rm
i	"e"	p**i**t
ī	"ee"	p**ee**l
u	"ooh"	p**u**t
ū	"ooooh"	sh**oe**

The second subgroup includes short and long vowels that are much less common and are more difficult to pronounce. In English, they would be considered consonants but in Vedic Sanskrit they are used as vowels.

ṛ	"r"	like a rolling r, ac**re**
ṝ	"rr"	same but lengthened
ḷ	"l"	like a rolling l, tab**le**
ḹ	"ll"	same but lengthened

The third subgroup consists of long vowels only. These vowels are pronounced by blending two vowel sounds from the first subgroup.

e	"ey"	h**ey**
ai	"eye"	p**ie**
o	"oh"	t**oe**
au	"ow"	d**ow**n

Vowel beats

Vowels may be short or long depending on the number of beats required to pronounce them. Short vowels use one beat while long vowels use two. A single beat can be roughly approximated between one-half to two-thirds of a second.

Short vowels	a	i	u
	ṛ	ḷ	

Long vowels	ā	ī	ū	
	ṝ	ḹ		
	e	ai	o	au

Vowel tones

Vowels can also be classified as monophthongs and diphthongs. These classifications refer to the tones used to pronounce the vowel.

Monophthongs are pronounced with a single, continuous tone. This tone does not change during the pronunciation of the vowel. Monophthongs may be short or long, being pronounced for one or two beats.

Diphthongs are pronounced by blending two vowel sounds into a single syllable. Pronunciation begins with one vowel tone and ends with a different one.

Examples of diphthongs in English include coin, loud and side.

All diphthongs are long vowels and require two beats for pronunciation.

Monophthongs

a ā i ī u ū

ṛ ṝ ḷ ḹ

Diphthongs

e ai o au

Specific rules are used to form diphthongs. The combine monophthong vowels to produce dual tone, long vowels. This joint sound is a combination of two distinct sounds so that diphthongs are pronounced as a blend.

Diphthong formation rules

a + i → e

ā + i → ai

a + u → o

ā + u → au

Vowel add-ons

Two vowel "add-ons" follow the vowels in the *Devanāgarī* alphabet.

Vowel add-ons can only be added onto an existing vowel. They extend the vowel's sound with a closing sound of "uhm" or "uh." They are pronounced according to the vowel that they are added to, along with their ending sound of "uhm" or "uh." In the following examples, the vowel add-ons are added to the "a" vowel.

The vowel add-ons are:

anusvāra:	aṁ
visarga:	aḥ

Anusvāra and *visarga* can only be added onto a vowel and cannot exist on their own. *Anusvāra* is a sound produced nasally as an "aṁ" (pronounced "um") or "mmm" sound, and is influenced by the vowel that precedes it.

Visarga can be pronounced in various ways, and is often influenced by the geographical region where the language is being used. In South India it usually sounds like an "aha" sound when preceded by "a." When it follows other vowels, it sounds like an echo of the preceding vowel, like "uhu" or "ihi." In some cases, it may be pronounced so subtly that it is barely noticed.

Variations in pronunciation

Throughout India, many variations exist in pronunciation of the Sanskrit *Devanāgarī* alphabet and the language in general. Even more variations exist among local languages and dialects that are related to the *Devanāgarī* alphabet.

For professional Āyurvedic practice in a Western environment, the goal is to memorize the standard, classical pronunciation of Vedic Sanskrit. Keep in mind that it is almost impossible for non-native Indians to do this at the level which natives would consider "perfect."

For native English speakers, the primary goal is to know how the sounds should be produced and explain their rules. Practicing pronunciation to perfect it can take years of study and often requires long-term access to classical Sanskrit teachers in India.

Memorization and recitation

The vowels and vowel add-ons of classical Vedic *Devanāgarī* are memorized and recited following one pattern. Follow the order in the table below to memorize these *akṣharas* completely.

***Devanāgarī*: The Sanskrit Alphabet in ĀYUT Transliteration**

Vowels	a	ā	i	ī	u	ū	ṛ	ṝ	ḷ	ḹ
	e	ai	o	au	aṁ	aḥ				
Consonants	ka	kha	ga	gha	ṅa					
	cha	chha	ja	jha	ña					
	ṭa	ṭha	ḍa	ḍha	ṇa					
	ta	tha	da	dha	na					
	pa	pha	ba	bha	ma					
Semivowels	ya	ra	la	va						
Sibilants	śha	ṣha	sa							
Aspirate	ha									

TEST YOURSELF

Learn, review and memorize key terms from this section.

anusvāra

aspirate

combined vowel

consonant

diphthong

long vowel

monophthong

semivowel

short vowel

sibilant

simple vowel

visarga

vowel

vowel add-on

Chapter 32: Review

ADDITIONAL READING

Utilize these references to expand your understanding of the concepts in this chapter.

CLASSICS	1st read	2nd read

REQUIRED READING	Chapters

OPTIONAL READING	Format
Applied Sanskrit for Āyurveda and Yoga, I, Jessica Vellela	Book

References

Kale, M. R. (1924). "A Smaller Sanskrit Grammar." Gopal Narayen & Co.

QUESTIONS & ANSWERS

Record your questions for this chapter here for further research and discussion.

Question:

Answer:

Question:

Answer:

Question:

Answer:

SELF-ASSESSMENT

1. An *akṣhara* is a
   a. diacritical mark
   b. letter
   c. syllable
   d. All of the above
   e. None of the above

2. Languages that are spoken as they are written and written as they are spoken have high
   a. phonemic ornithology
   b. phonemic orthography
   c. phonemic orthostatic
   d. phonemic pronunciation
   e. None of the above

3. "Schwa" is distinctly identified in all *aḳsaras* except
   a. aspirate
   b. consonants
   c. semivowels
   d. sibilants
   e. vowels

4. The classical Vedic *Devanāgarī* alphabet includes
   a. 14 *akṣharas*
   b. 25 *akṣharas*
   c. 47 *akṣharas*
   d. 49 *akṣharas*
   e. 51 *akṣharas*

5. Diacritical marks _____ and _____ the Roman alphabet.
   a. abbreviate and simplify
   b. condense and modify
   c. expand and modify
   d. neutralize and contain
   e. shorten and compress

6. Which of the following vowels is a diphthong?
   a. ā
   b. ī
   c. o
   d. ṛ
   e. u

7. Vowel add-ons can only be used
   a. at the beginning of a word
   b. at the end of a word
   c. in conjunction with a semivowel
   d. on an existing vowel
   e. None of the above

8. Which combination produces a diphthong?
   a. a + e
   b. a + u
   c. ā + e
   d. i + u
   e. o + u

9. Applying *virāma* stops an inherent
   a. schwa
   b. semivowel
   c. *visarga*
   d. vowel
   e. vowel add-on

10. Monophthongs can be
    a. half beat
    b. one beat
    c. one or two beats
    d. two beats
    e. All of the above

Chapter 33 : Advanced Devanāgarī

KEY TERMS

aspirate	guttural	palatal	sibilant
aspirated	labial	retroflex	unaspirated
consonant	nasal	semivowel	velar
dental			

The entire group of consonants is called *vyañjana* and it consists of 25 consonants, 4 semivowels, 3 sibilants and 1 aspirate.

All consonants are connected with a vowel by default in order to produce a syllabic sound. In the *Devanāgarī* alphabet, this default vowel is the "a," the first, short "uh" sound. When each consonant is pronounced, it is followed by the "uh" sound. This is the inherent schwa of Sanskrit.

All forms of consonants produce their sound by stopping, restricting, interrupting or changing the outward flow of air as they are being pronounced.

This is distinct from vowels which are produced through an open, unimpeded passage of air. Semivowels, sibilants and the aspirate have variations in their specific pronunciations.

CONSONANTS

The 25 true consonants are classified as non-aspirated, aspirated and nasal depending on their method of pronunciation. Non-aspirated consonants are pronounced as they appear. Typically, they correspond to their standard usage in English.

Aspirated consonants, however, are pronounced with a slight extension of breath or aspiration to produce a soft "ha" sound. This sound is generated by forcing a small amount of air from the lungs with a pronounced exhalation or aspiration. Nasal consonants are produced by sending the exhaled air up through the nasal cavity.

The 25 true consonants are always listed in order as five rows with five columns. Non-aspirated and aspirated sounds alternate and are followed by the nasal.

All of the consonants included in one row are produced with the position of the tongue originating from the same place in the mouth or throat.

Each row is used to distinguish this method of pronunciation, making it easier to remember because all consonants on the same row have a similar sound production method.

Row	Name	Pronunciation
1st	Velar	from the throat
2nd	Palatal	from the inner surfaces of all the teeth
3rd	Retroflex	from the roof of the mouth
4th	Dental	from the back of the front teeth
5th	Labial	from the lips

Aspiration methods

Additionally, the 25 true consonants are classified based on their aspiration method as non-aspirated, aspirated or nasal.

Non-aspirated consonants are pronounced without additional exhalation effort. This typically corresponds to their usage in English.

Aspirated consonants, however, are pronounced with a slight extension of breath or aspiration to produce a soft "ha" or breath sound with the consonant.

This sound is generated by forcing a small amount of air from the lungs with a pronounced exhalation or aspiration.

Nasal consonants are produced by redirecting the exhaled air up through the nasal cavity. When done correctly, it creates a subtle reverberation and resonance throughout the skull.

In each consonant row, the non-aspirated and aspirated sounds alternate by column. The first and third columns are always unaspirated. The second and fourth columns are always aspirated. And the fifth column is always produced as the nasal sound.

Review the 25 true consonants below with their aspiration methods.

Aspiration methods:

UN = Unaspirated

AS = Aspirated

NA = Nasal

	UN	AS	UN	AS	NA
1st	ka	kha	ga	gha	ṅa
2nd	cha	chha	ja	jha	ña
3rd	ṭa	ṭha	ḍa	ḍha	ṇa
4th	ta	tha	da	dha	na
5th	pa	pha	ba	bha	ma

Practice reading all 25 consonants while pronouncing them. Work with one row at a time. When all rows become easy to pronounce, they will also be easy to memorize.

1st row: Velar consonants

These are pronounced by pressing the back of the tongue against the soft palate at the back of the mouth near the throat. The letter "k" in English is pronounced in a similar way.

These are also called guttural.

Cons	Sound	Asp	Example
ka	"kuh"	UN	"papri**ka**"
kha	"k-huh"	AS	"thic**k h**ull"
ga	"guh"	UN	"sa**ga**"
gha	"g-huh"	AS	"**gh**astly"
ṅa	"nguh"	NA	"hu**ng**, su**ng**"

2nd row: Palatal consonants

These are pronounced by pressing the outer edge of the tongue against the inner surfaces of all the teeth simultaneously and spreading the lips slightly wide. The letter "ñ" ("enye") in Spanish is pronounced in a similar way.

Cons	Sound	Asp	Example
cha	"chuh"	UN	"**chu**g"
chha	"ch-huh"	AS	"mu**ch h**oney"
ja	"juh"	UN	"**ju**st"
jha	"j-huh"	AS	"ra**j h**oney"
ña	"nyuh"	NA	"o**nio**n"

3rd row: Retroflex consonants

These are pronounced by curling the tip of the tongue up to touch the roof of the mouth or sit in between the two ridges of the hard palate. With the mouth open, create the sound.

There is no exact English equivalent for this, but the tongue can be held in that position while pronouncing the following examples to understand its production method.

These are also called lingual or cerebral.

Cons	Sound	Asp	Example
ṭa	"tuh"	UN	"Borsch**t** **a**gain"
ṭha	"t-huh"	AS	"Borsch**t** **h**oney"
ḍa	"duh"	UN	"a**du**lt"
ḍha	"d-huh"	AS	"re**dh**ead"
ṇa	"nuh"	NA	"ge**n**tle"

4th row: Dental consonants

The tip of the tongue is pressed against the backs of the upper and lower front teeth with the mouth slightly open, and then the sound is created.

The English word "late" is pronounced in a similar manner by pressing the tip of the tongue against the back of the front teeth when starting to produce the "l" sound.

Cons	Sound	Asp	Example
ta	"tuh"	UN	"**te**a"
tha	"t-huh"	AS	"boa**t-h**ouse"
da	"duh"	UN	"**d**art"
dha	"d-huh"	AS	"bloo**d-h**ound"
na	"nuh"	NA	"**n**ine"

5th row: Labial consonants

These are pronounced by pressing the lips together, curling them slightly inwards, and then creating the sound. The letter "p" in English is pronounced the same way.

Cons	Sound	Asp	Example
pa	"puh"	UN	"**pu**p"
pha	"p-huh"	AS	"cu**p** **h**ook"
ba	"buh"	UN	"**bu**tter"
bha	"b-huh"	AS	"a**bh**or"
ma	"muh"	NA	"**me**ss"

The consonant "pha" is rarely pronounced with a "p" sound. Instead, it is pronounced like "ph" in English as in "phone." It is possible that this phonetic deviation was influenced from cultures in Central Asia and Persia.

Semivowels

The four semivowels behave grammatically like consonants but their pronunciation is similar to vowels. Semivowels blend consonant and vowel pronunciation requiring that the mouth and lips be partially open.

Semi-vowel	Sound	Examples
ya	"yuh"	"**yu**p"
ra	"ruh"	"**ru**b"
la	"luh"	"**lu**g"
va	"vuh" or "wuh"	"**Vu**lcan" or "**wh**at"

The semivowel "ya" is the most common *akṣhara* to slightly alter its pronunciation when following other vowels.

Consider the Sanskrit term "āyu," meaning

life or life span (as in the word Āyurveda). The long "ā" precedes the semivowel "y" which is followed by the short vowel "u." The combination of the long "ā" with the "y" creates a sound almost identical to the long, diphthong vowel "ai."

This may appear to be an exception to pronunciation rules, but it is not. Pāṇini's complex grammatical rules include explanations for blends of conjoined sounds such as this.

The semivowel "va" can be pronounced like a "v" or a "w" as in "va" or "wah" depending on its position in the word.

Regional Indian languages and dialects can have a noticeable influence on the pronunciation of Sanskrit.

Sibilants

The three sibilants are pronounced by making a hissing sound. The English sounds "shhh" and "ssss" are near equivalents for two of the three Sanskrit sibilants.

The first "sh" sound (śha) is pronounced like "shhhh" in English, by laying the tongue flat, pulling it up along the side teeth and then pushing air through the front teeth.

The second "sh" sound (ṣha) is different and is created by curling the tip of the tongue up and slightly back to just barely contact the ridges on the hard palate, while pushing air through the front teeth.

The third "sa" sound (sa) is pronounced more like a hiss than the other two, with the tongue completely flat and pushing air through the teeth.

Sibilants	Sound	Examples
śha	"shuh"	"**sh**ut"
ṣha	"shuh"	**sh**ine
sa	"suh"	"**su**pper"

Aspirate

The aspirate is pronounced by exhaling while making a "ha" (or "huh") sound. It requires slightly forced exhalation to produce the sound. It is like breathing out while making the sound.

Aspirate	Sound	Examples
ha	"huh"	"**huh**"

Memorization and pronunciation

The full *Devanāgarī* should always be memorized in a specific order, with vowels first, then consonants, followed by semivowels, sibilants and the aspirate.

Use the following table to review the complete ĀYUT transliterated *Devanāgarī*. The entire alphabet is in order of memorization and recitation.

Use the additional charts to practice pronunciation until the entire alphabet is memorized.

Devanāgarī: The Sanskrit Alphabet in ĀYUT Transliteration

Vowels	a	ā	i	ī	u	ū	ṛ	ṝ	ḷ	ḹ
	e	ai	o	au	aṁ	aḥ				
Consonants	ka	kha	ga	gha	ṅa					
	cha	chha	ja	jha	ña					
	ṭa	ṭha	ḍa	ḍha	ṇa					
	ta	tha	da	dha	na					
	pa	pha	ba	bha	ma					
Semivowels	ya	ra	la	va						
Sibilants	śha	ṣha	sa							
Aspirate	ha									

Vowels

a	"uh"
ā	"uuh"
i	"e"
ī	"ee"
u	"ooh"
ū	"ooooh"
ṛ	"r"
ṝ	"rr"
ḷ	"l"
ḹ	"ll"
e	"ey"
ai	"eye"
o	"oh"
au	"ow"
aṁ	"uhm"
aḥ	"uh" or "uh-huh"

Consonant Key

1st = Velar - from the throat
2nd = Palatal - from the back of the palate
3rd = Retroflex - from the roof of the mouth
4th = Dental - from the back of the teeth
5th = Labial - from the lips

UN = Unaspirated AS = Aspirated

NA = Nasal

Consonants

	UN	AS	UN	AS	NA
1st	ka	kha	ga	gha	ṅa
2nd	cha	chha	ja	jha	ña
3rd	ṭa	ṭha	ḍa	ḍha	ṇa
4th	ta	tha	da	dha	na
5th	pa	pha	ba	bha	ma

Semivowels

ya	"yuh"
ra	"ruh"
la	"luh"
va	"vuh" or "wuh"

Sibilants

śha	"sh-huh"	"**sh**ut"
ṣha	"sh-huh"	**sh**ine
sa	"suh"	"**su**pper"

Aspirate

ha	"huh"

TEST YOURSELF

Learn, review and memorize key terms from this section.

aspirate

aspirated

consonant

dental

guttural

labial

nasal

palatal

retroflex

semivowel

sibilant

unaspirated

velar

Chapter 33: Review

ADDITIONAL READING

Utilize these references to expand your understanding of the concepts in this chapter.

CLASSICS	1st read	2nd read

REQUIRED READING	Chapters

OPTIONAL READING	Format
A Smaller Sanskrit Grammar, MR Kale	

References

Kale, M. R. (1924). "A Smaller Sanskrit Grammar." Gopal Narayen & Co.

QUESTIONS & ANSWERS

Record your questions for this chapter here for further research and discussion.

Question:

Answer:

Question:

Answer:

Question:

Answer:

SELF-ASSESSMENT

1. Which consonant row is pronounced by pressing the back of the tongue to the soft palate?
   a. dental
   b. labial
   c. palatal
   d. retroflex
   e. velar

2. Which dental consonant is pronounced nasally?
   a. ṅa
   b. ña
   c. ṇa
   d. na
   e. ma

3. What consonant is found in Row 2 Column 4?
   a. da
   b. dha
   c. ga
   d. jha
   e. tha

4. Which *akṣhara* behaves grammatically like a consonant but is pronounced like a vowel?
   a. da
   b. ma
   c. pa
   d. ta
   e. va

5. Which of the following is not a sibilant?
   a. ha
   b. śha
   c. ṣha
   d. sa
   e. None of the above

6. Which *akṣhara* is found in Row 4 Column 3?
   a. da
   b. dha
   c. ja
   d. na
   e. tha

7. Which *akṣhara* is a semivowel?
   a. aḥ
   b. aṁ
   c. ma
   d. ra
   e. śha

8. Sibilants are pronounced by creating
   a. a double beat
   b. a guttural sound
   c. a hissing sound
   d. an aspiration on exhalation
   e. pursed lips

9. Which of the 25 main consonants does not follow normal phonetic pronunciation rules?
   a. da
   b. ka
   c. ma
   d. na
   e. pha

10. Which semivowel is often pronounced as "wa?"
    a. la
    b. ra
    c. va
    d. ya
    e. None of the above

Chapter 34 : Word formation and dissection

KEY TERMS			
dhātu	schwa	schwa deletion	virāma
√ duṣh			

AKṢHARA MECHANICS

Out of the 49 *akṣharas* in the complete, Vedic *Devanāgarī* alphabet, only certain *akṣharas* are able to change their inherent syllabic sound. The *akṣharas* which cannot change their syllabic sounds are the 14 vowels and 2 vowel add-ons. These vowels and vowel add-ons remain static or unchanged when compared to the remaining groups of consonants.

Instead of the vowels changing their syllabic sounds, they can be combined onto existing consonants to alter the sound of the consonant. These combinations can occur in two forms, simple and conjunct, depending on the type of consonant.

First, it is important to understand the basic state of consonants in their standard syllabic form. This is the same format that the consonants appear in the alphabet. All consonants include an inherent schwa in Sanskrit which is often modified to create complex sounds and words.

Schwa and *virāma*

In the *Devanāgarī* alphabet, the 25 consonants, 4 semivowels, 3 sibilants and 1 aspirate are each listed in order and followed by the letter "a" in their ĀYUT transliterated form.

This "a" is called schwa. It is the inherent single syllable "a" vowel that is naturally attached to each consonant in its base form in the alphabet. This "a" is the first vowel of the complete alphabet.

Schwa is defined by the Oxford Learner's Dictionary as a noun used in phonetics (Schwa, n.d.).

Schwa is a vowel sound in parts of words that are not stressed, for example the 'a' in about or the 'e' in moment; the phonetic symbol for this, /ə/.

Its origin is from late 19th century German, and earlier from the Hebrew šĕwā'.

Schwa is the natural "a" or "uh" sound that is attached to each consonant in the *Devanāgarī* alphabet. This sound is required to be connected to any of the consonants in their base form in the alphabet so that they may be pronounced completely.

When consonants combine to form words, the schwa may be stopped by a *virāma*. In the original *Devanāgarī* script, the *virāma* is represented by a small diagonal line that is placed below the *akṣhara* on the right side and drawn downward and away from the *akṣhara* at a 45-degree angle.

In ĀYUT transliteration, the *virāma* is not required to be written or represented. Instead, the trailing "a" of the consonant is simply removed from the Roman alphabet representation.

Review the following examples to see schwa and *virāma* in both the original *Devanāgarī* script and the ĀYUT transliterated form.

Words that naturally contain a *virāma*

Devanāgarī script	ĀYUT Transliteration	Translation
भिषक्	*bhiṣhak*	Āyurvedic Doctor
स्रोतस्	*srotas*	Channel
अप्	*ap*	Water
ओजस्	*ojas*	*Ojas*
क्षुत्	*kṣhut*	Hunger
शरत्	*śharat*	Post-monsoon season

In each of the previous examples, the *virāma* can be seen in the first column with the *Devanāgarī* script. It is the small, diagonal line placed below the last *akṣhara* pointing downward toward the rigth at a 45-degree angle.

Let's look at the first word, *bhiṣhak*, in its original *Devanāgarī* script form to see the *virāma.*

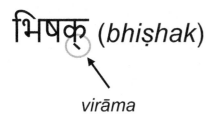

भिषक् (*bhiṣhak*)

virāma

Notice that the *virāma* mark must be included in the original *Devanāgarī* script in order to stop the inherent schwa.

However, in ĀYUT transliteration, the *virāma* mark is not required. Instead, the trailing "a" is omitted. Without the "a" the sound is not pronounced when the word is spoken.

In all of the examples cited above, the *virāma* appears at the end of the term. This is not a requirement. A *virāma* can appear anywhere within the word as well, depending on the *akṣharas* used and any conjunct consonants. When consonants combine, they may be written in several ways in the original *Devanāgarī* script. One of these ways includes using the *virāma*. Review the various types of *akṣhara* combinations to see these rules in action.

TEST YOURSELF

Learn, review and memorize key terms from this section.

schwa

virāma

AKṢHARA NOTATION

When working with the *Devanāgarī* alphabet, it is important to be able to identify specific *akṣhara* accurately. *Akṣhara* notation allows all of the true consonants to be identified by row and column position. It also allows semivowels, sibilants and the aspirate to be identified by type and position.

These notations are used in further study for word dissection exercises.

For true consonants, any *akṣhara* can be expressed as its row:column position and aspiration method. For example, the first and second rows of *akṣharas* are notated as:

ka	1:1 UN	cha	2:1 UN
kha	1:2 AS	chha	2:2 AS
ga	1:3 UN	ja	2:3 UN
gha	1:4 AS	jha	2:4 AS
ṅa	1:5 NA	ña	2:5 NA

UN is unaspirated. AS is aspirated and NA is nasal. These indicate the breath regulation required to produce each sound.

Each remaining true consonant row is notated in the same way.

For semivowels and the sibilants, the type and position must be notated to determine their correct identification.

Because each has only one row, the type is stated instead of row, followed by the position.

ya	SV 1	śha	SB 1
ra	SV 2	ṣha	SB 2
la	SV 3	sa	SB 3
va	SV 4		

There is only one aspirate, and its notation is aspirate alone.

ha	aspirate

AKṢHARA COMBINATIONS

Recall that an *akṣhara* is any syllable which may be a vowel or consonant. The *Devanāgarī* alphabet is composed of *akṣharas* which combine in various ways to form words.

These can be grouped into simple and complex combinations. Simple combinations are composed of a single consonant plus any vowel. Complex combinations are composed of conjunct consonants plus any vowel.

To fully understand these formations, practice the exercises of word dissection and word formation. This allows each word to be deconstructed to its most basic components and then recombined to fully understand its structure.

First, review regular and half consonants. Then step through the process of creating simple combinations of a single consonant plus a vowel, and conjunct consonants.

Regular and half consonants

Regular and half consonants include all 25 consonants, the semivowels, sibilants and aspirate. In their most basic forms, regular consonants are the same as their normal forms in the *Devanāgarī* alphabet. Each of these contain a natural schwa in their regular form, and their pronunciation sounds like it ends in "uh." Because the schwa is a short "a" (ie, the first vowel), it is held for one beat when pronounced.

To form a half consonant, start with any of the regular, base consonants. Then apply *virāma* to stop the inherent schwa sound. By stopping the schwa, the normal, single beat of pronunciation is reduced to a half beat. Additionally, as the consonant is pronounced it must be cut short so as to omit the schwa.

Review the following examples.

Regular consonants			Half consonants		
Devanāgarī	ĀYUT	Pronunciation	*Devanāgarī*	ĀYUT	Pronunciation
क	ka	papri**ka**	क्	k	tri**ck**
च	cca	**chu**tney	च्	ch	ou**ch**
प	pa	**pu**p	प्	p	yu**p**
ल	la	**lu**ll	ल्	l	lu**ll**
स	sa	**su**pper	स्	s	fu**ss**

The examples above include various consonants, semivowels and aspirates. Any type of consonant can be used to create a half consonant and its pronunciation must be shortened accordingly.

However, in regular use, certain consonants, like the aspirate *ha*, are rarely used in half consonant form. As a general rule, this helps to differentiate the final "*h*" that is often found at the end of terms. Notice that this "*h*" almost always has the diacritical dot below it. This indicates that it is "*ḥ*" or the *visarga* (vowel add-on) instead of the aspirate.

Half consonants are the smallest, shortest forms of syllabic sounds that can be created in the Sanskrit alphabet. Creating half consonants is a required first step in the next type of formation where consonants combine with vowels.

Consonant and vowel combinations

Consonant and vowel combinations occur in every word in the Sanskrit language. These combinations can be created from any consonant (including semivowels, sibilants and the aspirate) plus one vowel.

Recall that vowels may be short or long, monophthongs or diphthongs, and depending on the type used, the final combination must follow that specific pronunciation.

All consonants can be combined with each of the 14 vowels plus two additional vowel add-ons. With each of the 14 base vowel combinations, the two vowel add-ons can only be appended to each form.

When traditionally learning the *Devanāgarī* alphabet and all of its forms of combinations, students practice recitation of every consonant and vowel form in sequence. This recitation starts with the "ka" consonant, applies *virāma*, and then methodically attaches each vowel to create the consonant and vowel combination.

Each of these combinations is recited in order. At the end of the sequence, the next consonant is recited in all of its forms. This continues until all of the consonant and vowel combinations have been pronounced in order.

Review a few of these consonant and vowel combination sequences. Practice reciting them aloud and improve memorization by continuing through the consonants beyond this example.

Consonant: ka

Consonant + vowel combination sequence:

ka kā ki kī ku kū kṛ kṝ kḷ kḹ

ke kai ko kau kaṁ kaḥ

Consonant: kha

Consonant + vowel combination sequence:

kha khā khi khī khu khū khṛ khṝ khḷ khḹ

khe khai kho khau khaṁ khaḥ

Consonant: ga

Consonant + vowel combination sequence:

ga gā gi gī gu gū gṛ gṝ gḷ gḹ

ge gai go gau gaṁ gaḥ

Consonant: gha

Consonant + vowel combination sequence:

gha ghā ghi ghī ghu ghū ghṛ ghṝ ghḷ ghḹ

ghe ghai gho ghau ghaṁ ghaḥ

Consonant: ṅa

Consonant + vowel combination sequence:

ṅa ṅā ṅi ṅī ṅu ṅū ṅṛ ṅṝ ṅḷ ṅḹ

ṅe ṅai ṅo ṅau ṅaṁ ṅaḥ

Complete the second row of consonants with their vowel combination sequence.

Consonant:

Consonant + vowel combination sequence:

Consonant:

Consonant + vowel combination sequence:

Consonant:

Consonant + vowel combination sequence:

Consonant:

Consonant + vowel combination sequence:

Consonant:

Consonant + vowel combination sequence:

Remember that in order to form each consonant and vowel combination, the inherent schwa must be stopped by first applying the *virāma*. Review the following example.

Consonant: ka

ka + *virāma* = k (half consonant)

With the half consonant, add any vowel to create a single or double beat, as follows.

k + a = ka (single beat)

k + ā = kā (double beat)

k + i = ki (single beat)

k + ī = kī (double beat)

This is repeated until all forms are created. Each vowel is added to the base half consonant.

Recall that the representation of the *virāma* mark is not actually written in ĀYUT transliterated Sanskrit. It is only required in the original *Devanāgarī* script.

Because of this, it is easy to forget that this mandatory step exists when creating consonant and vowel combinations. When reading and writing Sanskrit only through the transliterated form, remember that the *virāma* has been applied to create all variations of combined consonants and vowels.

Conjunct consonants

Knowing, recalling and understanding the existence of this process is just as important in the formation of conjunct consonants. Stopping schwa by applying *virāma* must occur in order to produce conjunct consonants. In many words, two or more consonants may be joined together to form the word.

Recall that the base consonants in the *Devanāgarī* alphabet all include the schwa as the single beat, inherent "a" vowel.

In order to allow these consonants to join without retaining the inherent "uh" sound between them during pronunciation, the schwa must be stopped by application of *virāma*.

Review the following examples.

Example #1: Double conjunct

Consonant: na

Consonant: ta

Join the "na" and "ta" to form "nta."

na + *virāma* = n (half consonant)

n + ta = nta (single beat)

This conjunct consonant, "nta" can be seen in the word *danta*, meaning tooth.

Example #2: Double conjunct

Consonant: ja

Consonant: va

Join the "ja" and "va" to form "jva."

ja + *virāma* = j (half consonant)

j + va = jva (single beat)

This conjunct consonant, "jva" can be seen in the word *jvara*, meaning fever.

Note the pronunciation in this example is always a "w" sound rather than a hard "v" sound. In loose forms of transliteration, this term will often be incorrectly transliterated as "*jwara*" instead of "*jvara*" based on phonetic usage.

Example #3: Triple conjunct

Consonant: ta

Consonant: ta

Consonant: va

Join the "ta" and "ta" and "va" to form "ttva."

ta + *virāma*	=	t (half consonant)
t + ta + *virāma*	=	tta (single beat)
t + t + va	=	ttva (single beat)

This conjunct consonant, "ttva" can be seen in the word *sattva*, meaning determination.

Note the pronunciation in this example should recognize the presence of each half consonant in the word. To hear this distinction, try pronouncing *sattva* as "sat-tva" with attention to enunciating the first "t" of the word. Then allow the rest of the conjunct consonant, "tva" to be pronounced subsequently. Maintain the tongue pressed against the back surfaces of the front teeth to catch the first half consonant "t" in "sat."

Like the previous example, the "va" in *sattva* is always pronounced as a "w" rather than a hard "v" sound. Similarly, this term is also incorrectly transliterated as "*sattwa*" based on phonetic usage.

Special conjunct consonants

A few conjunct consonants are considered special because their combined forms in *Devanāgarī* script are written quite differently from their base components. These special conjunct consonants are often listed separately in transliteration tables found at the beginning of most Āyurvedic classical texts and scholarly works.

While these special conjunct consonants must be memorized in *Devanāgarī* script, they do not appear differently in ĀYUT transliteration.

Devanāgarī	ĀYUT	Pronunciation
क्ष क् + ष	kṣha k + ṣha	bac**k-sh**eet
ज्ञ ज् + ञ	jña j + ña	**in-y**a

Conjunct consonants with any vowel

Up to this point, examples have only demonstrated use of the first, simple vowel, *a,* which has one beat. However, conjunct consonants can be formed with any vowel.

The use of different vowels with conjunct consonants depends on the way the word itself is formed. Certain conjunct consonants naturally use certain vowels in their combinations. In other situations, the final vowel or ending appended to a word depends on the grammatical usage of the term in the complete sentence.

For example, a term used as a subject, direct object, indirect object, in a prepositional phrase or other construct, along with its gender and number, will require a specific case ending.

Additionally, certain words may be written with a final short or long *a* and retain the same meaning.

These variations and exceptions can be confusing at first. Always remember that when learning Sanskrit for Āyurveda, proper usage of ĀYUT transliteration will help to greatly reduce if not eliminate confusion. Careful and consistent usage of ĀYUT transliteration is a requirement for smooth, clear and concise communication.

Review a few examples of conjunct consonants using other vowels.

Example #1: Double conjunct with long vowel

Consonant: da
Consonant: dha
Vowel: ā

Join the "da" and "dha" and "ā" to form "ddhā."

da + *virāma* = d (half consonant)
d + dha = ddha (single beat)
d + dha + a = ddhā (double beat)

OR

d + dha + *virāma* + ā = ddhā (double beat)

This conjunct consonant, "ddhā" can be seen in the word *siddhānta*, meaning law or principle.

Example #2: Double conjunct with diphthong vowel

Consonant: śha
Consonant: la
Vowel: e

Join the "śha" and "la" and "e" to form "śhle."

śha + *virāma* = śh (half consonant)
śh + la = śhla (single beat)
śh + la + *virāma* + e = śhle (double beat)

This conjunct consonant, "śhle" can be seen in the word *śhleṣhma*, which is a synonym for kapha.

Example #3: Double conjunct with ṛ vowel

Consonant: sa
Consonant: ma
Vowel: ṛ

Join the "sa" and "ma" and "ṛ" to form "smṛ."

sa + *virāma* = s (half consonant)
s + ma = sma (single beat)
s + ma + *virāma* + ṛ = smṛ (single beat)

This conjunct consonant, "smṛ" can be seen in the word *smṛti*, meaning remembered.

Note in this example the "ṛ" is the vowel. This is often incorrectly transliterated as "ri" or "ru." Without knowing the *Devanāgarī* alphabet and the term thoroughly, it would be very easy to confuse the "ṛ" vowel for an "r" consonant plus either "i" or "u" as the vowel.

WORD DISSECTION AND FORMATION

The next step of combining consonants and vowels is to produce words. In order to understand how words are formed and to know their component *akṣharas*, review the following exercises of word dissection and formation.

Word dissection breaks each word down to its base *akṣharas* and identifies the specifics of each *akṣhara*.

For vowels, note the following:

1. Short or long vowel
2. Monophthong or diphthong
3. Anusvara or visarga

For consonants, note the following:

1. Row number
2. Column number
3. Unaspirated, aspirated or nasal

For semivowels, note the following:

1. Semivowel number (1-4)

For sibilants, note the following:

1. Sibilant number (1-3)

And for the aspirate, it only needs to be identified as such because there is only one aspirate.

Example #1: Kapha

kapha		→	ka	+	pha				
	ka	=	1:1 UN, includes schwa (short *a*)						
	pha	=	5:2 AS; includes schwa (short *a*)						

Example #2: Pitta

pitta		→	pi	+	t	+	ta		
		→	pa + *virāma*	+	i	+	ta + *virāma*	+	ta
	pa	=	5:1 UN; includes schwa (short *a*), apply *virāma*						
	i	=	short vowel, monophthong						
	ta	=	4:1 UN; includes schwa (short *a*), apply *virāma*						
	ta	=	4:1 UN; includes schwa (short *a*)						

Example #3: Vāta

vāta		→	vā	+	ta		
		→	va	+	a	+	ta
	OR	→	va + *virāma*	+	ā	+	ta
	va	=	SV 4; includes schwa (short *a*), apply *virāma*				
	ā	=	long vowel, monophthong				
	ta	=	4:1 UN; includes schwa (short *a*)				

Example #4: Āyurveda

āyurveda		→	ā	+	yu	+	r	+	ve	+	da
		→	ā + ya + *virāma* + u + ra + *virāma* + va + *virāma* + e + da								
	ā	=	long vowel, monophthong								
	ya	=	SV 1; includes schwa (short *a*), apply *virāma*								
	u	=	short vowel, monophthong								
	ra	=	SV 2; includes schwa (short *a*), apply *virāma*								
	va	=	SV 4; includes schwa (short *a*), apply *virāma*								
	e	=	long vowel, diphthong								
	da	=	4:3 UN; includes schwa (short *a*)								

Example #5: Doṣha

doṣha	→	do	+	ṣha				
	→	da + *virāma*	+	o	+	ṣha		

da	=	4:3 UN; includes schwa (short *a*), apply *virāma*
o	=	long vowel, diphthong
ṣha	=	SB 2; includes schwa (short *a*)

Example #6: Dhātu

dhātu	→	dhā	+	tu				
	→	dha + *virāma*	+	ā	+	ta + *virāma*	+	u

dha	=	4:4 AS; includes schwa (short *a*), then apply *virāma*
ā	=	long vowel, monophthong
ta	=	4:1 UN; includes schwa (short *a*), then apply *virāma*
u	=	short vowel, monophthong

Example #7: Vaidya

vaidya	→	vai	+	d	+	ya		
	→	va + *virāma*	+	ai	+	da + *virāma*	+	ya

va	=	SV 4; includes schwa (short *a*), then apply *virāma*
ai	=	long vowel, diphthong
da	=	4:3 UN; includes schwa (short *a*), then apply *virāma*
ya	=	SV 1; includes schwa (short *a*)

Example #8: Lakṣhaṇa

lakṣhaṇa	→	la	+	kṣha	+	ṇa		
	→	la	+	ka + *virāma*	+	ṣha	+	ṇa

la	=	SV 3; includes schwa (short *a*)
ka	=	1:1 UN; includes schwa (short *a*), then apply *virāma*
ṣha	=	SB 2, includes schwa (short *a*)
ṇa	=	3:5 NA; includes schwa (short *a*)

Example #9: Vṛddhi

vṛddhi		→	vṛ + d + dhi
		→	va + *virāma* + ṛ + da + *virāma* + dha + *virāma* + i
	va	=	SV 4; includes schwa (short *a*), then apply *virāma*
	ṛ	=	short vowel, monophthong
	da	=	4:3 UN; includes schwa (short *a*), then apply *virāma*
	dha	=	4:4 AS; includes schwa (short *a*), then apply *virāma*
	i	=	short vowel, monophthong

Example #10: Kṣhaya

kṣhaya		→	kṣha + ya
		→	ka + *virāma* + ṣha + ya
	ka	=	1:1 UN; includes schwa (short *a*), then apply *virāma*
	ṣha	=	SB 2, includes schwa (short *a*)
	ya	=	SV 1; includes schwa (short *a*)

Word dissection allows any known word to be broken down and reduce it to its most basic components. This allows the word and its specific meaning. to be understood in detail. Word dissection is an excellent tool when reading complex, combined lines of Sanskrit which are commonly seen in the Āyurvedic classics.

Word formation is the opposite of word dissection. It combines the base components of any word. It is especially useful when *sandhi* is applied. In classical Āyurvedic literature, multiple terms are often combined in sequence in prose and poetry.

Word dissection examples

Use the following terms to practice word dissection and formation.

Srotas

Ojas

Āyuḥ

Veda

Ahitāyu

Sukha

Duḥkha

Agni

Ṛtu

Hita

Jñāna

Śhākha

Kāma

Mokṣha

Śhruti

Smṛti

Anādi

Aṣhṭa

Śhiṣhya

Kṣhatriya

Āgama

Yukti

Āpta

Pratyakṣha

Deśha

GRAMMATICAL DHĀTUS

Bringing consonants and vowels together is the first step in forming words. Most words in Sanskrit derive from a verbal root called a *dhātu*.

Various Sanskrit scholars claim differing numbers of *dhātus*, ranging from 1,200 to 2,000. Each *dhātu* can be considered a cluster of consonants and vowels with a specific meaning.

Note that when writing a *dhātu*, it is preceded by the " √ " sign. This square root sign indicates that this is the root form which acts as the base word form.

Learning a few common *dhātus* can be helpful for deriving meanings of words in later study. For example, the word *doṣha* derives from the *dhātu* √ *duṣh*.

The Monier-Williams Sanskrit Dictionary defines √ *duṣh* as "to become bad or corrupted, to be defiled or impure, to be ruined, or to perish." Understanding the word's *dhātu* gives insight into the meaning of its derived word, *doṣha*.

On this base, various modifications can be applied using prefixes, suffixes and even other words. Each *dhātu* can take many forms. Their subsequent meanings can be altered or customized based on the combination with other prefixes, syllables and modifiable endings.

Altered and expanded *dhātus* can morph into any type of word form, including verbs, nouns, adjectives, adverbs, etc.

Prefixes are often added to *dhātus* to influence the final meaning. With formed words, endings are frequently modified based on the grammatical context of the word in the sentence.

Sanskrit grammar functions like Latin, German and Malayalam, and uses declensions for nouns and verbs rather than additional words like pronouns and prepositions to construct sentences.

Examples of common *dhātus* can be found in the Monier Williams Sanskrit English dictionary.

√ *ag*

to move tortuously, wind, go

√ *as*

to be, live, exist, be present, take place, happen

√ *ās*

to sit, sit down, rest, lie, be present, exist

√ *bandh*

to bind, tie, fix, fasten, chain

√ *char*

to move one's self, go, walk, move, stir, roam about, wander

√ *dhā*

to hold, put, maintain, give, bear

√ *dip*

to shine, burn, be illustrious

√ *kṛ*

to do, make, perform, accomplish, cause, effect, prepare, undertake

√ vā

to go, blow, hurt, injure, kill, move

√ *vid*

to know, understand, perceive, learn, become or be acquainted with, be conscious of, have a correct notion of

Each of these *dhātus* is commonly used in classical Āyurveda and Yoga. When combined with various prefixes, suffixes and other word parts, the final meaning can become very specific.

For example, the *dhātu* √ *kṛ* develops into the terms *prakṛti*, *vikṛti*, *saṁskṛta* and *kṛta*.

TEST YOURSELF

Learn, review and memorize key terms from this section.

dhātu

√ duṣh

AKṢHARA MEANINGS

Sanskrit is a prolific, highly developed language. Even its most basic *akṣharas* in the *Devanāgarī* alphabet have individual meanings. Each single *akṣhara* can be translated in numerous ways depending on the term where it is used and the context.

This type of knowledge that is naturally embedded in the language provides students with yet another tool for learning. Each *akṣhara* can be researched in the dictionary and its meanings can be memorized. When constructing words, these inherent *akṣhara* meanings can be utilized to provide a better understanding of any given term.

Use the Monier-Williams Sanskrit dictionary online, or the Spoken Sanskrit dictionary online to research a few *akṣharas*.

A simple example is the word *khaga* which means bird. By applying word dissection, we can see that this word is composed of two basic consonants:

khaga > kha + ga

Kha refers to space or sky, while *ga* refers to going or moving. Thus, *khaga* is the one who goes or moves around in the sky, or a bird.

DISTINCTIONS IN DEVANĀGARĪ USAGE

The *Devanāgarī* script covered here originates from the older, Vedic Sanskrit. This provides the foundations for today's varied usage in several Indian languages, including Hindi. However, the current *Devanāgarī* used in Hindi contains a slightly smaller number of *akṣharas*, and the pronunciation rules are significantly different.

It should be noted that many native Hindi speakers will tend to use Hindi pronunciations for Sanskrit terminologies in Āyurveda. This causes confusion for those beginning to learn Sanskrit as these minor differences may appear significant.

Variations in spelling, in transliteration schemes and in regional Indian dialects are the most common sources for confusion. For example, the word "Āyurveda" (Sanskrit) is pronounced "Āyurved" in Hindi, as if a *virāma* had been applied to the final consonant in the word.

This is called schwa deletion. Schwa exists in Sanskrit and only a few common Indian languages like Malayalam. Schwa deletion, or syncope, occurs in most major Indian languages including Hindi, Urdu, Bengali, Punjabi and Gujarati.

Unlike Sanskrit, Hindi does not recognize the

inherent "ah" sound, or schwa in each consonant. This means that any Sanskrit term which naturally ends in "a" (the inherent schwa) will lose it's "ah" sound when pronounced by native Hindi speakers.

Additionally, conjunct consonants tend to be pronounced where they would not actually exist in Sanskrit because of the same absence of schwa in Hindi. Although the pronunciation and transliterated word may appear to be different, the intended meaning generally remains the same.

The word "Devanāgarī" (Sanskrit form) is a good example, because its Hindi transliteration is written "Devanāgri" (notice the dropped "a" at between the g and r). When pronounced, however it may sound different enough to appear to be a different word.

There are many examples to demonstrate this. Common Āyurvedic terms such as *doṣha*, *vāta*, *pitta*, and *kapha* turn into shortened forms when pronounced by many native Hindi speakers. They become "doṣh," "vāt," "pitt," and "kaph" with the trailing "ah" sound conspicuously absent.

Because of the non-existence of schwa in these languages, native speakers read Sanskrit *Devanāgarī* and apply schwa deletion. This removes the "a" vowel from the end of words so they sound shortened. This type of pronunciation is not considered classical Sanskrit and should be avoided in Āyurveda. These pronunciations are correct when used in Hindi.

Examples of Hindi pronunciation can include:

Sanskrit	**Hindi**
Āyurveda	Āyurved
Doṣha	Doṣh
Vāta	Vāt
Pitta	PItt
Kapha	Kaph

Any term that ends with an inherent schwa will typically be shortened by native speakers of other Indian languages where schwa does not exist.

In Malayalam and Tamil, two predominant South Indian languages which are influenced by Dravidian roots, there is a tendency to add an "mmm" sound onto the end of many common Āyurvedic terms.

With these native speakers, terms like *doṣha*, *vāta*, *pitta*, and *kapha* are pronounced as "doṣham," "vātam," "pittam," and "kapham." Although these regional phonetic differences do not change the underlying meaning of the terms, they can present confusion for people who are not native speakers of an Indian language.

TEST YOURSELF

Learn, review and memorize key terms from this section.

schwa deletion

Chapter 34: Review

ADDITIONAL READING

Utilize these references to expand your understanding of the concepts in this chapter.

CLASSICS	1st read	2nd read

REQUIRED READING	Chapters

OPTIONAL READING	Format

References

"duṣh." Monier-Williams Sanskrit-English Dictionary, 1899, http://www.sanskrit-lexicon.uni-koeln.de/scans/MWScan/2014/web/webtc/indexcaller.php

Kale, M. R. (1924). "A Smaller Sanskrit Grammar." Gopal Narayen & Co.

Monier Williams Sanskrit-English Dictionary (2008 revision). (n.d.). Retrieved from https://www.sanskrit-lexicon.uni-koeln.de/monier/

Schwa. (n.d.). Retrieved from https://www.oxfordlearnersdictionaries.com/us/definition/english/schwa?q=schwa

QUESTIONS & ANSWERS

Record your questions for this chapter here for further research and discussion.

Question:

Answer:

Question:

Answer:

Question:

Answer:

SELF-ASSESSMENT

1. Word dissection identifies
   a. *akṣharas*
   b. base syllables
   c. conjunct consonants
   d. vowels
   e. All of the above

2. To stop an inherent schwa, apply the
   a. *akṣhara*
   b. aspirate
   c. ellipse
   d. *virāma*
   e. *visarga*

3. Which modern Indian language commonly applies schwa deletion?
   a. Gujarati
   b. Hindi
   c. Malayalam
   d. Tamil
   e. Urdu

4. *Virāma* is never visibly applied in
   a. *akṣharas*
   b. complete Sanskrit terms
   c. conjunct consonants
   d. *Devanāgarī*
   e. transliteration

5. Which of the following is a half consonant?
   a. *ā*
   b. *cha*
   c. *da*
   d. *m*
   e. *tha*

6. Which of the following is a special conjunct consonant?
   a. *aṁ*
   b. *ddhā*
   c. *kī*
   d. *kṣha*
   e. *ttva*

7. When performing word dissection, consonants must be identified by their
   a. aspiration
   b. consonant number
   c. row number
   d. nasal pronunciation
   e. All of the above

8. Sanskrit *dhātus* number between
   a. 800 to 1,000
   b. 1,000 to 1,000
   c. 1,000 to 1,200
   d. 1,200 to 2,000
   e. 1,200 to 2,400

9. The Sanskrit *dhātu* √ *duṣh* means
   a. to become bad
   b. to become corrupted
   c. to become impure
   d. to be ruined
   e. All of the above

10. The *akṣhara* "ga" means
    a. to be or become
    b. to fly
    c. to go or move
    d. to make complete
    e. None of the above

Chapter 35 : Numerals, prefixes and suffixes

Learning common numerals, prefixes and suffixes is a helpful way to quickly grasp basic Sanskrit language concepts. Use the information in this chapter to practice basic reading, pronunciation and recognition of simple terms and components. Prefixes and suffixes are especially helpful to expand vocabulary early in studies.

NUMERALS

Numbers and their numeral forms are used frequently in Āyurvedic study and practice. Review this entire list and become familiar with numbers 0 to 25.

Cardinal	Sanskrit	Cardinal Sanskrit	Cardinal Transliteration	Ordinal	Ordinal Sanskrit	Ordinal Transliteration
0	०	शून्य	śhūnya	n/a	n/a	n/a
1	१	एकम्	ekam	1st	प्रथम अग्रिम आदिम	prathama agrima ādima
2	२	द्वि	dvi	2nd	द्वितीय	dvitīya
3	३	त्रि	tri	3rd	तृतीय	tṛtīya
4	४	चतुर्	catur	4th	चतुर्थ	caturtha
5	५	पञ्च	pañca	5th	पञ्चम	pañcama
6	६	षष् षड् षट्	ṣhaṣh ṣhaḍ ṣhaṭ	6th	षष्ठ	ṣhaṣhṭha
7	७	सप्त	sapta	7th	सप्तम	saptama
8	८	अष्ट	aṣhṭa	8th	अष्टम	aṣhṭama
9	९	नवम्	navam	9th	नवम	navama
10	१०	दश	daśha	10th	दशम	daśhama
11	११	एकादश	ekādaśha	11th	एकादश	ekādaśha
12	१२	द्वादश	dvādaśha	12th	द्वादश	dvādaśha
13	१३	त्रयोदश	trayodaśha	13th	त्रयोदश	trayodaśha

14	१४	चतुर्दश	caturdaśha	14th	चतुर्दश	caturdaśha
15	१५	पञ्चदश	pañcadaśha	15th	पञ्चदश	pañcadaśha
16	१६	षोडश	ṣhoḍaśha	16th	षोडश	ṣhoḍaśha
17	१७	सप्तदश	saptadaśha	17th	सप्तदश	saptadaśha
18	१८	अष्टादशन्	aṣhṭādaśhan	18th	अष्टादश	aṣhṭādaśha
19	१९	नवदश	navadaśha ekonaviṁśhati ūnaviṁśhati ekānnaviṁśh ati	19th	नवदश एकोनविंश	navadaśha ekonaviṁśha ekonaviṁśhatitama ūnaviṁśha ūnaviṁśhatitama ekānnaviṁśha ekānnaviṁśhatitama
20	२०	विंशति	viṁśhati	20th	विंश विंशतितम	viṁśha viṁśhatitama
21	२१	एक-विंशति	ekaviṁśhati	21st	एकविंश एकविंशतितम	ekaviṁśha ekaviṁśhatitama
22	२२	द्वाविंशति	dvāviṁśhati	22nd	द्वाविंश द्वाविंशतितम	dvāviṁśha dvāviṁśhatitama
23	२३	त्रयो-विंशति	trayoviṁśhati	23rd	त्रयोविंश त्रयोविंशतितम	trayoviṁśha trayoviṁśhatitama
24	२४	चतुर्विंशति	caturviṁśhati	24th	चतुर्विंश चतुर्विंशतितम	caturviṁśha caturviṁśhatitama
25	२५	पञ्चविंशति	pañcaviṁśhati	25th	पञ्चविंश पञ्चविंशतितम	pañcaviṁśha pañcaviṁśhatitama

PREFIXES

Prefixes are commonly used in Sanskrit on many types of words (verbs, nouns, adjectives, etc). Understanding common prefixes is helpful to better understand the specific meaning of the term. Review this entire list and practice using these prefixes (Prefixes, 2011).

Transliterated prefix	Original Sanskrit	Meaning
a	अ	not, negative
ā	आ	completely, in total
abhi	अभि	to, against
adhi	अधि	above, over, on
an	अन्	not, negative; used before a vowel
anu	अनु	after, following
apa	अप	away, off
api	अपि	on, close on
ati	अति	across, beyond, surpassing, past
ava	अव	down, away, off
du	दु	bad, difficult, hard
ni	नि	down, into
nir	निर्	free from, absent of
nis	निस्	out from, without
parā	परा	away
pari	परि	around, about
pra	प्र	forward, in front of
sam	सम्	proper, well done
su	सु	good
sva	स्व	own, one's own
ud	उद्	up, up out

upa	उप	towards, near

SUFFIXES

Suffixes are commonly used in Sanskrit for Ayurveda as shortened forms of indicating common concepts. Understanding these regularly used suffixes is helpful for faster comprehension. Review this entire list and practice using these suffixes.

Transliterated suffix	Original Sanskrit	Meaning
atva	अत्व	-ness
ghna	घ्न	decreasing
ja	ज	born of or produced by
ka	क	action of
kara	कर	increasing
la	ल	of, producing, belonging to
ta	त	the one having something done to it

Chapter 35: Review

ADDITIONAL READING

Utilize these references to expand your understanding of the concepts in this chapter.

CLASSICS	1st read	2nd read

REQUIRED READING	Chapters

OPTIONAL READING	Format
Sanskrit Grammar, http://www.learnsanskrit.org/grammar	

References

"Prefixes" (2011, July 20). http://www.learnsanskrit.org/references/lists/prefixes

"Sanskrit Grammar" (2011, July 20). http://www.learnsanskrit.org/grammar

QUESTIONS & ANSWERS

Record your questions for this chapter here for further research and discussion.

Question:

Answer:

Question:

Answer:

Question:

Answer:

SELF-ASSESSMENT

1. Which of the following represents the number 315?
   a. ३१५
   b. ३१५
   c. ३१७
   d. ३९४
   e. ३१२

2. Which of the following represents the number ४९८?
   a. 367
   b. 498
   c. 594
   d. 782
   e. 867

3. The three *doṣhas* are termed
   a. *aṣhṭa doṣhas*
   b. *dvi doṣhas*
   c. *pañca doṣhas*
   d. *sapta doṣhas*
   e. *tri doṣhas*

4. The suffix "ja" indicates
   a. born of, or produced by
   b. decreasing
   c. going away from
   d. increasing
   e. None of the above

5. The suffix "ghna" indicates
   a. around
   b. decreasing
   c. down
   d. hard
   e. increasing

6. The prefix "a" indicates
   a. above, over, on
   b. completely, in total
   c. negation
   d. on, close on
   e. own, one's own

7. Which prefix indicates being in front of, or forward?
   a. *abhi*
   b. *du*
   c. *pra*
   d. *sam*
   e. *sva*

8. The term *saṁskṛta* contains which prefix?
   a. *a*
   b. *aṁ*
   c. *an*
   d. *sa*
   e. *saṁ*

9. To indicate that something is increasing, which suffix should be added?
   a. *ghna*
   b. *ja*
   c. *ka*
   d. *kara*
   e. *ta*

10. The meaning of the term *sukha* is indicated by
    a. its prefix *sa*
    b. its prefix *su*
    c. its suffix *ha*
    d. its suffix *kha*
    e. None of the above

Chapter 36 : Sandhi

KEY TERMS

avagraha sandhi

Sandhi is a widely used concept in Sanskrit, especially in the Āyurvedic classics. The word itself literally means joint. In the context of Sanskrit, it specifically refers to the act of joining two words together. It allows two words to modify their conjoining letters by altering the ending syllable of the first word and the beginning syllable of the second word. This makes the pronunciation smoother.

While this concept does not formally exist in English, there are a few examples where it is found in speech. A common example is the word "cupboard" which is not pronounced "cup-board" but rather "cubboard." This alteration allows it to be pronounced quickly and easily.

The rules of *sandhi* in Sanskrit are large and complex. There are dozens of potential combinations which each have their own specific names and classical examples cited by the father of Sanskrit grammar, Pāṇinī. A formal study of Sanskrit requires that the student learn each *sandhi* combination, memorize the names of formations and memorize their corresponding classical examples.

Here a few references are provided to better understand the concept and its implications. The main tool for creating and breaking *sandhis* is a *sandhi* chart. At the introductory level start with *sandhis* that occur with vowels only. When these are easy to recognize, break and form, then move on to the *sandhis* with consonants, semivowels, sibilants and the aspirate.

The charts can be used in two ways:

1. To create a *sandhi* by joining two words together
2. To break a *sandhi* at its joint and separate the two original words

Creating a *sandhi* is generally easier at first. Breaking *sandhis* becomes easier as one's vocabulary increases.

The rules of *sandhi* in Sanskrit are large and complex. There are dozens of potential combinations which each have their own specific names and classical examples cited by the father of Sanskrit grammar, Pāṇinī. A formal study of Sanskrit requires that the student learn each *sandhi* combination by memorizing formation names and their corresponding classical examples in original *śhloka* (verse) form

Sandhis form in various ways depending on the type of *akṣhara* found at the end of the first word and at the beginning of the second word.

When the *akṣharas* join in a *sandhi*, they are replaced by a specific *akṣhara* or *akṣhara* combination. Generally, the replacement produces a smoother version of the two sounds coalesced into a single sound.

When pronounced, most *sandhis* sound so smooth that they are barely discernable as transitions from one word to the next. This feature of Sanskrit allows it to be easily used for writing in poetic meter.

Combinations and their replacements are listed in the following table.

Ending *akṣhara*	Starting *akṣhara*	Replaced by
Vowel	Vowel	Vowel Or, semivowel plus vowel
Consonant	Vowel, semivowel, sibilant or aspirate	Consonant Or, consonant plus sibilant
Consonant	Consonant	Consonant Or, *anusvāra* (aṁ) Or, nasal consonant Or, *anusvāra* (aṁ) plus sibilant
Visarga (aḥ)	Vowel, semivowel or sibilant	Vowel Or, semivowel r(a)
Visarga (aḥ)	Consonant	Vowel Or, vowel plus sibilant Or, semivowel r(a) Or, sibilant

VOWEL *SANDHIS*

There are several types of vowel plus vowel combinations, depending on the vowels being short or long, and monophthong or diphthong.

Each of these combinations can be seen in the vowel *sandhi* chart. The final *akṣhara* of the first word is listed on the left. The starting *akṣhara* of the second word is listed on the top.

The chart should be read from left to right. First find the ending *akṣhara* then move right across the row to find the starting *akṣhara*. The intersection point is the replacement *akṣhara*.

Unshaded rows and columns indicate short vowels. Shaded rows and columns indicate long vowels.

Note that three *akṣharas* from the classical Vedic *Devanāgarī* alphabet are not listed here (ṝ, ḷ, ḹ). Because these are so rarely used, they are omitted from standard *sandhi* charts.

Wherever two *akṣharas* are listed as the replacement, it indicates that one or the other may be used. This flexibility allows greater versatility for poetic meter.

Unshaded rows and columns indicate short vowels. Shaded rows and columns indicate long vowels.

Note that three *akṣharas* from the classical Vedic *Devanāgarī* alphabet are not listed here (ṝ, ḷ, ḹ). Because these are so rarely used, they are omitted from standard *sandhi* charts.

Final *akṣhara*: First word	Starting *akṣhara*: Second word										
	a	**ā**	**i**	**ī**	**u**	**ū**	**ṛ**	**e**	**ai**	**o**	**au**
a	ā	ā	e	e	o	o	ar	ai	ai	au	au
ā	ā	ā	e	e	o	o	ar	ai	ai	au	au
i	ya	yā	ī	ī	yu	yū	yṛ	ye	yai	yo	yau
ī	ya	yā	ī	ī	yu	yū	yṛ	ye	yai	yo	yau
u	va	vā	vi	vī	ū	ū	vṛ	ve	vai	vo	vau
ū	va	vā	vi	vī	ū	ū	vṛ	ve	vai	vo	vau
ṛ	ra	rā	ri	rī	ru	rū	ṝ	re	rai	ro	rau
e	e ‘	a ā	a i	a ī	a u	a ū	a ṛ	a e	a ai	a o	a au
ai	ā a	ā ā	ā i	ā ī	ā u	ā ū	ā ṛ	ā e	ā ai	ā o	ā au
o	o ‘	avā	avi	avī	avu	avū	avṛ	ave	avai	avo	avau
au	āva	āvā	āvi	āvī	āvu	āvū	āvṛ	āve	āvai	āvo	āvau

CREATING A *SANDHI*

To create a *sandhi* with a vowel plus a vowel combination, begin by identifying the *akṣhara* at the end of the first word. Confirm that it is a vowel. Then match it using the previous chart by finding the vowel in the leftmost column, “Final *akṣhara*: First word.”

Then, identify the *akṣhara* at the start of the second word. Confirm that it is a vowel. Then match it in the chart in the top row, “Starting *akṣhara*: Second word.”

Follow the top column down to where it meets the row from the left. That intersection point is what will replace the *akṣhara* at the end of the first word and the *akṣhara* at the beginning of the second word.

Example #1: Short plus long vowel

ām**a** + **ā**śhaya → ām**ā**śhaya

The ending short *a* + the beginning long *ā* are replaced by a long *ā*.

Example #2: Short plus short vowel

dhāt**u** + **a**gni → dhāt**va**gni

The ending short *u* + the beginning short *a* are replaced by the semivowel *va*.

Note here that vowel combinations may combine to form long or longer vowels (ie, two beats) or they may convert into semivowels.

The possible changes that can occur through *sandhi* combinations can generally be categorized as easy, medium and difficult.

Easy *sandhis* will often occur when two short vowels of the same type combine, such as *a* plus *a*, or *i* plus *i*, or *u* plus *u*.

Medium *sandhis* will often occur when monophthongs (short or long vowels) combine to form a diphthong or semivowel.

Difficult *sandhis* will often occur when different types of consonants combine to form other consonants. These are challenging to create, identify and break at an introductory level.

Gaining proficiency with *sandhis* requires long-term study and practice. Students with larger vocabularies will find it much easier to identify *sandhis* quickly through word recognition.

TEST YOURSELF

Learn, review and memorize key terms from this section.

sandhi

BREAKING A *SANDHI*

To break a *sandhi*, first identify the location of the *sandhi* in the conjoined words. This can be tricky if the base words are unfamiliar. However, with practice, even unknown words can be separated easily, especially when using the dictionary as a reference tool.

Once the *sandhi* has been identified, look through the body of the charts to find it, and then follow the column up to the top to locate the original ending of the first word. Then follow the row to the right to find the original beginning of the second word. You can use the same examples above to practice this, just working with the charts in the opposite way.

CONSONANT *SANDHIS*

Sandhis also commonly occur at junctions between consonants, semivowels and the *visarga* (aḥ). The combinations are generally medium or difficult to recognize and split.

Consonant *sandhis* can require multiple changes to reach their final form. Several passes split them to their original base terms. With grammatical changes due to case endings, this rectification process can be complicated.

Proficiency in splitting complex *sandhis* takes considerable practice. It also requires an extensive vocabulary and a basic working knowledge of grammar.

Consonant *sandhis* follow the same rules as vowel *sandhis* to create and break them. Use the following charts to identify the ending *akṣhara* of the first word, and the starting *akṣhara* of the second word.

Consonant plus vowel, semivowel, sibilant or aspirate

		Starting *akṣhara*: Second word								
		Vowels	**y**	**r**	**l**	**v**	**śh**	**ṣh**	**s**	**h**
Final akṣhara: First word	**k**	g	g	g	g	g	g			g(gh)
	ṭ	ḍ	ḍ	ḍ	ḍ	ḍ				ḍ(ḍh)
	t	d	d	d	l	d	ch(chh)			d(dh)
	p	b	b	b	b	b				b(bh)
	ṅ	ṅṅ								
	n	nn			ṁl		ñ(śh/chh)			
	m		ṁ	ṁ	ṁ	ṁ	ṁ	ṁ	ṁ	ṁ

Example #1: Consonant plus vowel

ru**k** + **a**dhiṣhṭhāna → ru**ga**dhiṣhṭhāna

The final consonant "-k" plus the starting short vowel "a-" are replaced by a "-g-" consonant plus the original starting short vowel.

śhara**t** + **ṛ**tu → śhara**dṛ**tu

The final consonant "-t" plus the starting short vowel "ṛ-" are replaced by a "-d-" consonant plus the original starting short vowel.

Example #2: Consonant plus semivowel

kṣhu**t** + **l**avaṇa → kṣhu**ll**avaṇa

The final consonant "-t" plus the starting semivowel "l-" are replaced by the consonant "-l-."

Example #3: Consonant plus sibilant

bṛha**t** + **śh**arīra → bṛha**chchh**arīra

The final consonant "-t" plus the starting semivowel "śh-" are replaced by the conjunct consonant "-chchh-" (from the *akṣharas* cha plus chha).

Example #4: Consonant plus aspirate

bṛha**t** + **h**ṛdaya → bṛha**ddh**ṛdaya

The final consonant "-t" plus the starting aspirate "h-" are replaced by the conjunct consonant "-ddhh-" (from the *akṣharas* da plus dha).

Consonant plus consonant

		Starting *akṣhara*: Second word										
		k kh	**g gh**	**ch chh**	**j jh**	**ṭ ṭh**	**ḍ ḍh**	**t th**	**d dh**	**p ph**	**b bh**	**n m**
Final *akṣhara*: First word	**k**		g		g		g		g		g	ṅ
	ṭ		ḍ		ḍ		ḍ		ḍ		ḍ	ṇ
	t		d	ch	j	ṭ	ḍ		d		d	n
	p		b		b		b		b		b	m
	ṇ											
	n			ṁśh	ñ	ṁṣh	ṇ	ṁṣh				
	m	ṁ	ṁ	ṁ	ṁ	ṁ	ṁ	ṁ	ṁ	ṁ	ṁ	ṁ

Example #1: Consonant plus consonant

ru**k** + **d**oṣha → ru**gd**oṣha

The final consonant "-k" plus the starting consonant "d-" are replaced by a "-g-" consonant plus the original starting consonant.

śhara**t** + **j**vara → śhara**jj**vara

The final consonant "-t" plus the starting consonant "j-" are replaced by a "-j-" consonant plus the original starting consonant.

Visarga (aḥ) plus vowel, semivowel or sibilant

		Starting *akṣhara*: Second word								
		Vowels	**y**	**r**	**l**	**v**	**śh**	**ṣh**	**s**	**h**
Final *akṣhara*: First word	**aḥ**	a o ‘	o	o	o	o				o
	āḥ	ā	ā	ā	ā	ā				ā
	?ḥ	r	r		r	r				r

Example #1: Visarga plus vowel, semivowel or sibilant

āyu**ḥ** + **v**eda → āyu**r**veda

The final visarga "-uḥ" plus the starting semivowel "v-" are replaced by a "-r-" semivowel plus the original starting semivowel.

pitta**ḥ** + **r**akta → pittorakta

The final visarga "-aḥ" plus the starting semivowel "r-" are replaced by an "-o-" vowel plus the original starting semivowel.

chakṣhuḥ + indriya → chakṣhurindriya

The final visarga "-uḥ" plus the starting vowel "i-" are replaced by a "-r-" semivowel plus the original starting vowel.

Visarga (aḥ) plus consonant

		Starting *akṣhara*: Second word										
		k **kh**	**g** **gh**	**ch** **chh**	**j** **jh**	**ṭ** **ṭh**	**ḍ** **ḍh**	**t** **th**	**d** **dh**	**p** **ph**	**b** **bh**	**n** **m**
Final *akṣhara*: First word	**aḥ**		o	aśh	o	aṣh	o	as	o		o	o
	āḥ		ā	āśh	ā	āṣh	ā	ās	ā		ā	ā
	?ḥ		r	śh	r	ṣh	r	s	r		r	r

Example #1: Visarga plus consonant

pitta**ḥ** + **ch**etana → pittaśhchetana

The final visarga "-aḥ" plus the starting consonant "ch-" are replaced by "-aśh-" plus the original starting consonant.

kaphā**ḥ** + **t**asya → kaphāstasya

The final visarga "-āḥ" plus the starting consonant "t-" are replaced by "-ās-" plus the original starting consonant.

AVAGRAHA

In the vowel *sandhi* chart, look at the intersections of the final vowels "-e" and "-o" with the starting vowel "a-." The replacement *akṣhara* for these combinations can be the *avagraha*, or ellipse. This is represented as an apostrophe (').

This is a special condition of *sandhi* where the vowels involved in the combination do not change to a replaced vowel. Instead, the ending vowel of the first word remains the same, and the starting vowel of the second word undergoes ellipsis.

Ellipsis is the removal of a syllable, so that the syllable is skipped when the combined words are pronounced.

Avagraha is written using an S-shaped character in *Devanāgarī* script. When transliterated, it is represented by a single apostrophe.

Avagraha (*Devanāgarī*) ऽ

Avagraha (ĀYUT) '

Review the following examples where *sandhi* produces the *avagraha*.

ĀYUT transliteration

eko + ayam → eko ' yam

Devanāgarī

एको अयम् → एकोऽयम्

The *avagraha* is not pronounced in recitation of Sanskrit verses and is often used in poetry to maintain meter. It essentially allows extra syllables to be included, but not pronounced.

In the example above, the phrase "eko ayam" is pronounced as "eko yam."

TEST YOURSELF

Learn, review and memorize key terms from this section.

avagraha

SANDHI EXAMPLES

Use the following examples to practice identifying and breaking *sandhis*. Utilize the *sandhi* charts to look for replacements of ending and starting *akṣharas*. With unknown terms, this may require several attempts.

Ahitāyu

Hitāyu

Āptopadeśha

Antarāgni

Vātādi

Bhūtāgni

Dehāgni

Dīrghāyu

Doṣhopakrama

Dvividhopakrama

Garbhotpatti

Ghrāṇendriya

Hiṅgvāṣhṭaka

Hṛdayopalepa

Samāgni

Viṣhamāgni

Vegāvarodha

Bṛhaccharīra

Chapter 36: Review

ADDITIONAL READING

Utilize these references to expand your understanding of the concepts in this chapter.

CLASSICS	1st read	2nd read

REQUIRED READING	Chapters
Lesson 3: Sandhi Charts, https://ubcsanskrit.ca/lesson3/sandhicharts.html	

OPTIONAL READING	Format

References

Aklujkar, Ashok. (2005). "Sanskrit: An Easy Introduction to an Enchanting Language." Svādhyāya, Vol. 1B pp. 64-66.

Lesson 3: Sandhi Charts. (n.d.). Retrieved from https://ubcsanskrit.ca/lesson3/sandhicharts.html

QUESTIONS & ANSWERS

Record your questions for this chapter here for further research and discussion.

Question:

Answer:

Question:

Answer:

Question:

Answer:

SELF-ASSESSMENT

1. Which of the following terms contains a *sandhi*?
   a. *amūrti*
   b. *bhūtāgni*
   c. *dhātumala*
   d. *mahābhūta*
   e. *pañcakarma*

2. *Sandhi* means
   a. added to
   b. between
   c. joint
   d. to make or do
   e. None of the above

3. Where is the *sandhi* in the term *puruṣhārtha*?
   a. *a*
   b. *ā*
   c. *ṣh*
   d. *u*
   e. None of the above

4. The term *dehāgni* can be broken by *sandhi* to create which two terms?
   a. de and hāgni
   b. deh and āgni
   c. deha and agni
   d. dehā and agni
   e. dehav and āgni

5. *Avagraha* is a/an
   a. *akṣhara*
   b. *anusvāra*
   c. ellipsis
   d. monophthong
   e. *navam*

6. The terms *garbha* and *utpatti* combine using *sandhi* to create the term
   a. garbhātpatti
   b. garbhetpatti
   c. garbhotpatti
   d. garbhutpatti
   e. garbhvatpatti

7. Where is the *sandhi* in the term *āptopadeśha*?
   a. a
   b. ā
   c. de
   d. e
   e. o

8. *Sandhi* is used to make
   a. pronunciation smoother
   b. words longer
   c. writing easier
   d. All of the above
   e. None of the above

9. When combining terms using *sandhi*, the final *akṣhara* of the first term is combined with
   a. the entire second term
   b. the first *akṣhara* of the second term
   c. the first letter of the second term
   d. the second *akṣhara* of the first term
   e. None of the above

10. Combining two of the same short vowels always results in
    a. an equivalent semivowel
    b. *avagraha*
    c. their long vowel
    d. "v" plus the same long vowel
    e. None of the above

Chapter 37 : Language and grammar

KEY TERMS

Anglicization

Sanskrit and English differ in almost every fundamental aspect of their languages and grammar. Sanskrit is much more similar to Latin and Greek because of its use of declensions and cases. English has evolved out of these more complex grammatical structures to become the analytic language used today (Wheeler, 2018).

In Sanskrit, case endings allow words to be placed in any order in a sentence. Prepositional phrases are not used and are instead represented by the case of the noun. Verbs also use more complex endings to indicate singular, dual and plural formats. These constructs do not exist in English.

ANGLICIZATION OF SANSKRIT

As Sanskrit becomes more popular in Western spheres, its usage will increase in spoken and written English. When integrating Sanskrit into another language, it is important to understand how it is being used.

Generally, Sanskrit terms represent concepts that are unfamiliar in languages or cultures outside of India. Because of this, there typically is no English language equivalent for the Sanskrit term or concept. Rather than translate the term insufficiently, it is preferable to use the original Sanskrit term in the context of spoken or written English.

When integrating Sanskrit terms into a different language in this way, the rules and grammar of the main language should be applied. Consider the following example of the concept of *agni*, which is broadly correlated to the power of digestion and metabolism in Āyurveda:

"Health depends on *agni*'s current state."

The Anglicization of the Sanskrit term *agni* in this example applies " 's " (apostrophe plus s) to the term to make it possessive. This shows possessive form using English grammatical rules, not those of Sanskrit.

Consider the following example of a plural form using the concept of *doṣha* (commonly written as "dosha" without the under-dot):

"The three *doṣhas* of the body are *vāta*, *pitta* and *kapha*."

The Anglicization of the Sanskrit term *doṣha* applies " -s " to the term to make it plural. This use of plural is based on English grammatical rules, not those of Sanskrit.

For Sanskrit terms that end in "-s," their plural form is created by adding the ending "-es" to the term. For example, "*srotas*," which roughly translates as channel, or network of channels in the human body, is Anglicized to a plural form as "*srotases*."

When creating possessive forms of Sanskrit terms ending in "-s" or "-es," add an apostrophe at the end of the term. Consider the following examples:

The *doṣhas'* states are all increased.

The *srotases'* size is minute.

Similarly other English grammatical rules can be applied to Sanskrit terms when they are Anglicized.

Chapter 37: Review

ADDITIONAL READING

Utilize these references to expand your understanding of the concepts in this chapter.

CLASSICS	1st read	2nd read

REQUIRED READING	Chapters
Declensions and Cases, https://web.cn.edu/kwheeler/declensions.html	
Starting Out, http://www.learnsanskrit.org/start	
Verb Basics, http://www.learnsanskrit.org/start/verbs	

OPTIONAL READING	Format
http://www.springer.com/us/book/9783642001543	

References

Wheeler, L. Kip. (1998-2018). "Declensions and Cases." https://web.cn.edu/kwheeler/declensions.html

"Starting Out" (2011, July 20). http://www.learnsanskrit.org/start

"Verb Basics" (2011, July 20). http://www.learnsanskrit.org/start/verbs

"Noun Basics" (2011, July 20). http://www.learnsanskrit.org/start/nouns

QUESTIONS & ANSWERS

Record your questions for this chapter here for further research and discussion.

Question:

Answer:

Question:

Answer:

Question:

Answer:

SELF-ASSESSMENT

1. Languages that use declension systems ignore
   a. case endings
   b. number (singular, plural)
   c. word meaning
   d. word order
   e. All of the above

2. Sanskrit is a/an _____ language.
   a. analytic
   b. complementary
   c. dead
   d. synthetic
   e. technical

3. Verbal number in Sanskrit recognizes
   a. dual
   b. plural
   c. singular
   d. All of the above
   e. None of the above

4. Which languages use declension systems?
   a. Greek
   b. Latin
   c. Malayalam
   d. Old English
   e. All of the above

5. By changing the ending of a word in Sanskrit, it usually changes its
   a. complete meaning
   b. punctuation
   c. root term
   d. usage in the sentence
   e. None of the above

6. Which two Sanskrit grammatical components can easily be confused?
   a. case endings and suffixes
   b. grammatical dhātus and single bars
   c. prefixes and suffixes
   d. suffixes and double bars
   e. All of the above

7. Modern English is a/an _____ language.
   a. active
   b. analytic
   c. declension-based
   d. phonetic
   e. synthetic

8. A subject of a sentence must be in
   a. accusative case
   b. genitive case
   c. nominative case
   d. verbal number
   e. verbal order

9. In Sanskrit, the pronoun “we” is
   a. dual case
   b. plural case
   c. singular case
   d. All of the above
   e. None of the above

10. A Sanskrit sentence that refers to “Charaka and Suśhruta” is in
    a. dual case
    b. plural case
    c. singular case
    d. All of the above
    e. None of the above

Chapter 38 : Reading and writing proficiency

KEY TERMS

adhyāya	line numbers	samhitā	sthāna
commentary	poetry	single bar	ṭikā
double bar	prose	śhloka	

The goal with learning basic Sanskrit is to be able to fluently read the Romanized, transliterated form aloud with awareness of the correct pronunciation. In order to do this, the transliterated *Devanāgarī* alphabet must be completely memorized so that it can be recited naturally and easily.

The next step is to practice reading and speaking words aloud so that their unique combination of *akṣharas* becomes fluid. Beyond this, new words and eventually sentences will gradually become easier to read.

To study the classics, remember that being able to translate complete sentences, especially in older Vedic Sanskrit, is a very advanced skill and not a requirement for entry-level Āyurvedic study. Reading, writing and vocabulary recognition (of transliterated script) are the skills that one should focus on and grow in the early stages of training.

To navigate the classics, it is also helpful to be familiar with how Sanskrit words and sentences are conveyed. This is accomplished classically through prose and poetry. Prose is more commonly used in the older classics to fully explain concepts and details using ordinary language and sentence structure without metrical form.

Poetry became more prevalent in later literature once the concepts were more widely known and well-evolved. Since fewer detailed explanations were needed to convey meanings, information could be presented in a somewhat abbreviated form. Various forms of poetic meter were used depending on the author, the geographical region and cultural and religious influences.

Both prose and poetry form are written in single lines known as a *śhloka* in Sanskrit. *Śhlokas* are found throughout Sanskrit literature and are not unique to Āyurveda.

Śhlokas can behave like sentences, statements, aphorisms, or poetic lines. There is very little punctuation used when writing *śhlokas*. Typically, only a vertical single bar "|" or double bar " || " is present at the end of a line to indicate an intermediate stop or full stop (like a period), respectively.

These bars do not necessarily mean that all words of a sentence are found together as a period would. They merely indicate the end of something and are more commonly used to count line numbers within the text.

It's easy to recognize the difference between prose and poetry in the classics. Review the following examples.

PROSE

Review this example from Cha. Sū. 30/23 (Śarmā, R. K., & Dāsa, B., 2016):

Definition of Āyurveda :

तदायुर्वेदयतीत्यायुर्वेदः; कथमिति चेत् ? उच्यते-स्वलक्षणतः सुखासुखतो हिताहिततः प्रमाणाप्रमाणातश्च; यतश्चायुष्याण्यनायुष्याणि च द्रव्यगुणकर्माणि वेदयत्यतोऽप्यायुर्वेदः। तत्रायुष्याण्यनायुष्याणि च द्रव्यगुणकर्माणि केवलेनोपदेक्ष्यन्ते तन्त्रेण ॥ २३ ॥

The science which imparts knowledge about life, with special reference to its definition, and the description of happy and unhappy life, useful and harmful life, long and short spans of life and such other material alongwith their properties and actions as promote and demote longevity will be described in the entire treatise. [23]

Some commentators derive the term वेदयति from the root '*vidl*' (विद्लृ लाभे), to get. But any such meaning cannot be accepted in the present context.

Figuratively, the term *āyuṣ*' indicates substances which both promote and demote longevity. Substances which are not conducive to longevity are not to be used and so they are to be discarded. Thus the knowledge of even such substances serves the useful purpose for the sustenance of life; hence they are described among others to mean life.

Scanned from: Śharmā, R. K., & Dāsh, B. Agniveśha's Charaka Saṁhitā. Varanasi: Chowkhamba Sanskrit Series Office; Reprint Edition. 2016. Cha. Sū. 1/41-42.

Here the *Devanāgarī* script is preceded by an italicized English heading, *Definition of Āyurveda*. This helps convey the *śhloka* contents and is usually added by the translator. Headings were not generally used in the original literature. Following the heading is the actual *śhloka* written in the original *Devanāgarī* script.

Notice the bar that runs over the top of many of the *akṣharas*. Sometimes this bar can indicate words that work together grammatically in a sentence, or words which the author wants to emphasize together. However, the top bar can have many uses, intentions and interpretations, and at times it may have no apparent significance at all.

Next, find the single bar "|" on the third line. This indicates some sort of separation, either in meaning or grammar, within the *śhloka* itself. Finally the *śhloka* ends with the double bar " || " followed by a numeral.

These numerals may be written in *Devanāgarī* numbers or Arabic numbers, depending on the translator and editor. This is followed by another double bar " || " to complete the *śhloka*.

The English printed in the larger font size immediately below the *Devanāgarī* script is the direct translation. Note that translators often take meaning and interpretation of the text as a higher priority over grammatical translation. This means that they try to capture the "sense" of the *śhloka* over focusing on matching the translation grammatically. Inconsistencies and irregularities in translation are common, especially in grammar, spelling and transliteration.

Initially most native English-language readers cannot understand the translations correctly. This is normal. It takes time, exposure and experience to be able to navigate the classics, even when they are presented in English.

Certain Sanskrit terms are often translated using a single English word which does not fully or properly convey the meaning, especially in variable contexts. Because of this, each *śhloka* must be broken down into its component words and understood before the entire meaning can be derived.

Although this is a time consuming process, it is one of the most effective ways to learn Āyurveda authentically and understand its true meanings.

A second section of translated English text in slightly smaller font can be found below the original translation. This is the translation of the relevant commentary section. Here, in Charaka's work, it is the commentary, or *ṭikā*, of Chakrapāṇi, from his work entitled Āyurveda Dīpika. This commentary provides explanations throughout the text about potentially controversial concepts, answers to controversies, and insightful interpretation, meaning and context. It is an invaluable reference for students and practitioners.

POETRY

Next, review this example of poetry from Cha. Sū. 1/41-42 (Śarmā, R. K., & Dāsa, B., 2016):

हिताहितं सुखं दुःखमायुस्तस्य हिताहितम् ।
मानं च तच्च यत्रोक्तमायुर्वेदः स उच्यते ॥ ४१ ॥

That (science) is designated as Āyurveda where advantageous and disadvantageous as well as happy and unhappy (states of) life alongwith what is good and bad for life, its measurement and life itself are described. [41]

Life is of four types viz., *hita* (useful or advantageous), *ahita* (harmful or disadvantageous), *sukha* (happy) and *duḥkha* (unhappy or miserable). All these will be subsequently explained in the *Arthedaśamahāmūlīya* chapter—cf. *Sūtra* 30:23–25. Thus, Āyurveda is a science which deals with all these four types of life, its wholesome and unwholesome habits and its span—short and long and the description of life itself. The various points relating to the span of life will be explained later (cf. Sūtra 30:25).

Thus, broadly speaking, Āyurveda stands for knowledge of life (*Veda* from √*Vid*—to know). Another meaning of the term *Veda* may be attainment, etc., (*Veda* from √*Vid*—to attain) but this is not intended here because attainment, etc. of life is not a direct object of Āyurveda—its direct object being just the knowledge of life.

शरीरेन्द्रियसत्त्वात्मसंयोगो धारि जीवितम् ।
नित्यगश्चानुबन्धश्च पर्यायैरायुरुच्यते ॥ ४२ ॥

The term *'āyus'* stands for the combination of the body, sense organs, mind and soul, and its synonyms are *dhāri* (the one that prevents the body from decay), *jīvita* (which keeps alive), *nityaga* (which serves as a permanent substratum of this body) and *anubandha* (which transmigrates from one body to another). [42]

4

Scanned from: Śharmā, R. K., & Dāsh, B. Agniveśha's Charaka Saṁhitā. Varanasi: Chowkhamba Sanskrit Series Office; Reprint Edition. 2016. Cha. Sū. 1/41-42.

Here the difference which can be noticed immediately is that the *Devanāgarī* script appears to be written in a fixed amount of space on the line.

It is in metrical form rather than freely written prose. The use of poetic meter allows these *śhlokas* to be chanted or recited in a musical way.

The short and long use of vowels accentuates the rise and fall of the syllables when recited correctly. This type of recitation can be learned easily once the *Devanāgarī* alphabet is mastered.

It can then take years of practice to recite fluidly because each line becomes memorized. This type of practice is not within the scope of learning elementary Sanskrit.

Notice that the first line ends with a single bar. With *śhlokas* in poetic meter, the single and double bars are much more meaningful. They indicate when the metrical line ends, so that the flow of pronunciation can be smooth during recitation.

Although the *śhloka* here is printed across two lines, it is actually considered to be only one line for counting purposes. The first line which ends in the single bar is technically a half line, and it requires the second line to be fully complete.

The numbering system is the same throughout the text, and the same as the previous example. Here, the *Devanāgarī* numerals are used at the end of the *śhloka*. Arabic numbers are used at the end of the translation but may not be printed consistently.

Sanskrit terms which are maintained in their original form are printed in italics so they can be recognized quickly throughout the text. When they appear for the first time in the text, the rough translation or known equivalent (i.e., the botanical name in the case of medicinals) is provided in parentheses. This only happens on the first occurrence of the term.

TEST YOURSELF

Learn, review and memorize key terms from this section.

double bar

____

poetry

____

prose

____

single bar

____

VOCABULARY AND CONTEXT

Sanskrit is a complex language with many details. Yet it can be simple and elegant at the same time. Classical authors utilized these special features of the language to encapsulate the knowledge of Āyurveda in a way which still cannot be matched by any other language today.

Because of the wide range of flexibility that the language offers, individual words and terms can be used in a variety of contexts to convey slightly different, or distinct meanings. Being able to understand and interpret these meanings appropriately in various contexts and in some cases with multiple interpretations provides an advantage to knowing deeper meanings of the classical texts.

To practice this skill and be able to ascertain multiple levels of interpretations, the student must memorize vocabulary terms and their meanings. Advancing further, one must regularly read the classics along with the commentary and consider what the author is trying to convey by understanding the context of the word in the *śhloka*, the *śhloka* in the *adhyāya*, the *adhyāya* in the *sthāna*, and the *sthāna* within the *saṁhitā*. This takes continued practice and dedicated effort over some period of time.

Once the student has considered the contextual meaning, questions naturally arise. These questions should be written down regularly and collected by each student. Once they have been answered, the text should be re-read thoughtfully with the answer in mind.

Often times, answers to questions are found in the text itself in another chapter or section. Additional insight from other authors should also be referenced for a more complete understanding of the topic. By studying and recognizing multiple perspectives and viewpoints, the question often clarifies itself.

This practice helps the student to gain a more open-minded approach towards the science and ultimately improves one's abilities later in practice. It is one of the key steps in transitioning the mind to function more like the traditional scholars and practitioners.

TEST YOURSELF

Learn, review and memorize key terms from this section.

adhyāya

---

commentary

---

line numbers

---

saṁhitā

śhloka

---

sthāna

ṭikā

Chapter 38: Review

ADDITIONAL READING

Utilize these references to expand your understanding of the concepts in this chapter.

CLASSICS	1st read	2nd read

REQUIRED READING	Chapters

OPTIONAL READING	Format

References

Śharmā, R. K., & Dāsh, B. Agniveśha's Charaka Saṁhitā. Varanasi: Chowkhamba Sanskrit Series Office; Reprint Edition. 2016.

QUESTIONS & ANSWERS

Record your questions for this chapter here for further research and discussion.

Question:

Answer:

Question:

Answer:

Question:

Answer:

SELF-ASSESSMENT

1. *Śhlokas* behave like
   a. aphorisms
   b. poetic lines
   c. sentences
   d. statements
   e. All of the above

2. In classical Āyurvedic literature, poetry is
   a. at the beginning of each text
   b. more common in later works
   c. the only type of writing style used
   d. All of the above
   e. None of the above

3. A double bar (" || ") at the end of a line indicates
   a. a full stop
   b. a half sentence
   c. poetry
   d. prose
   e. None of the above

4. The term *adhyāya* refers to a
   a. chapter
   b. large, voluminous work
   c. line of poetry
   d. section of the text
   e. single verse

5. The *ṭikā* of a classical text is its
   a. chapter
   b. commentary
   c. section
   d. translation
   e. transliteration

6. A *sthāna* refers to a
   a. chapter
   b. commentary
   c. complete text
   d. section
   e. translation

7. Line numbers are generally counted in poetry based on the position of
   a. commentary
   b. double bars
   c. long bars over the original script
   d. single bars
   e. standard chapters

8. Visually, poetry can be distinguished easily from prose in the original *Devanāgarī* script because it appears
   a. as commentary in a different font size
   b. numbered by Arabic numerals
   c. to be written in a fixed amount of space
   d. with heading before each section
   e. with single and double bars

9. English translations of classical Āyurvedic literature are generally
   a. clear and concise
   b. easy to navigate
   c. easy to understand on the first read
   d. presented in user-friendly formats for the student
   e. None of the above

10. One of the most famous commentaries in classical Āyurvedic literature is
   a. Chakrapāṇi's Āyurveda Dīpika
   b. Charaka's Saṁhitā
   c. Ḍalhaṇa's Nibandha Saṅgraha
   d. Suśhruta's Saṁhitā
   e. All of the above

Unit Review

ORAL EXAM QUESTIONS

Use these questions to prepare answers for the oral examination. You may create written statements or cue cards to memorize the key points that should be included in your response. Scoring is based on your accuracy, brevity, clarity (ABC), use of Sanskrit terms and concepts, and confidence.

1. Name at least three languages which use a script different from the Roman alphabet in English. Give an example of a letter or character that is not found in the Latin alphabet.
2. Using the vocabulary terms in this chapter, what do you notice about how they're written?
3. Explain the concepts of translation and transliteration in your own words.
4. Explain the differences between Sanskrit and *Saṁskṛta* in your own words and write an example sentence for each.
5. Using the example of ambiguous transliteration above with the terms *vata*, *vāta* and *vaṭa*, identify the differences in the transliterated forms of the terms and the differences in the *Devanāgarī* forms. How do these differences affect pronunciation?
6. Use the Monier-Williams dictionary online and the Spoken Sanskrit dictionary online to look up any five Sanskrit terms that you learned so far. Which tool is easier to use? Which is more accurate?
7. Sanskrit is a language with high phonemic orthography. That means it is ________________ and it is ______________________ .
8. Practice writing and reciting the vowels of the *Devanāgarī* alphabet accurately from memory.
9. List the monophthongs and diphthongs and give five example words of each using any Vocabulary Terms.
10. Practice writing and reciting the entire *Devanāgarī* alphabet accurately from memory.
11. Write 15 examples of words with conjunct consonants using any Vocabulary Terms and identify the conjunct consonant formation(s) in each word. Note if any of the conjunct consonants include the two special conjunct characters which are written differently in the original *Devanāgarī*.
12. What are the most common examples of terms that appear differently when spoken or written by native Hindi speakers that you have seen in Āyurvedic contexts? What was your initial understanding or misunderstanding of the usage of the term(s)?
13. Use any ten Vocabulary Terms to practice word dissection. Take each term and break it down completely.
14. Using the Monier-Williams dictionary, find synonyms, antonyms and sets of words which belong together categorically.
15. Write two sentences demonstrating the use of cardinal and ordinal forms of Sanskrit numbers.
16. Find any three Vocabulary Terms that use any prefix or suffix. Dissect the terms, identify the prefix or suffix and explain the meaning.
17. Explain the concept of *sandhi* in your own words. What purposes could it have served to benefit Sanskrit in its spoken and written forms? Are there any similar constructs in English that might serve a similar purpose?
18. Identify three English words that use the concept of *sandhi*.

Appendix 1

Health care systems and therapies

A brief review of select Whole Medical Systems and Single Component Therapies is included here for reference. Their status of licensed or unlicensed refers to the state of the discipline in the United States at the time of this writing. Readers are advised to check the board or governing body's website for the latest information.

WHOLE MEDICAL SYSTEMS

Traditional Chinese Medicine

Licensed (most states), founded in 1982, National Certification Commission for Acupuncture and Oriental Medicine.

http://www.nccaom.org/

The National Certification Commission for Acupuncture and Oriental Medicine (NCCAOM) is the only national organization that validates entry-level competency in the practice of acupuncture and Oriental medicine (AOM) through professional certification. NCCAOM manges certification and recertification, NCCAOM exam development and development of the profession.

Tibetan Medicine

Unlicensed

https://atiyogafoundation.net/en/studies/tibetan-medicine/

The Tibetan name for this holistic healing system is Sowa Rigpa, which means the science of healing. This system is strongly influenced by Tibetan Buddhism and focuses on therapeutic management for three bodily humors, rLung (blood circulation, nervous system, and thoughts), mKhris-pa (thermoregulation, metabolism, and liver function) and Bad-kan (digestion, joint health and mental stability).

Western Medicine

Licensed - (all states)

Western Medicine is widely practiced worldwide, and is also referred to Conventional or Allopathic Medicine. Qualifying physicians possess the United States degree of doctor of medicine (MD) or doctor of osteopathic medicine (DO), or a recognized international equivalent.

Since 1933, the American Board of Medical Specialties has built a solid national system of standards for recognizing medical specialists and providing information to the public.

http://www.abms.org/

Since 2015, the National Board of Physicians and Surgeons (NBPAS) is committed to providing certification that ensures physician compliance with national standards and promotes lifelong learning.

https://nbpas.org/

Homeopathy

Unlicensed, founded in 1982, Accreditation Commission for Homeopathic Education in North America.

http://achena.org/

The Accreditation Commission for Homeopathic Education in North America (ACHENA). It is the primary Council on Homeopathic Education (CHE), it's an independent accreditation agency that assesses the educational standards of homeopathic schools and programs.

Naturopathy

Licensed (some states), since 1981, American Naturopathic Medical Certification Board http://www.anmcb.org/

American Naturopathic Medical Certification Board (ANMCB) is a non-profit worldwide organization registered in Washington, DC that administers certification for natural health care professionals. The mission of the American Naturopathic Medical Certification Board has been to first and foremost protect the health and welfare of the public.

Osteopathy

Licensed, founded in 1949, American Osteopathic Association https://osteopathic.org/

The American Osteopathic Association mission is to advance the distinctive philosophy and practice of osteopathic medicine and to be the professional home for all physicians who practice osteopathically.

Herbalism

Unlicensed, founded in 1989, The American Herbalist Guild https://www.americanherbalistsguild.com/

The American Herbalists Guild promotes clinical herbalism as a viable profession rooted in ethics, competency, diversity, and freedom of practice. The American Herbalists Guild supports access to herbal medicine for all and advocates excellence in herbal education.

SINGLE COMPONENT THERAPIES

Midwifery

Licensed (some states), founded in 2001, North American Registry of Midwives registry board http://meacschools.org/

NARM's mission is to provide and maintain an evaluative process for multiple routes of midwifery education and training; to develop and administer a standardized examination system leading to the credential "Certified Professional Midwife" (CPM) and to identify best practices that reflect the excellence and diversity of the independent midwifery community as the basis for setting the standards for the CPM credential.

Massage Therapy

Licensed, founded 1992, Board Certification in Therapeutic Massage and Bodywork http://www.ncbtmb.org/

The National Certification Board for Therapeutic Massage & Bodywork (NCBTMB) is an independent, private, nonprofit organization. The mission of NCBTMB is to define and advance the highest standards in the massage therapy and bodywork profession. In support of this mission, NCBTMB serves the profession through Board Certification, Specialty Certificates, Approved Providers, and Assigned Schools.

Chiropractic

Licensed, founded 1974, National Board of Chiropractic Examiners certification board http://www.nbce.org/about/certification_licensure/

The National and International Board of Chiropractic Examiners is the international testing agency for the chiropractic profession. The NBCE develops, administers and scores standardized exams that assess knowledge, higher-level cognitive abilities and problem-solving in various basic science and clinical science subjects.

Dietician

Licensed, founded 1969, Commission on Dietetic Registration certification board https://www.cdrnet.org/

The Commission on Dietetic Registration oversees human nutrition and the development and modification of the human diet. A dietitian alters a person's diet based on their medical condition and individual needs. Dietitians are registered, licensed health care professionals who diagnose and treat nutritional problems. In some states it is illegal to perform individual diet counseling without being a licensed dietician.

Nutritional Therapy

Licensed (most states), founded 2013, Nutrition Specialists certification board https://nutritionspecialists.org/

The Board for Certification of Nutrition Specialists (BCNS) is the certifying body for the Certified Nutrition Specialist (CNS), and the Certified Nutrition Specialist-Scholar (CNS-S) credentials. The CNS certification is the gold standard credential for advanced clinical nutrition professionals, and the CNS-S certification recognizes advanced knowledge, scholarly work and experience in the field of nutrition in the areas of research, academia or industry.

Health and Wellness Coaching

Unlicensed, founded 2010, National Board for Health & Wellness Coaching certification board http://ichwc.org/

The mission of the National Board for Health & Wellness Coaching (NBHWC) is to support individuals in improving their health and well-being, preventing and managing chronic disease, making important health decisions and optimizing their lifestyles to achieve their best possible overall well-being.

Polarity Therapy

Unlicensed, founded 1984, Polarity Therapy certification board http://www.polaritytherapy.org/

The American Polarity Therapy Association has provided a foundation for the practice of polarity. Polarity Therapy is a unique wellness practice that involves touch. It was developed by Dr. Randolph Stone, (1889-1981), an Osteopathic physician and Chiropractor with a passion for natural healing. Unlike massage or physical therapy, whose purpose is re-educating the body to align with gravity, the purpose of Polarity Therapy is personal transformation.

Yoga

Unlicensed, founded 1997, Yoga Alliance certification board https://www.yogaalliance.org/

Yoga Alliance is the largest nonprofit association representing the yoga community. Their mission is to promote and support the integrity and diversity of the teaching of yoga. Yoga teachers who complete a 200 or 500 hour teacher training at a Registered Yoga School may apply for registration and use of the RYT credential.

Yoga Therapy

Unlicensed, founded in 1989, IAYT certification board https://www.iayt.org/

The International Association of Yoga Therapists (IAYT) supports the research and education of yoga therapy. IAYT serves as a professional organization for yoga teachers and yoga therapists worldwide. Their mission is to establish yoga as a recognized and respected therapy.

Made in the USA
Middletown, DE
10 August 2021

45703964R00199